SITES OF PAIN
Their possible significance

Pain is nature's warning sign of wrong functioning or disease. It is a valuable indicator in the detection of ailing parts. Persistent, localized pain should never be ignored. It calls for thorough medical investigation.

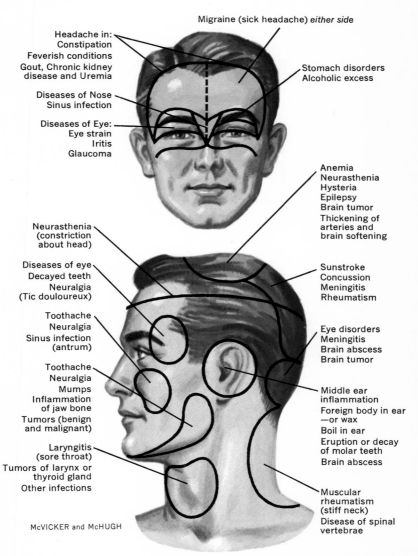

Migraine (sick headache) *either side*

Headache in:
Constipation
Feverish conditions
Gout, Chronic kidney
disease and Uremia

Stomach disorders
Alcoholic excess

Diseases of Nose
Sinus infection

Diseases of Eye:
Eye strain
Iritis
Glaucoma

Anemia
Neurasthenia
Hysteria
Epilepsy
Brain tumor
Thickening of
arteries and
brain softening

Neurasthenia
(constriction
about head)

Diseases of eye
Decayed teeth
Neuralgia
(Tic douloureux)

Sunstroke
Concussion
Meningitis
Rheumatism

Toothache
Neuralgia
Sinus infection
(antrum)

Eye disorders
Meningitis
Brain abscess
Brain tumor

Toothache
Neuralgia
Mumps
Inflammation
of jaw bone
Tumors (benign
and malignant)

Middle ear
inflammation
Foreign body in ear
—or wax
Boil in ear
Eruption or decay
of molar teeth
Brain abscess

Laryngitis
(sore throat)
Tumors of larynx or
thyroid gland
Other infections

Muscular
rheumatism
(stiff neck)
Disease of spinal
vertebrae

McVICKER and McHUGH

HEADACHES AND PAINS OF FACE AND NECK

Sites

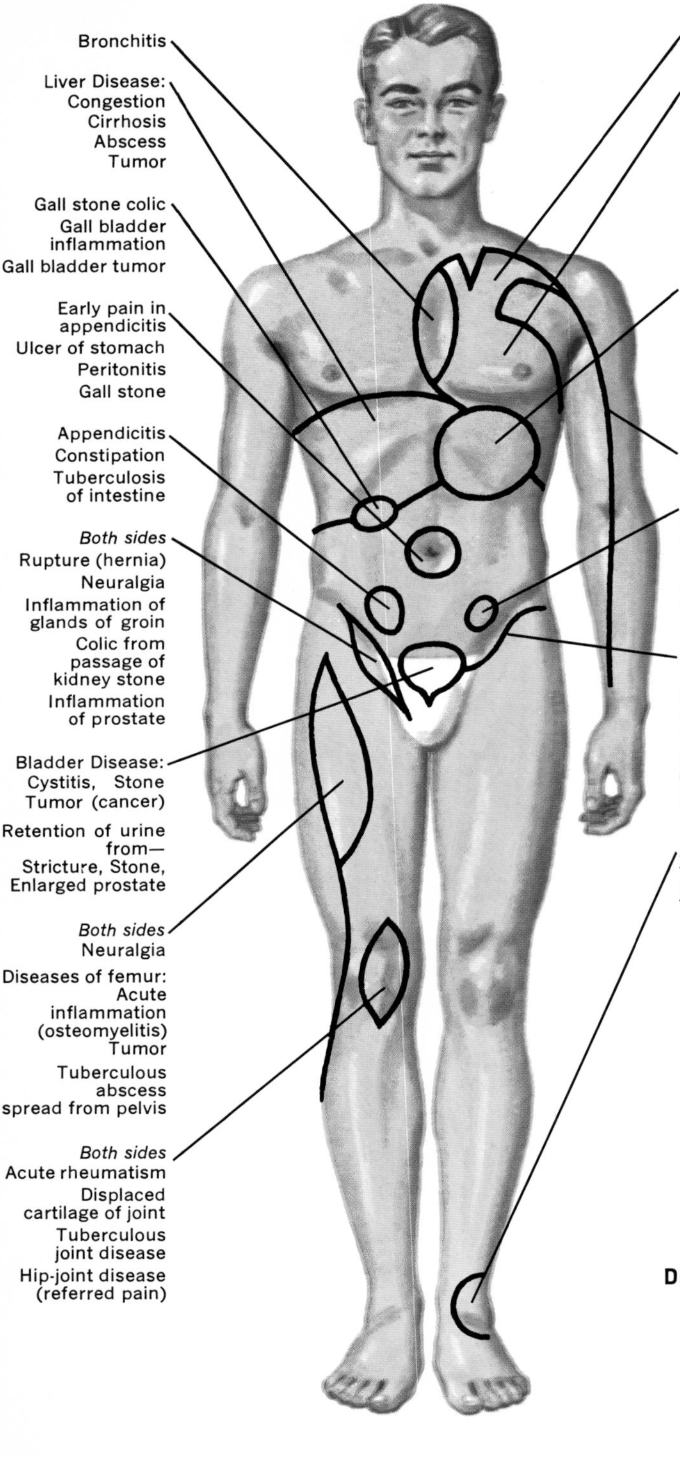

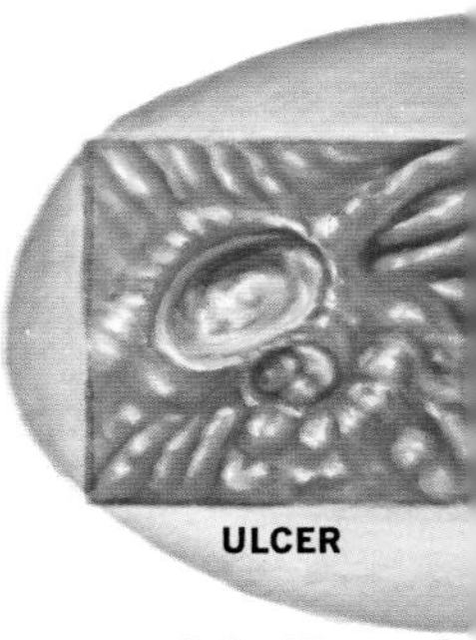

Bronchitis

Liver Disease:
Congestion
Cirrhosis
Abscess
Tumor

Gall stone colic
Gall bladder
inflammation
Gall bladder tumor

Early pain in
appendicitis
Ulcer of stomach
Peritonitis
Gall stone

Appendicitis
Constipation
Tuberculosis
of intestine

Both sides
Rupture (hernia)
Neuralgia
Inflammation of
glands of groin
Colic from
passage of
kidney stone
Inflammation
of prostate

Bladder Disease:
Cystitis, Stone
Tumor (cancer)

Retention of urine
from—
Stricture, Stone,
Enlarged prostate

Both sides
Neuralgia

Diseases of femur:
Acute
inflammation
(osteomyelitis)
Tumor
Tuberculous
abscess
spread from pelvis

Both sides
Acute rheumatism
Displaced
cartilage of joint
Tuberculous
joint disease
Hip-joint disease
(referred pain)

Angina pectoris

Disease of aortic
heart valve
Disordered rhythm
of heart action
Pericarditis
Angina pectoris
Pains of emotional
origin

Stomach Disease:
Dyspepsia—gas
Ulcer
Gastritis
Dilation
Cancer
Duodenal ulcer

Angina pectoris

Constipation
Twisting of
intestine (volvulus)
Drooping of
abdominal organs
(visceroptosis)

Both sides
Muscular strain
Colic from passage
of kidney stone
Tortuous
spermatic veins
(varicocele)
Intestinal colic

Acute rheumatism
Tuberculous
joint disease

ULCER

Diseases of the Stomach

On the left are two
gastric ulcers; on
the right, inflam-
mation of the lin-
ing of the stomach

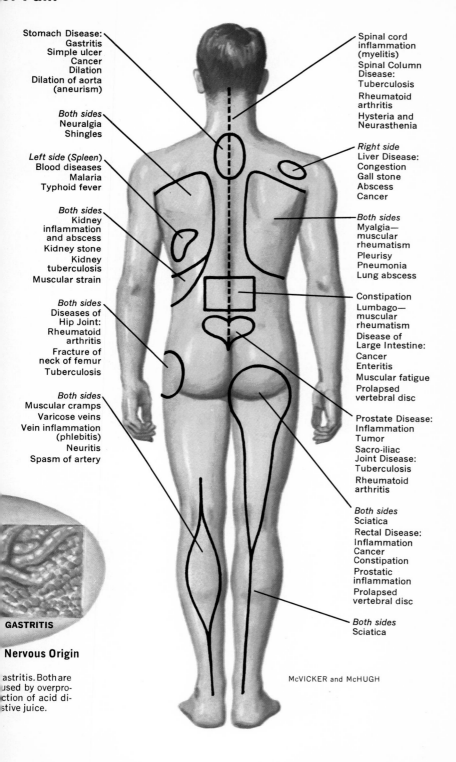

Stomach Disease:
Gastritis
Simple ulcer
Cancer
Dilation
Dilation of aorta
(aneurism)

Both sides
Neuralgia
Shingles

Left side (Spleen)
Blood diseases
Malaria
Typhoid fever

Both sides
Kidney
inflammation
and abscess
Kidney stone
Kidney
tuberculosis
Muscular strain

Both sides
Diseases of
Hip Joint:
Rheumatoid
arthritis
Fracture of
neck of femur
Tuberculosis

Both sides
Muscular cramps
Varicose veins
Vein inflammation
(phlebitis)
Neuritis
Spasm of artery

Spinal cord
inflammation
(myelitis)
Spinal Column
Disease:
Tuberculosis
Rheumatoid
arthritis
Hysteria and
Neurasthenia

Right side
Liver Disease:
Congestion
Gall stone
Abscess
Cancer

Both sides
Myalgia—
muscular
rheumatism
Pleurisy
Pneumonia
Lung abscess

Constipation
Lumbago—
muscular
rheumatism
Disease of
Large Intestine:
Cancer
Enteritis
Muscular fatigue
Prolapsed
vertebral disc

Prostate Disease:
Inflammation
Tumor
Sacro-iliac
Joint Disease:
Tuberculosis
Rheumatoid
arthritis

Both sides
Sciatica
Rectal Disease:
Inflammation
Cancer
Constipation
Prostatic
inflammation
Prolapsed
vertebral disc

Both sides
Sciatica

McVICKER and McHUGH

GASTRITIS

Nervous Origin

astritis. Both are
used by overpro-
ction of acid di-
stive juice.

Sites of Pain

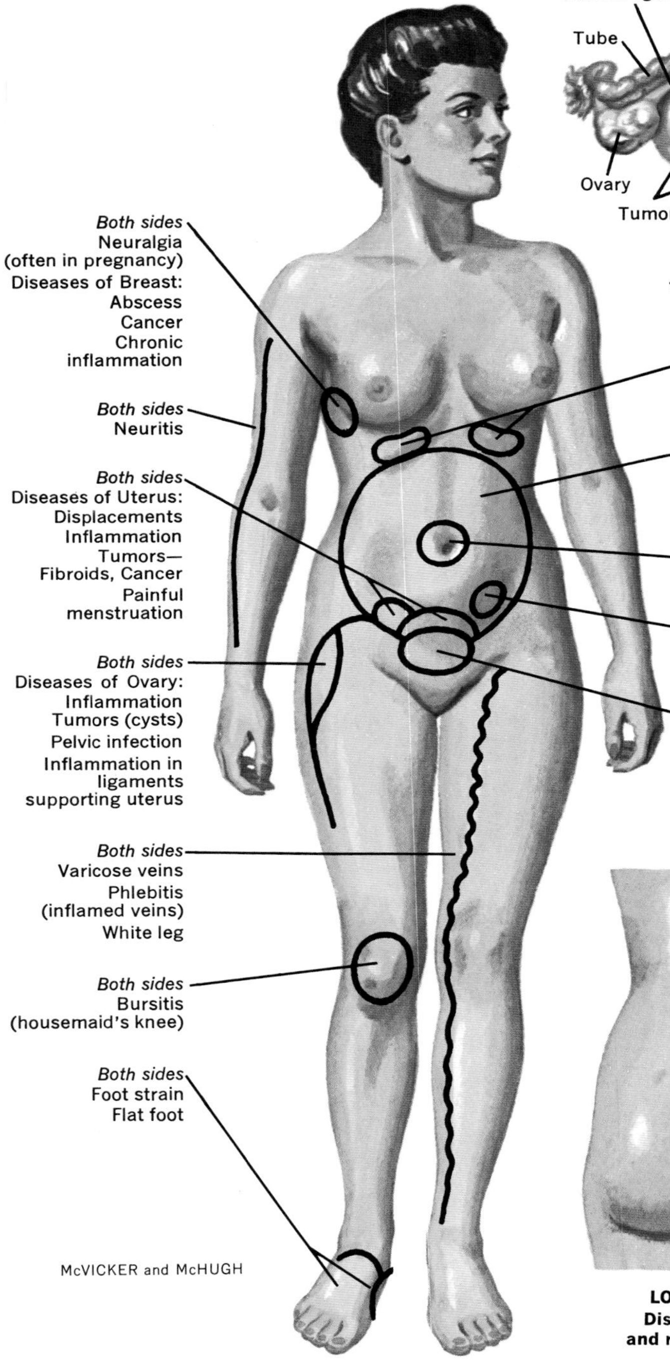

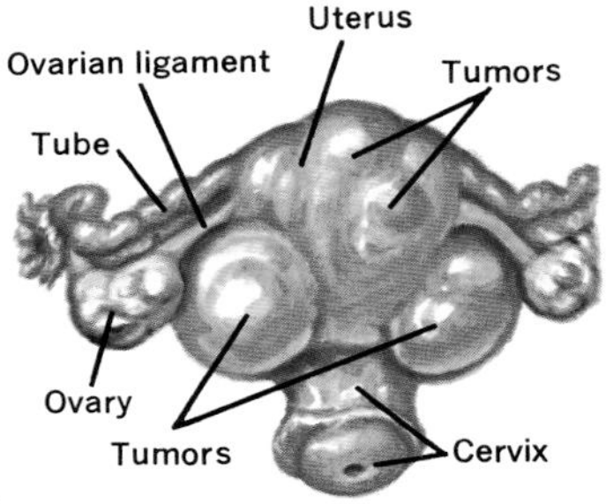

Uterus
Ovarian ligament
Tumors
Tube
Ovary
Tumors
Cervix

Fibroid Tumors of the Uterus (womb)

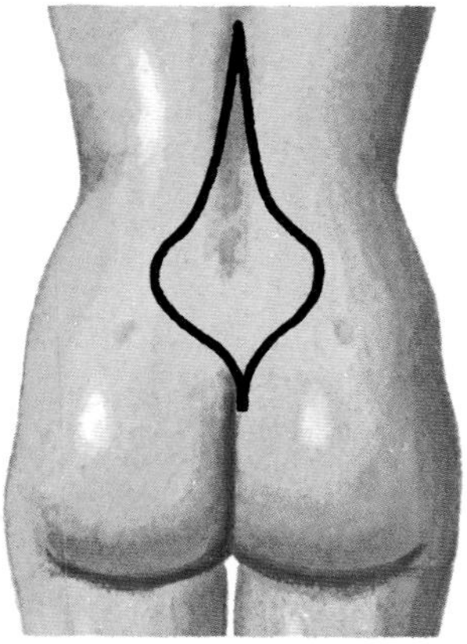

Both sides
Neuralgia
(often in pregnancy)
Diseases of Breast:
Abscess
Cancer
Chronic
inflammation

Both sides
Neuritis

Both sides
Diseases of Uterus:
Displacements
Inflammation
Tumors—
Fibroids, Cancer
Painful
menstruation

Both sides
Diseases of Ovary:
Inflammation
Tumors (cysts)
Pelvic infection
Inflammation in
ligaments
supporting uterus

Both sides
Varicose veins
Phlebitis
(inflamed veins)
White leg

Both sides
Bursitis
(housemaid's knee)

Both sides
Foot strain
Flat foot

Both sides
Diseases of Uterus
(referred pain)

Constipation
Abdominal
inflammation
Floating kidney

Umbilical hernia
Gall stones

Both sides
Inflammation of
Fallopian tubes

Bladder disease:
Cystitis
(inflammation)
Stone
Tumor

McVICKER and McHUGH

LOW BACK PAIN
Diseases of uterus
and related structures

FISHBEIN'S
ILLUSTRATED
MEDICAL
and HEALTH
ENCYCLOPEDIA

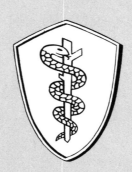

COMPLETE IN
4
VOLUMES

4

PELVIS

ZYME
INDEX

FISHBEIN'S

ILLUSTRATED

MEDICAL
and HEALTH
ENCYCLOPEDIA

THE *A*UTHORITATIVE HOME MEDICAL GUIDE WITH
MODERN RESEARCH REPORTS AND ADVICE
ON THE CAUSES, SYMPTOMS, TREATMENT
AND PREVENTION OF DISEASE

HOME LIBRARY EDITION

H. S. STUTTMAN CO., INC. *Publishers*
NEW YORK, N.Y. 10016

PELVIS, the bony basin at the bottom of the trunk which joins the lower spine and the thigh bones. The gaps in the two pelvic bones are closed with attached muscles and membranes. The pelvic cavity contains the sexual organs.

The female pelvis requires special examination in pregnancy to determine whether it is large enough for normal childbirth or so contracted that a Cesarean section is necessary. The measurements are taken by *pelvimetry*, using an instrument shaped like calipers to measure the front-to-back and lateral diameters.

Pain in the back part of the female pelvis is usually attributable to uterine disorders. The cramps of *dysmenorrhea* (painful and difficult menstruation) are often relieved by rest in bed, hot drinks, and use of a heating pad. Severe pelvic pain does not respond to aspirin and may require a prescription analgesic. *See also* SKELETAL SYSTEM.

Pelvis—This important framework of the body includes the ilium, ischium and pubis sections of each hip bone, plus the sacrum and coccyx at the bottom of the spinal column. The ilium and sacrum are joined at the sacroiliac, a joint receiving great stress from the body's weight pushing down and the legs and pelvis pushing up. In addition to the sexual organs, the pelvic cavity contains the rectum and bladder. The acetabulum of each hip bone is the depression into which the thigh bones fit. This attaches the legs to the trunk and forms the hip joints.

The Pelvis

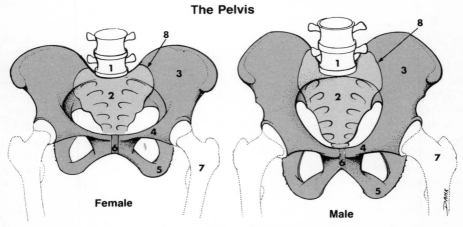

Female

Male

1. 5th Lumbar Vertebra
2. Sacrum
3. Ilium
4. Pubis
5. Ischium
6. Symphysis
7. Femur
8. Sacroiliac Joint

PEMPHIGUS, a rare acute or chronic skin disease characterized by successive crops of large blisters, cause unknown. The complications are infection of the blisters and thickening and shedding of the surface cells (*acanthosis*).

Formerly almost all victims died of the disease. The drugs *cortisone* and *ACTH* have revolutionized the treatment of pemphigus. For treatment of infected blisters, *tetracycline,* a broad-spectrum antibiotic, is generally used. Most victims are bedridden and their skin must be protected from friction against rough sheets, sometimes by continuous immersion in a bath. Large blebs are punctured with a sterile needle and itching may be relieved by a *benzocaine* or *dibucaine* ointment. *See also* BLISTERS.

PENICILLIN, the first and still most widely used antibiotic, discovered by Sir Alexander Fleming through a laboratory accident. Its various forms are specific for the germs of blood poisoning, pneumonia, meningitis, infection of the heart lining, septic sore throat, boils, syphilis, gonorrhea, and other bacterial diseases. Penicillin is derived from a bread mold. *See also* ANTIBIOTICS; INFECTION.

PENIS, the male sexual and urinary organ that transports semen from the prostate and ejaculatory ducts to the vagina and ejects urine from the bladder through the urethral tube.

The penis is composed of three columns of erectile tissue which become hard and erect when filled with blood as occurs during sexual excitement. The two larger columns—which erect the penis for the sexual act—are called the *corpora cavernosa;* the smallest column—which surrounds the urethra—the *corpus spongiosum.* The conical cap at the end of the penis—the *glans*—is partitioned from the corpora cavernosa behind by a ring, and covered in front by the loose *foreskin* (*prepuce*). The operation of *circumci-*

sion (removal of the foreskin) is performed as a religious rite shortly after birth in some cultures and also for hygienic reasons.

There are two congenital malformations of the penis: *hypospadias,* in which the urinary opening is on the under side of the penis; and *epispadias,* in which it occurs on top. The penis is vulnerable to such venereal diseases as *gonorrhea,* the hard chancre of *syphilis,* and chancroid; all are preventable by venereal prophylaxis, and all can be cured with antibiotics. *See also* CHORDEE; CIRCUMCISION; EJACULATORY SYSTEM; FORESKIN; IMPOTENCE; PRIAPISM; REPRODUCTIVE SYSTEM; URETHRA; URETHRITIS *and* **medigraphs** GONORRHEA; STERILITY; SYPHILIS; TRICHOMONAS; UNDESCENDED TESTICLES.

PEP PILLS, *amphetamines* used for artificial stimulation. Taken in excessive dosage, they produce excitement and an abnormal sense of well-being. *See also* **medigraph** AMPHETAMINE ABUSE.

PEPSIN, an enzyme secreted by the mucous membrane of the stomach which digests protein. *See also* DIGESTION.

PEPTIC ULCER, an ulcer of the *stomach* or *duodenum.* The duodenum is the first 10 inches (25.4 centimeters) of the small intestine. About one person in ten gets an ulcer of this sort. It is four times as frequent in men as in women, is likely to afflict someone between 20–40 and reaches its highest incidence in people between 45–55. The duodenum is involved ten times more often than the stomach.

Nervous tension—producing an excessive secretion of hydrochloric acid—is believed to be the most important cause of ulcers. Contributory causes include irregular eating habits, lack of rest, and excessive smoking and drinking. In addition, certain drugs, including aspirin, tend to precipitate a peptic ulcer.

The key symptom is intermittent gnawing pain in the upper abdomen after eating, lasting from one-half to several hours or until relieved by food or an antacid. Often, the pain strikes between midnight and 3 A.M. Associated symptoms include nausea, vomiting, loss of appetite, constipation, and anemia when the ulcer bleeds extensively.

The principal complication is bleeding, appearing as bloody or tarry stools. *Occult blood* in the stools—obscure blood that is not visible—can be found by a simple chemical test. Sometimes the amount of blood lost is sufficient to cause *anemia.* Other complications are perforation of the ulcer with shock and internal hemorrhage; obstruction from contraction of the walls surrounding the ulcer; jaundice due to obstruction of the bile ducts; and the postoperative *dumping syndrome,* in which food and liquid are evacuated rapidly into the small intestine, distending the bowel and causing nausea and abdominal distress 20–30 minutes after eating.

The most important part of treatment is rest and relaxation, including tranquilizers and sedatives when needed (but never reserpine). To diminish the acid secretion in the stomach, *belladonna* or its alkaloid *atropine* are commonly prescribed. The diet must exclude alcohol, spices, cabbage, lettuce, coffee, tea and other irritants. The *Sippy diet,* consisting of a milk-cream mixture every hour or two and before retiring, has been modified to include eggs, toast, cereal, crackers, strained fruits and vegetables and supplements of the recommended daily allowances of essential vitamins and minerals. An antacid provides immediate temporary relief of pain. Sodium bicarbonate acts fastest but its use is followed by an acid rebound. Other substances help protect the ulcer and surrounding area against the acid gastric juice. When such measures do not help, an operation called *gastroenterostomy* is performed, linking the stomach to a part of the small intes-

tine and thereby by-passing the ulcer area and allowing it to heal in the absence of the irritating hydrochloric acid. *See also* ABDOMINAL PAIN; ALUMINUM HYDROXIDE; DUMPING SYNDROME; DUODENUM; JEJUNAL ULCER; STOMACH; ULCERS *and* **medigraphs** GASTRITIS; ULCERS OF THE DIGESTIVE TRACT.

PERCUSSION, a diagnostic procedure whereby the physician places a finger over a part of the chest wall or other organ and taps it sharply with a finger of the other hand, thereby producing a sound comparable to a light drumbeat. A resonant sound—over the lung, for example—indicates adequate or excessive air beneath the area; a dull or flat sound indicates an airless area. The liver and spleen areas may be outlined by their overlying flat note as compared with the resonance of the intestinal area which is inflated with gas. The size of the heart may be outlined by its flat-note area on percussion as contrasted with the resonant lungs. The physician learns by experience the degree of resonance and flatness which follows the customary percussion technique. *See also* DIAGNOSIS.

PERFORATED EARDRUM, usually the result of rupture or surgical incision to drain pus, following a middle ear infection. Before the advent of penicillin, perforations of the eardrum were common. They impair hearing in the affected ear and also disturb swimmers by permitting water to accumulate in the middle ear cavity, causing dizziness. *See also* EAR.

PERIARTERITIS NODOSA, a disease of the small and medium-sized arteries with inflammation of the outer coats of the arteries and small lumps and hemorrhagic areas. Its cause is unknown. It may occur at any age, tends to recur, and is frequently fatal when the affected arteries break down. *See also* POLYARTERITIS NODOSA.

Pericarditis

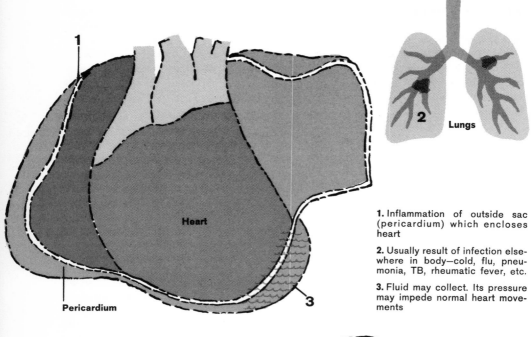

1

Heart

Pericardium

2 Lungs

3

1. Inflammation of outside sac (pericardium) which encloses heart

2. Usually result of infection elsewhere in body—cold, flu, pneumonia, TB, rheumatic fever, etc.

3. Fluid may collect. Its pressure may impede normal heart movements

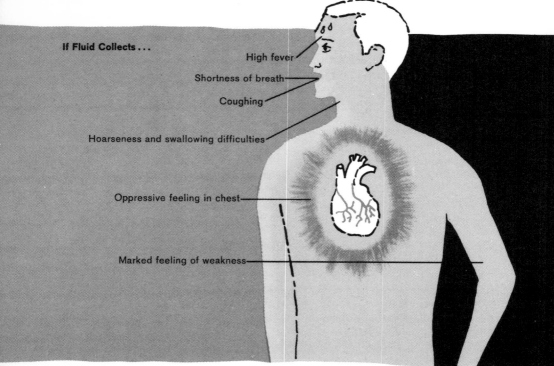

If Fluid Collects...

High fever

Shortness of breath

Coughing

Hoarseness and swallowing difficulties

Oppressive feeling in chest

Marked feeling of weakness

PERICARDITIS

PERICARDITIS IS AN inflammation of the *pericardium,* the membranous sac in which the heart is enclosed. The pericardium is composed of two layers separated by a capillary space in which a thin film of lubricating fluid assists the heart in moving freely in relation to contiguous structures. The outermost pericardial layer is made up of fibrous tissue. Thus, inflammation may involve the accumulation of fluid, or it may be dry and fibrinous, leading to a hardening and scarring of tissue.

causes

Acute pericarditis is usually a result of bacterial infection elsewhere in the body, such as pneumonia, osteomyelitis, or lung abscess; of a specific heart disorder; or a circulatory disorder, such as coronary thrombosis. It may accompany a tumor or be the consequence of a chest wound. *Nonspecific pericarditis* is a primary infection by a virus. Either of these forms of the disease may be "wet" and characterized by fluid accumulation, or "dry" and fibrinous. In *chronic pericarditis*—which is usually *constrictive* and may follow acute pericarditis or be associated with tuberculosis—fibrous deposits and adhesions form to constrict the space surrounding the heart and interfere with its movement. The accumulation of fluid between the pericardial layers in other forms of the disease also impedes heart action.

symptoms

Although symptoms of acute pericarditis vary with the underlying cause, almost all cases involve chest pains and shortness of breath. Pain may also spread to the back, shoulders and abdomen. A persistent cough is not uncommon. In constrictive pericarditis, there is also swelling of the ankles, liver enlargement and bulging of the veins in the neck.

treatment

The treatment for acute pericarditis is directed at the underlying disorder. Since this is likely to be caused by bacteria, antibiotics are prescribed, together with aspirin to relieve pain and bed rest to ensure recovery of normal strength. Nonspecific pericarditis involving fluid accumulation may respond favorably to cortisone therapy, although in some cases, it is necessary to drain the fluid by a surgical procedure that punctures the chest wall with a needle. Treatment for constrictive pericarditis involves surgical removal of the surrounding scar tissue to reestablish free movement for the heart.

PERICARDIUM, the tough membranous sac surrounding the heart and large arteries and veins. It lies behind the breastbone, the cartilages of the 3rd–7th ribs on the left side, and occupies a large part of the *mediastinum* (space between the two lungs). *See also* **medigraph** PERICARDITIS.

PERICHONDRITIS, inflammation of the membrane which covers the surface of a *cartilage.*

PERINATAL MEDICINE, *perinatology,* the specialization concerned with care of the unborn and the newborn, from conception through the first four weeks of life—and as much as the first year and beyond, if necessary. Special emphasis centers on high-risk mothers-to-be, the critically ill or premature newborn, and the detection, treatment and possible prevention of birth defects.

Mothers considered at high risk are the poor and very young (as they are often malnourished), those who have had previous pregnancies end in spontaneous abortion or miscarriage, the drug addicted (in addition to the handicaps from their mothers' poor health, addicts' babies are often born with the addiction and must undergo withdrawal in their first days of life), those with infectious diseases such as gonorrhea, and women whose families have a history of an inherited disease or abnormality.

Good nutrition is stressed in prenatal care so that the unborn child will receive the nourishment so crucial to physical and mental development during the nine months of gestation. Since low birth weight (less than five-and-a-half pounds) is the basic or contributing cause of half the infant deaths in the United States, inadequate or faulty diet during pregnancy—and even before conception—is one of the chief targets of perinatal medicine. Other important concerns include determining as early in pregnancy as possible the possibility of multiple birth, Rh factor incompatibility between the baby's and the mother's blood, the need for Cesarean delivery, or premature birth. A growing number of nurses certified as midwives are further aiding perinatal medicine's efforts to reach *all* pregnant

women with proper educational and medical services.

In addition to research and various forms of therapy, an important part of the fight to control birth defects is the program of genetic services and counseling, which seeks to provide and interpret information for prospective parents or pregnant women who risk having a child with some birth defect because of family history, evidence that one or both parents are carriers of an inheritable disease, or advanced maternal age. Prenatal diagnostic studies through x-ray, ultrasound, blood tests and amniocentesis (withdrawing a small amount of the amniotic fluid surrounding the fetus in the uterus for analysis) can now detect the presence (or assure the absence) of many defects, and at least a few disorders can be treated and corrected while the child is still in the womb. Where pregnancy has not yet occurred, tests can identify carriers of nearly 60 distinct metabolic defects enabling couples to make the choice not to have children if

Perinatal Medicine—Specialized care of high-risk newborn infants and research into their disorders is a major concern of perinatal medicine. This nursery is part of a center designed to offer maximum services in those areas. The room has no windows, lighting is controlled in intensity, and air quality, temperature and humidity are carefully controlled. Each incubator is equipped to continuously monitor an infant's heart rate, body temperature and lung function.

Courtesy, National Institutes of Health

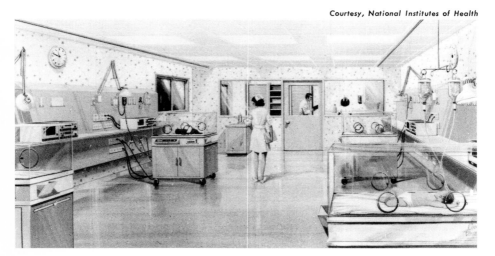

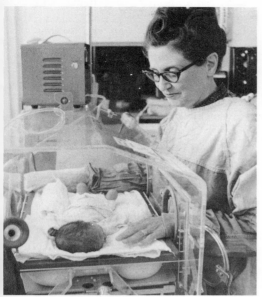

Courtesy, National Institutes of Health

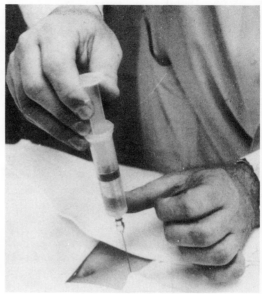

Courtesy, National Institutes of Health

Perinatal Medicine—A researcher observes a premature infant asleep on an oscillating waterbed. Waterbeds significantly reduce the temporary stop-breathing episodes common in premature babies. They were designed to compensate for the stimulation of floating in the uterus that an infant is deprived of by premature birth. Water in the bed is kept warm with a heater.

Perinatal Medicine—Analysis of fetal cells in amniotic fluid can reveal the presence of many genetic disorders before birth. In a procedure called amniocentesis, a long needle penetrates the woman's abdomen and into the uterus. A small sample of the fluid surrounding the fetus is then withdrawn for testing. Amniocentesis is performed 12–14 weeks after conception.

there is a strong possibility that a seriously incapacitating or potentially fatal disease or abnormality might be passed on to a child. *See also* BIRTH DEFECT; GENETIC COUNSELING; PREGNANCY.

R_{ESEARCH} *follows* ASTHMA; HYPOTHERMIA; THALASSEMIA.

○ R_{ESEARCH}
     REPORT

○   HEPATITIS B IN THE NEWBORN   ○
          PREVENTED BY ANTIBODY
○   TREATMENT   ○

○   Antibody treatment within 2–6 days
○ after birth of four infants whose   ○
     mothers had hepatitis prevented the
○ chronic infection of the newborn, ac- ○
     cording to physicians at the UNIVER-
○ SITY OF COLORADO MEDICAL CENTER.   ○
     The infants who were treated with

○   the specific human antibody to the   ○
     hepatitis antigen revealed no sign of
○   the disease antigen in tests conducted ○
     until they were 16 months old.
○   The Denver doctors suggest that the ○
     reservoir of chronic hepatitis B virus
○ infections would be reduced if preg-   ○
     nant women were tested at term so
○ that the offspring of antigen-positive ○
     mothers could be given prompt pro-
○ phylactic antibody treatment. NIH425   ○

PERINEPHRITIC ABCESS, an abscess located in the tissues surrounding the kidney. *See also* KIDNEY.

PERINEUM, the part of the body located in the pelvic outlet which is bounded in front by the arch of the two pubic bones, behind by the coccyx, and at the sides by the two large bony prominences

1151

surmounted by the buttocks. In the male, it is occupied by the root of the penis and the rectal opening; in the female, by the vaginal opening, the root of the *clitoris* (sensitive sexual organ), and the urinary and rectal openings.

In difficult childbirth, the perineal muscles and membranes are often torn and must be sewn up by the obstetrician. Such tears, unless repaired, may cause trouble later, particularly in subsequent childbirths. *Perineal tears* can frequently be prevented by an operation before delivery of the child called *episiotomy*, in which the size of the vaginal opening is enlarged by surgical incisions, which heal faster than perineal tears. *See also* EPISIOTOMY.

PERIODIC DISEASE, one that recurs at more or less regular intervals. In *tertian malaria,* the paroxysms occur every other day; in *quartan malaria,* every third or fourth day.

PERIODIC SYNDROME, a set of characteristic symptoms recurring together at more or less regular intervals—for example, the symptoms of peptic ulcer such as the pain after meals.

PERIODONTAL DISEASE, a disorder affecting the tissues that surround the teeth, specifically the gums. *Gingivitis* and *pyorrhea* are the two most common afflictions. *See also* DENTISTRY; TEETH.

RESEARCH **R**EPORT

CONNECTION ESTABLISHED BETWEEN INFLAMED GUMS AND BONE LOSS

A better understanding of the processes that culminate in *periodontal disease* and the resulting loss of teeth is provided by new evidence that the inflammation of gum tissue is directly related to the destruction of bone tissue. Scientists sponsored by the NATIONAL INSTITUTE OF DENTAL RESEARCH have shown that a substance called *prostaglandin E* (PGE), one of a family of fatty acids manufactured in the tissues, occurs at high levels in inflamed gums, and when cultured in tissue, PGE can cause bone to disappear or resorb.

Other related experiments indicate that the activation of *complement* at the surfaces of certain cells can trigger PGE synthesis which then destroys bone. Complement is a family of proteins that act in series. Activation, which is triggered by antibody-antigen complexes, results in various immunological responses, including the destruction of certain cells.

When the researchers cultured rat bones with complement inactivated by heat or deficient in one component, they found no increase in PGE or in bone loss. Since this type of bone loss differs from that which is caused by hormone imbalance, these recent findings may provide a new approach to some types of arthritis and other diseases of bone and connective tissue.   NIH914

PERIPHERAL ARTERIOSCLEROSIS

THIS IS A CONDITION in which the narrowing of the walls of the arteries blocks the nourishing blood supply to the legs, thus impairing their function.

It is often related to diabetes, overweight and other factors that result in hardening of the arteries, such as fatty diet and insufficient exercise.

causes
Peripheral arteriosclerosis (also known as *arteriosclerosis obliterans*) is a degenerative disorder that accompanies aging.

symptoms
Stiffness of the leg muscles, cramps in the calves (especially during the night) and discomfort caused by cold feet are among

Peripheral Arteriosclerosis (Arteriosclerosis Obliterans)

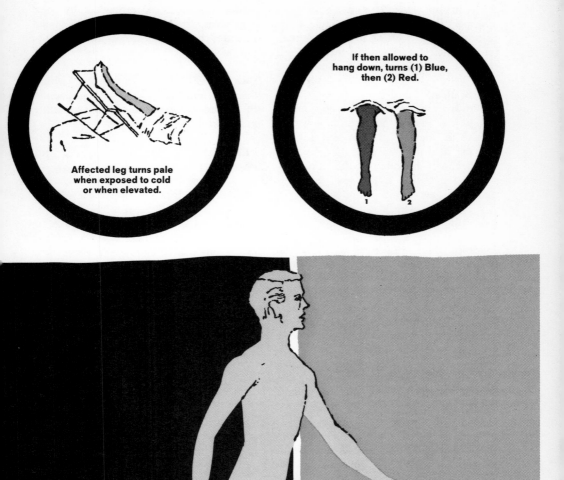

Affected leg turns pale when exposed to cold or when elevated.

If then allowed to hang down, turns (1) Blue, then (2) Red.

1   2

Affected leg is colder than other one.

Exercise causes pain in calf (claudication).

Shooting pains up and down leg sometimes occur at night.

Arteries to leg narrow—can no longer bring in sufficient blood, oxygen, food.

Skin becomes thin, shiny, easily infected. Gangrene may develop.

the common signs. If one leg is more affected than the other, it is likely to be paler and slightly bluish in skin tone than the healthier leg. The skin texture itself changes, becoming thin and shiny.

complications

Ulceration may result from even a minor wound or injury. Skin infections are harder to control; neuritis and accompanying pain may develop. If the condition becomes so acute that the blood supply to the tissues is too low, gangrene may occur, necessitating amputation.

treatment

Although there is no overall cure for the condition, there are several ways in which it can be relieved. Surgery can redirect blood supply to less obstructed blood vessels in the legs. Rest and relaxation combined with prescribed diet and exercise can sometimes prevent the arterial hardening from becoming acute. Properly fitted footwear is essential if further circulatory constriction is to be avoided. Feet should be protected from cold and damp, and any infection in the area must be brought to a doctor's attention without delay.

PERISTALSIS, the wormlike series of movements of the 23 feet of small intestine, beginning usually after a meal, which propels the liquefied food to the colon. Often, one is conscious of the peristaltic movement, which may produce a gurgling sound. When peristalsis is excessive, the colon becomes irritable; when it is deficient, *atonic constipation* may result. Peristalsis is promoted by raw vegetables, fruits and bulk laxatives and inhibited by certain drugs. *See also* DIGESTION.

PERITONEUM, the membrane which lines the abdominal walls and surrounds the contained organs. *See also* ABDOMEN; PERITONITIS.

PERITONITIS. *See* APPENDICITIS AND PERITONITIS.

PERLECHE, inflammation at the corners of the mouth with resulting *fissures,* common in children. It can be due to a deficiency of vitamin B$_2$ (*riboflavin*), often complicated by secondary infection with a fungus. The treatment is with therapeutic doses of vitamin B$_2$ and locally with a fungicide. *See also* CHEILOSIS.

Perleche

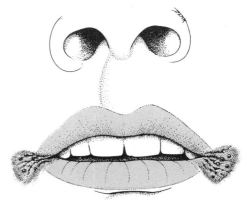

Perleche—The sores caused by this disease are often invaded by fungus infections.

PERNICIOUS ANEMIA

PERNICIOUS ANEMIA is a form of anemia in which the stomach does not secrete the substances essential for the absorption of vitamin B$_{12}$, without which red blood cells fail to mature properly in the bone marrow. The disease, which rarely occurs before the age of 35, appears to have a hereditary tendency. It is more common among persons of northern European origin who are blue-eyed

Pernicious Anemia
(Lack of red blood cells)

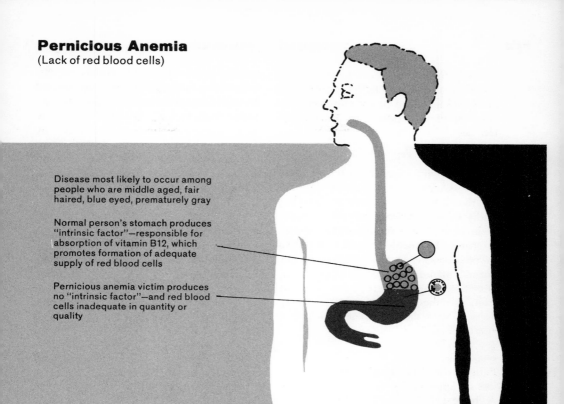

Disease most likely to occur among people who are middle aged, fair haired, blue eyed, prematurely gray

Normal person's stomach produces "intrinsic factor"—responsible for absorption of vitamin B12, which promotes formation of adequate supply of red blood cells

Pernicious anemia victim produces no "intrinsic factor"—and red blood cells inadequate in quantity or quality

Frequent Symptoms

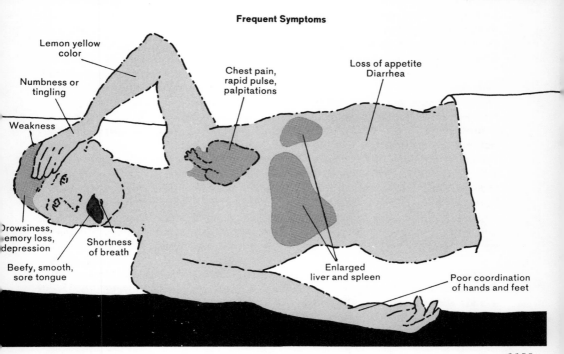

Lemon yellow color

Numbness or tingling

Weakness

Chest pain, rapid pulse, palpitations

Loss of appetite
Diarrhea

Drowsiness, memory loss, depression

Beefy, smooth, sore tongue

Shortness of breath

Enlarged liver and spleen

Poor coordination of hands and feet

and fair-haired than among a random selection of the population. Some cases are mild enough to be without symptoms (*asymptomatic*); others are fatal if untreated.

causes

The underlying cause of pernicious anemia is assumed to be a genetic disability of the autoimmune system involving faulty antigen-antibody response. The immediate cause is a failure of the stomach to secrete hydrochloric acid and the so-called *intrinsic factor* essential for the normal manufacture of red blood cells. Sometimes the deficiency disease results from extreme vegetarianism or from adherence to a diet completely lacking in vitamin B_{12}.

symptoms

Fatigue, breathlessness, palpitations and loss of appetite slowly become apparent. A typical indication of the disease is thickening and soreness of the tongue which becomes smooth, red and beefy-looking. The skin turns pale yellow. The victim becomes depressed, and memory loss combines with drowsiness to produce an effect of withdrawal from reality.

complications

If the disease is not diagnosed by blood tests and the deficiency goes uncorrected, complications occur which involve the nervous system. Vitamin B_{12} is essential for the preservation of the *myelin sheath* that covers the nerve fibers, and when this sheathing deteriorates, the victim experiences various neurological disorders beginning with tingling in the extremities and leading to loss of the sensations of pain and touch.

treatment

Pernicious anemia was truly a pernicious (fatal) disease until the 1920's when it was discovered that symptoms were relieved by feeding victims large amounts of liver and liver extract. Today, the disorder is simply and successfully treated by replacement doses of vitamin B_{12} injected intramuscularly. After the more acute symptoms have been reduced by large doses, injections are usually administered once a month for the person's lifetime. No other medications, special diets, or restriction of activities are necessary for the person's well-being.

PERNIO. *See* CHILBLAINS.

PEROXIDE, hydrogen peroxide solution, local antiseptic for application to minor cuts, scratches and abrasions, also used in dilution as a hair bleach. Its usefulness depends on the release of oxygen, which destroys microbes. Diluted with an equal volume of water, it is employed as a gargle for minor sore throat. Diluted with one or more parts of water, it serves as a vaginal douche. *See also* ANTISEPTICS.

PERSONALITY, the totality of an individual's characteristics as they concern his relations with others. The personality is of special importance to psychiatrists. A warm outgoing personality indicates an *extrovert,* which in extreme degree may be a *manic* symptom. A cold overcautious personality indicates an *introvert,* which when excessive indicates a suspicious nature and may possibly be a *paranoid* symptom. A grandiose personality suggests an *inferiority complex,* compensated for by a tendency toward exaggerated self-esteem. A *dual personality* (the Dr. Jekyll-and-Mr. Hyde type) is an alternation between a truly kind personality and an evil attitude springing from the subconscious mind. An *aggressive personality* is manifested by temper tantrums and harsh words or threatening gestures; an *inadequate personality,* by lack of social and emotional adaptability, ineptitude, poor judgment, and lack of physical and emotional stamina; a *neurotic personality,* by an evasive manner in meeting situations; and a *schizoid personality,* by a split mentality, seclusiveness, introversion, emotional indifference, and unsociable behavior. A person's true personality is largely manifested by his facial expressions in relation to the topic of conversation. *See also* BEHAVIOR; EMOTION; MENTAL HEALTH; NEUROSIS; PARANOIA; SCHIZOPHRENIA.

PERSPIRATION, *sweat,* composed of water (98–99 percent), salt, urea, and small amounts of other ingredients excreted from the body. The cooling effect of sweat evaporated on the skin helps regulate the body temperature. Perspiration is secreted by the sweat glands situated in the deepest of the several skin layers and reaching the surface through corkscrew-shaped ducts. The areas which sweat most profusely are the palms of the hands, the soles of the feet, and the armpits. The amount of water exuded in the sweat daily is about 1–1½ pints— more in hot weather and in the tropics. The chemical reaction is normally acid, alkaline when profuse.

Sensible perspiration can be seen and felt on the skin as wetness and small beads; *insensible perspiration* evaporates before it has time to show dampness. Profuse perspiration produces thirst due to loss of water and also fatigue and weakness due to loss of salt. Both must be replaced. Normally, perspiration is increased by nervous excitement and reduced by cold. During an exciting activity, such as watching a football game, the amount of sweat may increase as much as 50 percent. Sweating under intensive questioning was one of the signs used by witch doctors in detecting guilty natives, related to the cold sweat of fear. Sudden chilling of the body while sweating profusely—for example, as when suddenly exposed to the draft from an air conditioner without drying the skin beforehand—causes a sudden lowering of the body temperature.

Bromhidrosis (*bromidrosis,* B.O.) is a condition in which excessive perspiration has an offensive odor. Sweat itself has no odor, but it dissolves fats on the skin to form odorous acids. *Chromidrosis* is a rare disorder in which the sweat turns black, blue, green, red and yellow. Authorities believe it is caused by an infection with specific microorganisms. *Anhidrosis* is a condition in which sweating is absent or deficient.

Certain diseases cause excessive sweating. These include tuberculosis (which causes night sweats), malaria, rickets, hyperthyroidism, rheumatoid arthritis, rheumatic fever, migraine, and fevers in the stage when the temperature falls. Spicy foods, certain drugs and drug withdrawal induce perspiration, belladonna and atropine check it. Sweaty feet contribute to the growth of fungi and the development of athlete's foot.

The inconvenience of excessive sweating is best controlled by frequent washing and drying, application of deodorant antiperspirants, and medicated powders containing salicylic acid, undecylenic acid or zinc undecylenate, which also kill fungi. *See also* BODY ODOR; DEODORANTS AND ANTIPERSPIRANTS; EXCRETION; GLANDS; HYPERHIDROSIS; SKIN *and* **medigraphs** AMPHETAMINE ABUSE; ENDOCARDITIS, SUBACUTE BACTERIAL; HEAT STROKE; HEROIN ABUSE; HODGKIN'S DISEASE; HYPERTHYROIDISM; HYPOGLYCEMIA; KIDNEY STONES; MALARIA; MENOPAUSE; MIGRAINE HEADACHES; NEUROCIRCULATORY ASTHENIA; PANCREATITIS; RHEUMATIC FEVER; RHEUMATOID ARTHRITIS; RICKETS; TUBERCULOSIS.

PERTUSSIS. *See* WHOOPING COUGH.

PES PLANUS, *flatfoot, fallen arch,* manifested by an outward pointing of the toes and a type of gait like that of a comedian in oldtime movies. It is more common in women, possibly because of their stylish but crippling shoes. People whose occupations require them to stand long hours suffer most. After a bath, the imprint of the foot on the floor or rug is flat without the normal arch gap. Walking is uncomfortable and the pain may be reflected upward to the ankle, calf muscles, knee, hip and lower back. Arch support shoes and plastic or metal arch supporters relieve the discomfort. In severe cases, a podiatrist should be consulted. *See also* FEET.

PESSARY, an appliance of varied forms placed in the vagina to support a corrected uterine displacement or *prolapse* (the fall of the uterus toward the cervix) and for other purposes.

PESTICIDES, chemicals that kill pests, especially insects. One of the best known pesticides is DDT, which is highly effective but subject to restrictions because of its destructive effects on the environment. In the United States, the Environmental Protection Agency banned two widely used pesticides—*aldrin* and *dieldrin*—because of a potential cancer risk determined by experiments with rats and mice. Earlier, another U.S. agency, the Food and Drug Administration, found measurable amounts of dieldrin residue in most of their samples of dairy products, garden fruits, meat, fish and poultry. *See also* DDT; INSECT CONTROL.

PETECHIA, a small round red hemorrhagic spot on the skin which is not raised above the surface and does not disappear on pressure. Later it may turn blue or yellow. It is a sign of *purpura,* a hemorrhagic disease. *See also* PURPURA.

PETIT MAL, "little illness," a milder form of *epilepsy* without convulsions occurring mainly in children and characterized by brief blackouts of consciousness recurring daily. An electroencephalogram is used to diagnose it. *See also* **medigraph** EPILEPSY.

PETROLATUM, *hydrophilic petrolatum,* an ointment base and protectant.

PETROSITIS, inflamation of the *petrous portion of the temporal bone* (a pyramidal wedge at the base of the skull which contains the essential parts of the organ of hearing). *See also* EAR.

PEYOTE, a mind-altering drug distilled from a Mexican cactus, used by the natives to produce a state of exhilaration with feelings of ecstasy. *See also* **medigraph** MESCALINE ABUSE.

PHAGOCYTE, a cell, such as a white blood cell, that engulfs and digests microbes, brokendown cells, and other foreign particles. The phagocytes have been called "the body's policemen" but are effective only in the presence of *opsonins,* antibodies that render the bacteria susceptible to *phagocytosis* (absorption by the white blood cells). Some phagocytes are fixed in their location; others are wanderers in the bloodstream. *See also* BLOOD.

PHALANGES, the 14 bones each of the fingers and toes, arranged in groups of three for each digit, except for the thumb and big toe, which contain only two phalanges. *See also* SKELETAL SYSTEM.

PHALLUS, in embryology, the primordial bud in the embryo from which the penis develops in the male and the clitoris in the female.

PHANTOM LIMB, sensation and sometimes pain felt in a limb that although amputated is felt to be a part of the body. Since sensation is perceived in the brain and relayed to various organs, irritation of the cut nerve end in an amputation stump is flashed as a message to the brain area which formerly served the nerve that is no longer present. The brain interprets this as a sensation or pain in that area, even though the limb is no longer attached. Stories about phantom limbs were common in the Civil War and in World War I and often dramatized the horrors of war injuries.

PHARMACOLOGY, the study of the actions of drugs, both therapeutic and toxic. In modern medicine, therapy is based on the physiological properties of drugs, which are often determined by experiments on animals.

PHARYNGITIS. *See* PHARYNX.

PHARYNX, the throat passage between the mouth and the gullet. It is a tube composed of muscle and membrane, about 5 inches (13 centimeters) long, larger from side to side, and acts as a sound resonator and passage for food.

The pharynx has three parts: *nasal, oral* and *laryngeal.* The nasal part lies behind the nose and communicates with the nasal cavities. It is the part involved in *postnasal drip* resulting from nasal catarrh. The oral part is equipped with muscles and its function is to swallow food that has been chewed. The laryngeal part is continuous with the gullet and guarded by the *epiglottis,* a cartilage which closes automatically while swallowing and opens while talking. The *uvula* is a tab of muscle covered by mucous membrane hanging down from the soft palate curtain.

Acute pharyngitis—minor sore throat —is generally a complication of a cold, the infection traveling from the nose. Usually, it goes away in a few days and the discomfort can be relieved by gargles. *Acute tonsillitis*—septic sore throat, in which the throat is sore and the crypts of the tonsils are apt to be filled with a puslike secretion—is usually accompanied by fever and may be the result of infection with a virulent streptococcus (dot-shaped germs arranged in chains). The best treatment for such infections is rest in bed, hot lemonade, a light diet,

The Pharynx

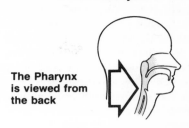

The Pharynx is viewed from the back

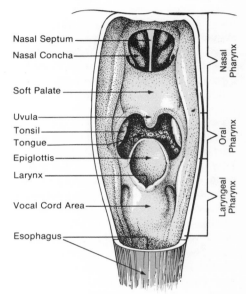

Nasal Septum
Nasal Concha
Soft Palate
Uvula
Tonsil
Tongue
Epiglottis
Larynx
Vocal Cord Area
Esophagus

Nasal Pharynx
Oral Pharynx
Laryngeal Pharynx

Pharynx—Air from the nose passes through the upper portion of the throat, the nasopharynx. The middle section, the oropharynx, receives food from the mouth and swallows it. In back of the larynx is the lower throat, the laryngopharynx.

aspirin if there is high fever, and penicillin or other antibiotics.

Chronic pharyngitis may be caused by smoking, inhalation of dust, or repeated attacks of cold, postnasal drip, or sinusitis. Its symptoms include a dry irritable throat and a hacking cough, usually without bringing up phlegm.

In *atrophic pharyngitis*—dry sore throat—thick crusts form in the throat and produce a foul odor. This condition is common in old age and as a complication of diabetes. If it spreads from the throat to the larynx, hoarseness and cough develop as symptoms. Another throat infection is *trench mouth* (*Vincent's angina*), with development of ulcers in the mouth and throat. It is due to a mixed infection, with a rod-shaped and a spiral germ that live in the absence of oxygen. It is best treated by a mouthwash that can provide oxygen, such as hydrogen peroxide.

The throat is the portal of entry for many systemic infections, so pharyngitis should not be considered lightly. To avoid future trouble, a victim should consult a physician. *See also* ADENOIDS; THROAT; TONSILS *and* **medigraphs** DIPHTHERIA; FLU; GERMAN MEASLES; MONONUCLEOSIS, INFECTIOUS; SCARLET FEVER; TONSILLITIS; TRENCH MOUTH.

PHENOBARBITAL, a long-acting barbiturate usually employed as a sedative, sleep aid, and anticonvulsant to control epileptic seizures. In addition to phenobarbital itself, the United States Pharmacopeia lists *phenobarbital elixir* and *phenobarbital tablets.* When tolerance develops with continued use, the dosage must be increased to get the same effect. Phenobarbital is habit-forming and leads to a psychological dependence. It has valuable uses in medicine but it is also one of the leading causes of drug abuse, poisoning and suicide. In the United States, the Food and Drug Administration reported that the use of phenobarbital to control epilepsy in pregnant women may be the cause of various birth defects. *See also* ANTICONVULSIVE.

PHENOL. *See* CARBOLIC ACID.

PHENOLPHTHALEIN, a cathartic drug, the active ingredient of many advertised laxatives. It acts in about six hours to make the colon evacuate its stool, irritates the colon with continued use, and ultimately leads to aggravation of constipation. Phenolphthalein should be used only for occasional constipation and never when abdominal pain or vomiting suggests the possibility of appendicitis. *See also* CATHARTICS; CONSTIPATION.

PHENYLKETONURIA, *PKU,* a rare genetic metabolic disorder caused by a deficiency of liver *phenylalanine hydroxylase,* and characterized by elevation of the levels of *phenylalanine* (an *amino acid*) in the blood. It is frequently associated with *mental retardation.* Symptoms in infancy include irritability, convulsive seizures, vomiting, and sometimes eczema, dry skin, and a mousy smell (due to *phenylacetic acid* in the sweat and urine). The urine may also contain *phenylketones.*

Treatment is by controlling the levels of blood phenylalanine by reducing the amounts of phenylalanine in the diet through a reduction in the intake of protein. Since protein is still an essential dietary element, synthetic preparations are given; these contain proteins low in phenylalanine and also vitamins and minerals. The diet is supplemented by fruits, vegetables and low-protein cereals. *See also* BIRTH DEFECT; GENETIC COUNSELING; MENTAL RETARDATION.

PHLEBITIS

P HLEBITIS IS INFLAMMATION of a vein, usually one of the superficially located veins of the lower leg. The condition is potentially more dangerous when it occurs in a more deeply situated blood vessel.

causes
The basic cause of phlebitis is not clearly defined. Generally, the inflammation is associated with some other disorder, such as varicose veins, arteriosclerosis and obesity.

Phlebitis

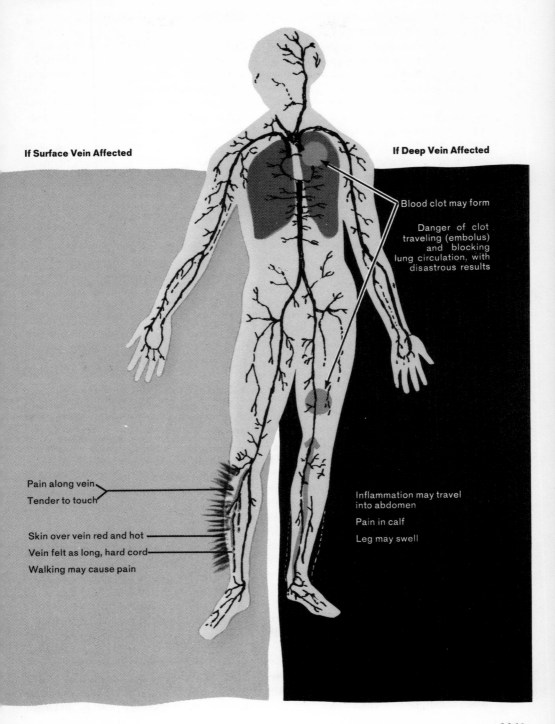

If Surface Vein Affected

If Deep Vein Affected

Blood clot may form

Danger of clot traveling (embolus) and blocking lung circulation, with disastrous results

Pain along vein
Tender to touch

Skin over vein red and hot
Vein felt as long, hard cord
Walking may cause pain

Inflammation may travel into abdomen

Pain in calf

Leg may swell

A serious injury to the area, surgery, or an infection such as pneumonia may also trigger a case of phlebitis. It can also occur in an elderly person who has been bedridden during a long illness and whose circulation has slowed down.

symptoms
The area surrounding the phlebitic vein becomes red, swollen and painful, and the nearby muscles become stiff. The pain may be acute during walking and as the inflammation increases. If phlebitis exists in the inner lining of a deeply situated vein, clotting may occur in the venous wall. This condition is called *thrombophlebitis.*

complications
The formation of clots may impede circulation, causing fluid accumulation, swelling and fever. If the clot breaks away from its original site and begins to circulate, it is called an *embolus.* The obstruction of a vital organ by an embolus is an emergency situation known as an *embolism.*

treatment
Superficial phlebitis is treated with painkillers and a supportive elastic bandage, but bed rest is not usually recommended since it increases the likelihood of clotting. When the inflammation is severe, or when deeper vessels are affected, anticoagulants are administered to reduce the risk of clot formation. Antibiotics may be prescribed to ward off the possibility of infection or abscess. If there is danger of an embolism, preventive surgery may be recommended.

PHLEBOTOMY, the opening of a vein for bleeding, practiced in the Middle Ages by physicians for many illnesses.

PHLEGM, a thick stringy mucus secreted by the mucous membrane of the nose, throat, or bronchial tubes.

PHLEGMON, inflammation of the connective tissue leading to ulceration or an abscess.

PHOBIAS, persistent abnormal fears of certain surroundings. There are many different phobias, the most common of which are *claustrophobia,* the fear of being confined in a small place such as an elevator or closet; *agoraphobia,* fear of large open spaces; *autophobia,* fear of being alone; *acrophobia,* the fear of heights; *necrophobia,* the fear of death and dead bodies; *mysophobia,* the fear of dirt; *photophobia,* intolerance of light; *coitophobia,* the fear of sexual intercourse; *gatophobia,* the fear of cats; *nyctophobia,* the fear of night; *hydrophobia,* the fear of water; *androphobia,* the fear of men; and *gynephobia,* fear of women. The nature of the phobia is indicated by the prefix, as for instance *cancerophobia* and *syphilophobia,* fears of cancer and syphilis. *See also* ANXIETY; FEAR; MENTAL HEALTH; NEUROSIS.

PHOSPHATE, a salt of phosphoric acid. *Calcium phosphate* comprises more than half of the weight of bones; *magnesium phosphate,* a small percent. Tooth enamel also contains a large amount of calcium phosphate and a small amount of magnesium phosphate. The phosphates play an important part in the biochemistry of the body. Phosphate depletion may cause certain bone diseases: *rickets, osteoporosis* (abnormally porous bones), and *osteomalacia* (softening of the bones). The calcium-phosphorus bone and blood ratios are regulated by the parathyroid glands. Phosphates are ingredients of many *enzymes* (substances that promote or induce actions in the body), including those used in the breakdown of fat and sugar. Certain relatively unstable compounds called *active phosphates* have a high potential energy content and release energy which is converted into muscular movement. Almost all energy obtained from food is either released as heat or stored as active phosphate. A high level of phosphorus in the blood combined with a low level of calcium is associated with disorders of the parathyroid glands.

Organic phosphates are distributed widely throughout the human body and are present in many foods. In mineral dietary supplements, the recommended daily allowance of phosphorus for adults and children four or more years of age is one gram; for pregnant and nursing women, two grams.

In medical treatment, inorganic phosphates are administered as blood calcium regulators in case of *hypercalcemia. Sodium phosphate* and *potassium phosphate* are cathartics. *Potassium bitartrate* is a mild saline laxative which produces a watery stool. *Phospho-Soda* is also used as a laxative. *See also* CALCIUM; PARATHYROID GLANDS *and* **medigraph** HYPERPARATHYROIDISM.

PHOSPHORUS, a poisonous and highly inflammable nonmetallic translucent element used in insecticides, rodenticides, matches and fireworks, and the manufacture of fertilizers. Balanced with calcium, phosphorus is an essential mineral and the recommended daily allowance in a supplement for adults or children four years of age or older is one gram. Therapeutically, phosphorus is used in the treatment of *rickets* and *osteomalacia* (softness of bones) and as a tonic.

Free phosphorus causes *fatty degeneration* of the liver, kidneys, and other organs, and *necrosis* of the lower jaw. The symptoms—which may not appear for several days after the phosphorus is ingested—include nausea, vomiting, diarrhea, jaundice, itching and abdominal tenderness. The mortality rate of acute poisoning is about 50 percent. If the victim is treated by the doctor within five hours of the poisoning, an antidote and nutrition usually are provided through a tube passed into the stomach. The antidote is *copper sulfate* which converts the phosphorus into insoluble *copper phosphide. See also* PHOSPHATE.

PHOTOPHOBIA, abnormal sensitivity to light. The condition is a symptom of *measles,* certain eye disorders—especially *pinkeye conjunctivitis*—and sometimes neurosis. The discomfort of photophobia can be relieved by wearing tinted glasses outdoors in bright sunlight, but such glasses should not be worn habitually in a dim light. *See also* EYE; PINKEYE *and* **medigraphs** CONJUNCTIVITIS; MEASLES; VITAMIN A DEFICIENCY.

PHOTOSENSITIVITY, the capacity of the eye to collect and react to light; also, the absorption of a certain portion of the solar spectrum by a substance such as *ergosterol,* which is thereby converted into *irradiated ergosterol* (vitamin D). *Photosensitization* is an abnormal condition of the skin which makes it hyperreactive to the ultraviolet radiation in sunlight.

PHTHISIS, an obsolete term for tuberculosis of the lungs, meaning a wasting away of the body, which is characteristic of advanced stages of the disease. *See also* **medigraph** TUBERCULOSIS.

PHYSIATRIST, a physician who specializes in the diagnosis and treatment of diseases with physical agents such as hydrotherapy, medicated baths, ultraviolet radiation, electrotherapy, colonic irrigation, and other mechanical measures. A *physiotherapist* is a licensed practitioner (not necessarily a physician) using such measures under medical supervision. *See also* PHYSICAL THERAPY.

PHYSICAL FITNESS, a normal condition of the human body; the body's ability to adapt itself to social matters and those of gainful employment. Physical fitness is evaluated by an annual medical checkup or, in the armed services, a routine examination to determine fitness for enlistment. *See also* EXERCISE.

PHYSICAL THERAPY, the treatment of disease and disability by physical means, including among other measures water, air, heat, cold, massage, exercises and electricity. Physiotherapy may restore function to paralyzed limbs and crippled joints and also help to relieve other disorders.

Hydrotherapy, utilizing water in tanks, pools or large baths, makes use of the buoyancy of water to treat paralyzed arms and legs. *Medicated baths* suitably heated provide an aid in the treatment of arthritis. The *whirlpool*—a special device in which water circulates in a whirling motion at any desired temperature—produces a mild massaging effect, and is useful in conditions in which blood circulation has been retarded. The *constant-flow bath*—in which an agitated person is placed in a canvas-type cradle with only his head above the surface—gently circulates warm water to soothe the nerves and to induce relaxation and sleep. In mental hospitals, violent patients under restraint are sometimes quieted down by the *continuous hot bath.* In chronic constipation, *colonic irrigation* evacuates the colon of retained feces and thus provides comfort, but its value for other purposes has been exaggerated.

Special exercises provide the best means of strengthening and training weak muscles. Ordinarily, walking, jogging and bicycle riding are recommended and special devices are also available including stationary bicycles, weight lifts and walkers. When the diaphragm is paralyzed and breathing is impaired (as in some cases of poliomyelitis), the *iron lung* supports breathing by alternating air pressure and a partial vacuum. *Occupational therapy* is an essential part of rehabilitation of disabilities, which not only requires the patient to use the incapacitated muscles but also trains him to develop new skills for gainful employment.

Massage is applied by rubbing, kneading, tapping, or stroking the body with the hands or special instruments for its stimulating effect on the underlying muscles and organs. The simplest method is superficial rhythmic stroking for relief of local pain and for relaxation. To promote flow of blood and lymph, the massage strokes are deeper and directed toward the center of the body. The kneading or squeezing type of massage pulls the tissue up and squeezes it between the fingers or hands, so as to get between the muscles and bones, thus stimulating the circulation and loosening adhesions. Another style of massage consists of tapping with the side of the hands or a special instrument in a hammerlike motion. Massage is also useful for relief of fatigue, muscular aches, stiff joints, sprains, and weak or paralyzed muscles. Massage of the gums every night is a routine part of oral hygiene. However, massage will not reduce weight.

Faradic and galvanic electrical currents are used in the treatment of paralyzed nerves and muscles. *Diathermy* utilizes an oscillating high-frequency electric current to generate local heat in the bodily tissues below the surface. It and the *infrared lamp* are used in the treatment of arthritis, bursitis, sinusitis, and other conditions where penetrating heat is useful.

Among the principal contributions of modern science to physical therapy are the life-saving *pacemaker, artificial heart-lung devices* which permit operations on the heart, and the instrumentation for *radioactive isotope scanning. See also* BATHING; DIATHERMY; HYDROTHERAPY; MASSAGE; OCCUPATIONAL THERAPY; PHYSIATRIST; SITZ BATH; WHIRLPOOL BATHS *and* **medigraphs** BELL'S PALSY; CEREBRAL PALSY; MULTIPLE SCLEROSIS; OSTEOARTHRITIS; PARKINSON'S DISEASE; RHEUMATOID ARTHRITIS; SCLERODERMA; STROKE; WHIPLASH INJURY OF THE NECK.

PHYSICIAN, a person who has established his qualifications to practice medicine and/or surgery by graduating from a recognized medical college, passing state or national examinations, and receiving a diploma and registration certificate accordingly. In exceptional cases, distinguished foreign physicians receive an honorary license and registration because of their generally recognized qualifications. Sometimes, foreign physicians practice under supervision. *See also* DOCTOR.

PHYSIOLOGY, the science that deals with the functions and actions of the organs, fluids and tissues of the body. It is distinguished from *anatomy,* which describes their physical structure and composition. In the medical curriculum, the three primary subjects are anatomy, physiology and chemistry.

PICA, a distorted craving to eat inedible substances such as chalk, hair, dirt or sand. In children, it is a recurrence of the infantile tendency to bring everything to the mouth. In adults, pica may occur during pregnancy and in *chlorosis* (a kind of anemia). *See also* APPETITE *and* **medigraph** LEAD POISONING.

PIEBALD SKIN, mottled white and black, a condition in which the skin pigment is not uniformly distributed but less in some areas, as in *vitiligo* (a skin disease in which smooth, light-colored patches form) and *leukoderma* (unnatural patches of white on the skin). Other than the unsightly appearance, these skin diseases are not serious and there is no recognized treatment for them. *See also* PIGMENTATION.

PIGEON BREAST, in children, a deformed chest with a prominent breastbone, usually due to *rickets.*

PIGEON-TOED, afflicted with a foot deformity in which the toes point inward—the reverse of flat feet. The condition is usually congenital and can be alleviated by wearing corrective shoes. *See also* FEET.

PIGMENTATION, the skin color as determined primarily by the distribution of *melanin,* which also colors the hair and eyes. Melanin distribution and skin pigmentation differ in the various human races: the *Caucasian* or white race; the *Mongolian* or yellow race; the *Malay* or brown race; the *American Indian* or red race; and the *Negro* or black race.

Melanin is an organic substance which absorbs ultraviolet light rays and heat from the sun. The denser the distribution of melanin, the darker is the skin. Some anthropologists have theorized that black skin has the greatest advantage in a hot and wet climate such as tropical Africa, brown skin in a hot and dry climate, and light skin in a cold and damp climate such as Europe and North America. Another theory is that the original human skin color was a medium brown and that other shades have evolved.

Metabolic pigment consists of melanin formed in the body. The two main bile pigments are *bilirubin* (red) and *biliverdin* (green). The red blood pigment is *hemoglobin,* from which the pigments *hemosiderin, methemoglobin, bilirubin* and *biliverdin* are derived.

Certain skin diseases manifest excessive or unevenly distributed pigment, including *freckles, liver spots, melanosis, vitiligo,* and *leukoderma;* also the systemic disorders *Addison's disease* (chronic adrenal cortical insufficiency) and *porphyria* (a metabolic disease). In sunburn, the skin darkens due to the ultraviolet rays of the sun. In the *albino,* melanin is absent. *See also* ALBINISM; FRECKLES; HAIR; JAUNDICE; LIVER SPOTS; MELANOSIS; PIEBALD SKIN; SKIN; VITILIGO *and* **medigraph** ADDISON'S DISEASE.

PILES. *See* HEMORRHOIDS.

Pilonidal Cyst

Cross Section of

Normal Skin

Pilonidal Cyst

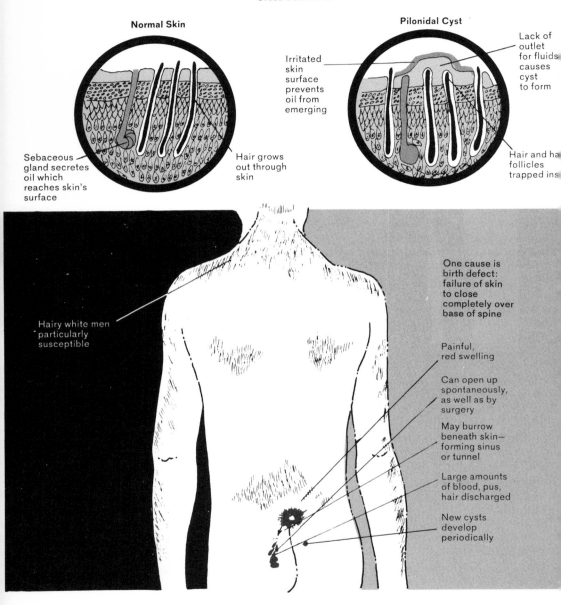

Irritated
skin
surface
prevents
oil from
emerging

Lack of
outlet
for fluids
causes
cyst
to form

Sebaceous
gland secretes
oil which
reaches skin's
surface

Hair grows
out through
skin

Hair and ha
follicles
trapped ins

Hairy white men
particularly
susceptible

One cause is
birth defect:
failure of skin
to close
completely over
base of spine

Painful,
red swelling

Can open up
spontaneously,
as well as by
surgery

May burrow
beneath skin—
forming sinus
or tunnel

Large amounts
of blood, pus,
hair discharged

New cysts
develop
periodically

PILONIDAL CYST

PILONIDAL CYST is a type of *retention cyst* that forms in the cleft between the buttocks at the base of the spine. Retention cysts develop when the outlet of a *sebaceous* (sweat) *gland* is plugged up but the gland continues to secrete sebum and other fluids. The pilonidal cyst can also be congenital.

causes

Pilonidal—which literally means "like a nest of hair"—cysts develop when a lapping over of the skin between the buttocks causes the fine hairs to grow inward, plugging up the pores through which the sweat gland ducts would normally exude their secretions. The retention of the accumulated secretions and ingrowing hairs blocks the duct and creates the cyst.

symptoms

The area becomes red and swollen, and because of the location, the cyst or cysts may be easily irritated. In some cases, the abscess may open and drain spontaneously, discharging a mixture of pus, hair and blood. Recurrence and remission are common in this type of cyst.

complications

In this particular disorder, abnormal pus-filled channels beneath the skin (*subcutaneous pilonidal sinuses*) may form through which infection may spread to surrounding tissue. In rare instances, osteomyelitis can develop.

treatment

If the cyst is comparatively small and infection is minimal, the only treatment necessary may be a few sessions in a warm *sitz bath* so that the cyst opens and drains. An antibiotic ointment may then be recommended as protection against invasion of bacteria. Where the condition is chronic or recurrent, surgery may be needed to remove damaged tissue.

PIMPLES, crops of small whitish or reddish lumps on the skin of the face, chest and back due to *acne,* usually accompanied by an oily skin and blackheads. The little lumps contain *comedones*—clumps of thickened oily secretion from the sebaceous glands, and also pus when infected. The underlying cause is believed to be overactivity of the sexual glands with excessive secretion of *testosterone* in males and of *progesterone* in females.

The disfigurement of pimples causes great mental distress in adolescence, but the disorder usually abates by the 20's. (Occasionally, acne may persist into the 30's.) Victims of acne should wash their skin thoroughly with soap and water to remove the thickened surface layers, and should avoid the use of creams and cosmetics which clog the sebaceous glands. *Sulfur* and *resorcinol* are useful local applications, and good results in both sexes have been reported with *estrone* (the female sex hormone) injections and ointments. However, too much estrone in boys gives them feminine characteristics. *See also* BLACKHEAD; COMEDONES *and* **medigraph** ACNE.

PINEAL GLAND. A gland the size of a pea which lies in a depression deep inside the *diencephalon* (the connection between the brain hemispheres and the midbrain). In early life, it has a glandular structure which seems to reach its greatest development at about the seventh year, after which it regresses and gradually disappears. Its physiological status is controversial, but it seems to be related to growth and sexual development. The supposition is that pineal extract slows down excessively rapid growth and retards overactivity of the sexual glands. Some authorities believe that it secretes a hormone which creates *melatonin,* a substance concerned with pigmentation. The results of animal experiments are contradictory.

From 25–30 percent of the cases of

pineal tumor are related to sexual precocity in boys. This disorder is often associated with increased pressure inside the skull resulting from compression of the aqueduct that connects the third and fourth ventricles, thus producing an accumulation of cerebrospinal fluid inside the brain. Surgical removal is difficult and the mortality rate is high because the tumor is difficult to get to without damaging nearby vital structures. The best treatment is x-ray radiation which affords a 60 percent five-year survival rate. An effective pineal extract for medical use has never been developed. *See also* GLANDS.

PINKEYE, the most prominent symptom of *epidemic contagious conjunctivitis* (inflammation of the membrane that lines the eyelids and covers the front of the eyeball). It may be transmitted by direct contact or the use of soiled towels. The eyes become red and the eyelids swollen and puffy. Often the lids are stuck together with pus when the victim wakes up in the morning. *Photophobia* (oversensitivity to light) is present and tinted glasses may be required for use outdoors. *Erythromycin ophthalmic ointment* one percent is an effective antibiotic for application to the eyelids, and *hydrocortisone* is also useful. In severe cases the eyelids may be brushed with *silver nitrate* one percent. An allergic form of the disease is called *vernal conjunctivitis,* which may be treated with antihistaminic drugs. *See also* **medigraph** CONJUNCTIVITIS.

PINS AND NEEDLES, a form of *paresthesia* (distorted sensation) related to nerve injuries or disorders.

PINWORM

PINWORMS—also called *threadworms* and technically known as *nematodes* —are the most common of all the worms that infect people, especially children in the United States. They are more of a nuisance than a serious disease. Infestation is highly contagious since the eggs can be inhaled or ingested. The mature worms live in the *cecum,* the pouch-like structure at the beginning of the large intestine.

causes
The adult female pinworm travels through the large intestine and lays her eggs on the skin of the buttocks around the anus. The skin begins to itch; the victim scratches and the eggs are picked up on the fingertips or lodge under the fingernails. The eggs may then be transmitted to the mouth or to the hands of someone else; or some of the eggs may adhere to the toilet seat, or to a towel used by another member of the family. The eggs are swallowed or breathed in and hatched into larvae in the small intestine. The larvae make their way to the cecum where they become adult pinworms. The mating process takes place, and the cycle is repeated.

symptoms
Infestation by pinworms causes itching around the buttocks, anus and vagina, especially at night when the worms themselves can actually be seen with the naked eye. They look like little pieces of white thread. Even if the worms themselves are not visible, the eggs will be apparent in a stool sample that the doctor may request for laboratory examination.

treatment
Medications are prescribed to relieve itching, and it is then recommended that everyone in the family take the medicines that will destroy the egg-laying females with which more than one member of the

Pinworm

Causes itching of anus—particularly at bedtime

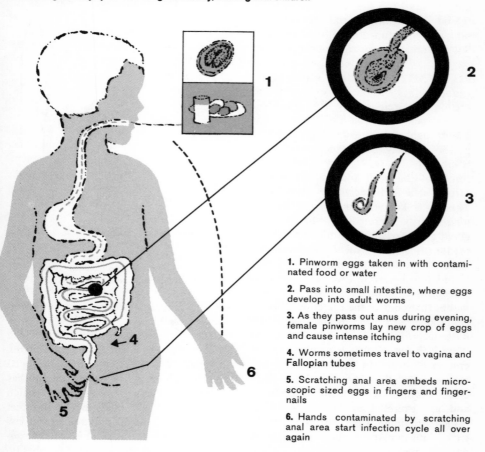

Pinworm generally spreads throughout family, starting with children

1. Pinworm eggs taken in with contaminated food or water

2. Pass into small intestine, where eggs develop into adult worms

3. As they pass out anus during evening, female pinworms lay new crop of eggs and cause intense itching

4. Worms sometimes travel to vagina and Fallopian tubes

5. Scratching anal area embeds microscopic sized eggs in fingers and fingernails

6. Hands contaminated by scratching anal area start infection cycle all over again

household is probably infected. The medication, which may have to be taken daily
for a week, causes minor side effects of
nausea and slight diarrhea. During the
course of the treatment, everyone must
be especially meticulous about not
scratching, keeping the fingernails short,
washing the hands before preparing or
eating food, and washing the hands after
going to the toilet.

prevention
Since pinworms are widespread and
highly contagious, there is no need to feel
especially unclean—or to make a child
feel guilty about dirty habits—if infestation occurs. The entire family may be
spared contagion if the itching anus
symptom is immediately brought to a
doctor's attention for treatment.

PITUITARY, the master gland of the
endocrine system (glands of internal secretion). It weighs only 7½ grains but
is a veritable storehouse of hormones, of
which eight are already known, and it
performs many important functions. It
is cradled in a small bony cavity in the
center of the skull and has an *anterior*
(front) lobe and a *posterior* (back) lobe.
The eight known *hormones* (chemical
messengers) secreted by the pituitary
gland and carried in the blood to distant
organs are: the *growth hormone;* the
thyroid-stimulating hormone; the *adrenal-
stimulating hormone* (ACTH); the *male
sex hormone stimulator;* two female hormones that control the secretion of *estrogen* and *progesterone* by the ovaries; the
milk secretory hormone; and the *anti-
diuretic hormone* which controls the secretion of urine. In pregnancy, the hormones regulating the female periodic
cycle become temporarily superfluous
and are excreted in the urine. When
urine containing such hormones is injected into immature rabbits or mice, the
animals mature in a few days, a result
which is diagnostic of pregnancy with

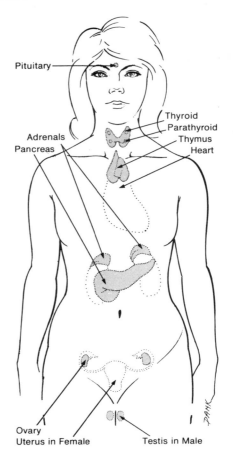

Pituitary—Hormones produced by the tiny pituitary gland regulate function of the other glands
shown here. They are all part of the endocrine
system. The pituitary also controls growth with
secretions of the hormone somatotrophin.

98–99 percent accuracy (*Aschheim-
Zondek test*).

The main diseases of the anterior lobe
of the pituitary gland include: *giantism,*
in which the skeleton is overdeveloped
and the subject is 6½–8 feet tall and has
a still greater span; *acromegaly,* in which
the bones of the face, hands and feet
are greatly enlarged and the lower jaw
protrudes; *pituitary basophilism (Cushing's syndrome),* characterized by obesity,
skin and muscular atrophy, softening of

PLASMA, the liquid part of the blood in which the red and white corpuscles are suspended. It contains a mixture of many proteins. Plasma should be distinguished from *serum,* which is the amber-colored fluid that exudes from coagulated blood when the clot shrinks. *See also* BLOOD.

PLASTIC SURGERY, reconstruction of deformed or absent tissue by special operations. Notable examples are the repair of *cleft palate* and *harelip* by closing the gap in the roof of the mouth and the upper lip; the operation for *spina bifida,* which closes a gap in the lower part of the spine; reconstruction of an unshapely nose by removing a hump or building up an absent or broken-down bridge; and removal of a *keloid* (a mass of overgrown scar tissue). Bone is sometimes chiseled out from the shin bone and implanted in a defective facial bone for cosmetic improvement. Plastic surgeons have become

expert in face-lifting operations to correct double chin and sagging features, thus providing a more youthful appearance. *See also* CLEFT PALATE; NOSE.

PLATELETS, thrombocytes, tiny circular or oval discs in the blood, numbering about 250,000 per cubic millimeter, concerned with the physiological processes of coagulation and contraction of a clot. *See also* BLOOD; BLOOD CONDITIONS; COAGULATION; PURPURA.
RESEARCH REPORT *follows* TRANSFUSION, BLOOD.

PLEURA, the moist membrane which lines one half of the chest cavity and is reflected over one lung and the corresponding half of the midriff, forming a sac whose cavity is known as the *pleural cavity*. Its moist secretion facilitates the movements of the lung in breathing. *See also* LUNGS *and* **medigraphs** LUPUS ERYTHEMATOSUS; PLEURISY; TUBERCULOSIS.

Platelets—From a unit of whole blood, a technician separates platelets to be transfused into leukemia victims to prevent hemorrhage. The remaining blood can then be transfused back into the donor. Potent antileukemic drugs cause leukemia patients to be temporarily unable to make their own platelets—the disc-shaped blood elements involved with coagulation.

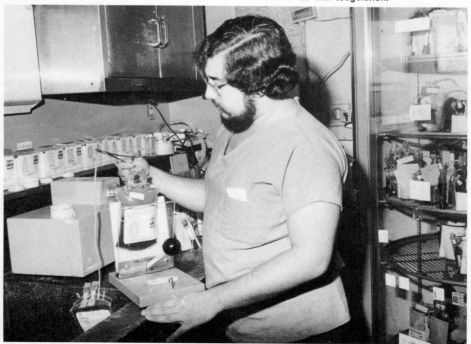

Pleurisy

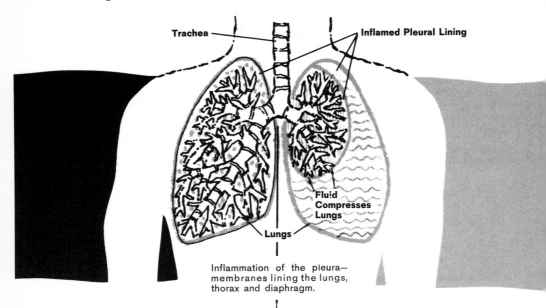

Trachea

Inflamed Pleural Lining

Fluid
Compresses
Lungs

Lungs

Inflammation of the pleura—
membranes lining the lungs,
thorax and diaphragm.

Dry Pleurisy
Painful inflammation of the
pleura lining, aggravated by
breathing, coughing, sneezing,
or anything else causing inflamed layers of lining to rub
together.

Wet Pleurisy
Inflammation plus accumulation of fluid, collapsing lung,
making breathing difficult.

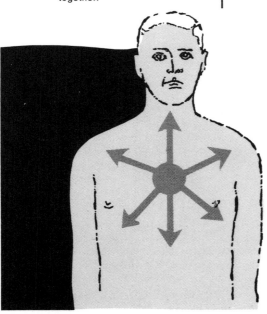

Most common symptom is severe
pain in chest, particularly when
breathing. Pain may radiate to abdomen, neck, shoulders or back.
Pleurisy can be a complication in
the wake of other diseases affecting
lungs, such as pneumonia, TB, flu,
etc.

PLEURISY

PLEURISY IS AN INFLAMMATION of the *pleura,* the two-layered membrane that encloses the lung and lines the cavity of the chest. Between the layers is a lubricating fluid. If, during an inflammation of the membranes, the fluid content is unaffected, the disorder is called *dry pleurisy.* When there is an abnormal increase in fluid, the condition is referred to as *wet pleurisy.* If the inflammation affects the pleural lining of the diaphragm, it is known as *diaphragmatic pleurisy.* This latter dry form of the disorder may be painful, but it is rarely serious and is likely to disappear within a few days.

causes
Pleurisy is usually the result of the spreading of infection from the lungs such as bacterial pneumonia, lung abscess, or influenza. It may also be caused by a tumor, or by an injury to the chest wall.

symptoms
Cough, sharp chest pain, shallow breathing, chills and fever are the typical symptoms. In dry pleurisy, the pain is caused by the fact that the inflamed membranes swell and rub against each other when the lungs fill up with air during breathing. Thus, the shallower the breathing, the less discomfort. The pain is usually less acute in wet pleurisy because there is no chafing of the membranes, but the accumulation of fluid hampers breathing by compressing the lungs.

complications
When the accumulated fluid of wet pleurisy becomes infected and pus-filled, the resulting condition, known as *empyema,* is a serious one. It is less common than it used to be, since antibiotic therapy usually forestalls it. When x-ray and other diagnostic evidence does indicate empyema, surgical drainage of the fluid may be necessary.

treatment
The treatment for pleurisy consists of antibiotics and bed rest. Heat applications and prescribed painkillers may alleviate some of the respiratory discomfort. Where the underlying cause is cancer or tuberculosis, other combination therapies are also involved.

prevention
Since pleurisy is a secondary complication in most cases, the effective way to prevent it is by giving prompt attention to all respiratory infections, by avoiding fatigue, and by maintaining good health.

PLEURODYNIA. *See* DEVIL'S GRIP.

PLEUROPNEUMONIA, pleurisy complicating pneumonia. *Pleurisy* is the most common complication of lobar pneumonia, accounts for the chest pain, and is accompanied by a small development of fluid in the chest cavity in almost 10 percent of cases. *See also* LUNGS *and* **medigraphs** PLEURISY; PNEUMONIA.

PLEXUS, a network or tangle of nerves, veins, or lymphatic vessels. The *brachial plexus,* formed by the four lower nerves from the neck and the highest nerve from the chest, distributes the branches that control the muscles of the arm and forearm. The *solar plexus* (which boxers try to punch) is the large network of nerves located deep in the upper abdomen and distributed to the abdominal organs.

PLUMBISM, lead poisoning, contracted mostly from inferior paints, old wallpaper, old plumbing, hair dyes, and painted cribs, carriages and toys. *See also* **medigraph** LEAD POISONING.

PNEUMOCONIOSIS, chronic inflammation of the lungs caused by inhalation of mineral dusts. Air contamination exposes everybody to the deposition of dust particles in the lungs. In most instances, various inborn mechanisms protect the body. Certain mineral dusts, however, damage the delicate lung structure and provide an occupational hazard for workers in industries where such dusts are present in the air. The most dangerous are *quartz (silica), asbestos, marble* and *beryllium.* Other inhaled dusts are *coal, iron, barium* and *wood.*

The most common form of pneumoconiosis is *anthracosis,* in which soot or carbon smoke blackens the lungs but does not cause any serious damage.

In *silicosis,* silica accumulates in the lungs over a period of 5–25 years and forms fibrous nodules, which coalesce, break down, and irritate the lungs. The main symptoms are shortness of breath, cough, expectoration of sputum containing silica particles, hoarseness, chest pains, and sometimes spitting up blood. In susceptible persons, asthma may result from any of the inhalants.

Bronchopneumonia, lung cancer, emphysema and pulmonary tuberculosis are all possible complications of these disorders.

Industries requiring work in dust-polluted places should provide protective masks for their employees. The work areas should be ventilated as thoroughly as possible, and collections of dust should be removed daily from the floors, walls and ceilings. In the United States, the Environmental Protection Agency has set standards to reduce air pollution from all causes. The Department of Health, Education and Welfare has published findings that occupational exposure to airborne asbestos can cause disease; and it has set standards limiting the amount of air contamination in surface coal mines. *See also* ASBESTOSIS; BERYLLIOSIS; DUST; INDUSTRIAL HEALTH; INHALING OF DANGEROUS SUBSTANCES; LUNGS *and* **medigraphs** ANTHRACOSIS AND ASBESTOSIS; EMPHYSEMA; LUNG CANCER; SILICOSIS; TUBERCULOSIS.

PNEUMONIA

ALTHOUGH THE TERM PNEUMONIA means any infection or inflammation of the lungs, its use is restricted to an acute and rapidly developing lung disease. One or both lungs may be involved —in the latter case it is called *double pneumonia*—and it may be a primary or a secondary infection. The type of pneumonia caused by *pneumococcus* bacteria, although much rarer than it once was and less of a threat because of antibiotics, is still a very serious illness, especially if the person is very old or very young. More prevalent is the lung inflammation known as "walking" (viral) pneumonia (*primary atypical pneumonia*).

causes
These pneumonias, which characteristically occur among young adults whose resistance may be low because of careless health habits, are caused by various viruses and other microorganisms that are smaller and less virulent than bacteria.

symptoms
The onset of these infections is gradual and the symptoms are less acute and less debilitating than those of bacterial pneumonia. There is a general feeling of fatigue accompanied by headache, pains in the joints, and a dry cough which eventually becomes loose enough to expel some of the congestive mucus. Symptoms are similar to those of influenza. A chest x-ray may be necessary for correct diagnosis.

complications
The chief danger of these comparatively mild pneumonias is that the person is

Pneumonia

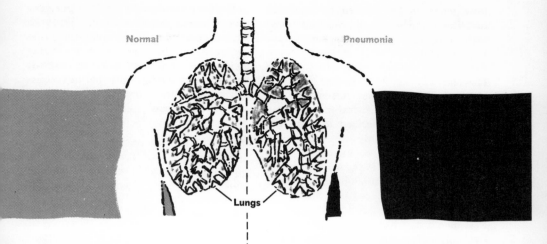

Normal   Pneumonia

Lungs

Lung is composed of millions of tiny little air cells surrounded by network of blood vessels. In normal breathing, lung flexibly contracts to force stale air out of cells, expands to bring in fresh air.

Lung is inflamed and congested by fluid or other material. This impairs ability of air cells to give off stale air, bring in fresh air.

Typical Symptoms of Virus Pneumonia

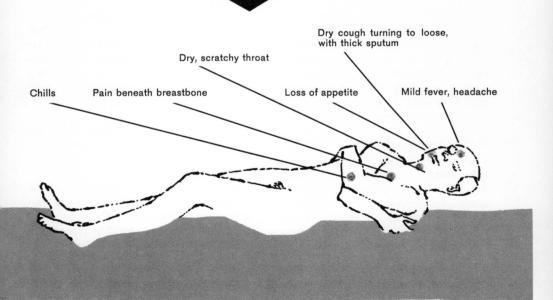

Dry cough turning to loose, with thick sputum

Dry, scratchy throat

Chills   Pain beneath breastbone   Loss of appetite   Mild fever, headache

more liable to be stricken by bacterial infection of the lungs and bronchial tubes. Such infections sometimes necessitate hospitalization.

treatment

Although antibiotics do not attack the organisms that cause viral pneumonia, they are usually prescribed to ward off bacterial infection during lowered resistance. Bed rest may be indicated, especially if there is a fever. All symptoms usually disappear in about a week if there are no complications.

prevention

The only safeguard against viral pneumonia is the maintenance of good health habits, with plenty of sleep, a wholesome diet and the avoidance of exposure to contagion.

PNEUMONIC PLAGUE. *See* PLAGUE.

PNEUMOTHORAX, a collection of air in the pleural sac, resulting from a stab wound or accidental surgical incision or from rupture of an abscess or tuberculous cavity. *Artificial pneumothorax* is employed in advanced tuberculosis to collapse the lung and give it a chance to heal by eliminating the strain and pressure of breathing. The other lung and the midriff take over the duty of respiration. The procedure of artificial pneumothorax is to insert a needle into the pleural cavity and inject sufficient air to compress the lung and stop its movement. *See also* ATELECTASIS; LUNGS; PLEURA *and* **medigraphs** BRONCHIECTASIS; EMPHYSEMA; LUNG ABSCESS; SILICOSIS; TUBERCULOSIS.

PODIATRY, diagnosis and treatment of diseases of the feet, formerly called *chiropody.* Podiatrists have a basic medical education and are licensed to prescribe such active drugs as may be needed and also to perform surgical operations on the feet. *See also* FEET.

POISONING. *See* FIRST AID.

POISON IVY, *dermatitis rhus,* a form of *contact dermatitis* resulting from touching poison ivy, poison oak or poison sumac by sensitized individuals. After a few hours, or even a few days, the hands or other contact areas become red and swollen; small and large blisters develop, which rupture and ooze and later form crusts. The itching is intense and may cause scratching and scars. To prevent recurrence, the sufferer should keep away from poison ivy, poison oak and poison sumac. *See also* ALLERGEN *and* **medigraph** CONTACT DERMATITIS.

POLIOMYELITIS

POLIOMYELITIS IS AN ACUTE contagious viral disease of the central nervous system that results in weakening and sometimes total loss of muscle function. Since the majority of its victims have traditionally been children under the age of ten, it has also been known as *infantile paralysis.* Effective immunization against this crippling disease was accomplished over a generation ago by the use of vaccines.

cause

The disease is caused by one of three different strains of the polio virus that attack the *motor nerve cells* in the spinal cord, thus disrupting the line of communication from the brain to the spinal cord to the muscle. The infectious agent may be present in the throat and in the intestinal tract, and is transmitted by food and water contaminated with human feces containing the virus, or by moisture from

Poliomyelitis (Infantile Paralysis)

After day or two of fever, headache and weakness, patient begins to develop such symptoms as:

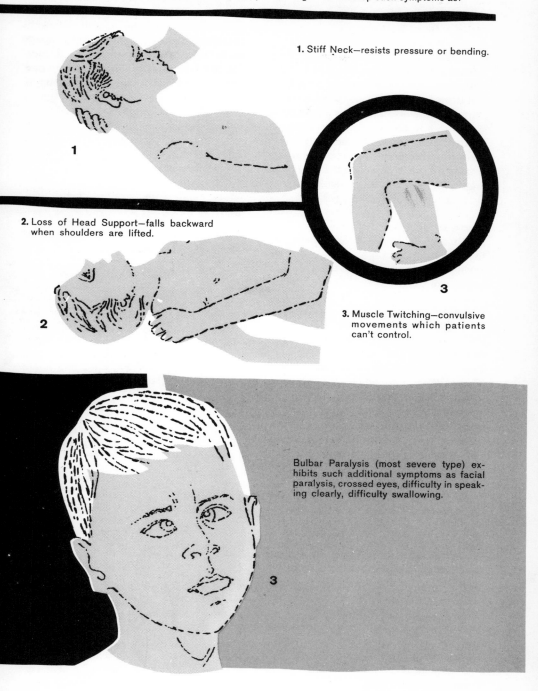

1. Stiff Neck—resists pressure or bending.

2. Loss of Head Support—falls backward when shoulders are lifted.

3. Muscle Twitching—convulsive movements which patients can't control.

Bulbar Paralysis (most severe type) exhibits such additional symptoms as facial paralysis, crossed eyes, difficulty in speaking clearly, difficulty swallowing.

the nose or mouth of a carrier or a person incubating the disease. Incubation period is from 7–10 days.

symptoms

The first symptoms are sore throat, vomiting, headache, fever, stiff neck and general drowsiness. In the *nonparalytic* form of the disease, symptoms usually subside in about a week and may never be accurately diagnosed. In *paralytic polio,* weakness of the muscles becomes evident around the ninth day after the first symptoms. Any or all of the muscles voluntarily controlled may be affected.

complications

If the disease attacks those nerves that control the muscles of breathing or swallowing, the patient may have to be placed in an iron lung. At any stage of the infection, lowered resistance to meningitis and other serious diseases increases the risks of permanent disability.

treatment

There is no cure for polio, but the stage of the disease at which treatment and close medical supervision begins is crucial to recovery and rehabilitation. Bed rest, proper diet and physical therapy for affected muscles during all phases are imperative. Some cases are mild enough to be handled at home; others require intensive care in a special hopsital unit.

prevention

Preferred immunization against polio consists of three oral doses of the *Sabin vaccine* starting at age two months and administered about two months apart. In communities where this is not routinely done, and enforced immunization does not take place until children are about to enter school, the most vulnerable victims of the disease are preschool-age youngsters. Wherever the vaccines have been used at the earliest time, poliomyelitis has practically disappeared.

POLLEN, the powdery male sex cells on the stamen of a flower, which are carried by the wind or by bees to distant flowers for fertilization. Certain pollens sensitize individuals, who subsequently develop allergies—specifically *hay fever* and *asthma.* The most common pollens of this type are *ragweed* (the fall type); *tree pollens* (the spring type); and *grass pollens* (the summer type). Since the pollen-bearing plants grow seasonally, a sufferer can avoid related allergies by moving temporarily to another area. *See also* ALLERGEN; ALLERGY; ANTIHISTAMINIC DRUGS *and* **medigraphs** BRONCHIAL ASTHMA; HAY FEVER.

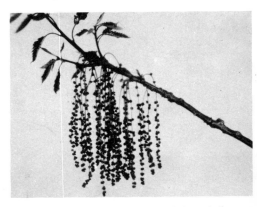

Pollen—The cottonwood (above) and the oak (below) are two of the trees that produce allergy-provoking pollen during April and May.

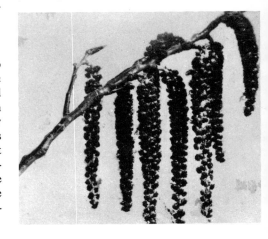

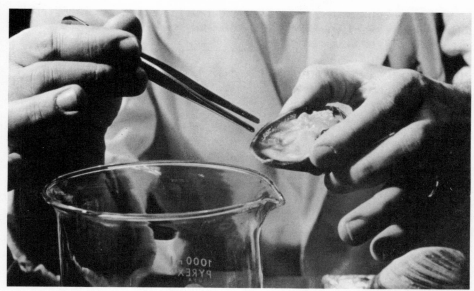

Courtesy, National Institutes of Health

Pollution—These clams will be carefully tested as part of a study of marine species that are sensitive to pollutants. If toxins are detected, authorities can be alerted to sources of potential human hazard. Industrial wastes and pesticides are two common causes of pollution.

POLLUTION, the contamination of the environment by such factors as chemicals, dusts, noise, toxic bacteria and radiation at harmful levels. There is a growing body of evidence that industrial wastes, pesticides, atomic radiation and other manmade pollutants—including such insidious threats as deadly chemicals mixed into animal feed and high mercury levels in fish—are replacing epidemics of infectious disease as the major determinants of life expectancy in the technologically advanced areas of the world. In the United States the Environmental Protection Agency has been established by Federal law to prevent further deterioration of the nation's air and water and to clean up such hazards as already exist. *See also* AIR POLLUTION; NOISE; POLYCHLORINATED BIPHENYLS; WATER POLLUTION *and* **medigraph** MERCURY POISONING.

R_{EPORT}ESEARCH *follows* POLYCHLORINATED BIPHENYLS.

POLYARTERITIS NODOSA, *Kussmaul-Maier disease,* a usually fatal disease of the blood vessels—most frequently those of the kidneys, but also of the heart, lungs, liver, gastrointestinal tract, eyes and joints. It is one of the group known as *collagen diseases.* Symptoms include necrosis (death) of segments of the vessels and inflammation of the arteries, causing functional impairment of the organs and tissues supplied by the affected arteries. The disease may be *acute,* with death occurring within a few months; or *chronic,* manifesting as a slow wasting disease. Other symptoms include fever, weight loss, abdominal and muscular pains, skin disturbances, and hypertension.

The cause is unknown. No cure is known, though *corticosteroids* may provide temporary relief. The disease usually occurs in middle age, and affects men three times as often as women.

Because *glomerulonephritis* is often

present, polyarteritis nodosa is believed to be a disease of *hypersensitivity. See also* COLLAGEN; VASCULAR SYSTEM.

POLYCHLORINATED BIPHENYLS

(PCBs), chemical compounds widely used in industry and considered a major environmental *pollutant* and *health hazard.* PCBs are similar in construction and toxicity to DDT and because they are highly stable and nonbiodegradable, they are carried by industrial waste into the air and water in their toxic form as a threatening contaminant. Workers exposed to PCBs on their jobs show symptoms of allergic dermatitis, eye and nasal irritation, and asthmatic bronchitis. In experiments with animals, PCBs have been shown to cause liver cancer and reproductive failure.

Tests sponsored by the U.S. Environmental Protection Agency indicate that PCBs have found their way into human milk and drinking water, as well as into fish and poultry. Since no area is considered immune to this threat, government agencies have ruled that temporary tolerance levels of PCBs in food for human consumption cannot exceed five parts per million for fish and poultry, 2.5 ppm for milk and dairy products and .5 ppm for eggs. Spot checks by official human monitoring programs calculate that approximately 40 percent of human fat tissue contains at least one part per million of PCBs. Moreover, a Canadian study found that human milk contained one ppm of PCBs—double the .5 ppm temporary tolerance level for infant and junior foods.

Ongoing research is being conducted to evaluate the cumulative effect of these chemicals as a threat to the nation's health. For example, it now appears that sludge is contaminated with PCBs and if the sludge is used to fertilize plants, the plants then become contaminated. This in turn can contaminate livestock and humans. *See also* AIR POLLUTION; IN-DUSTRIAL HEALTH; POLLUTION; PUBLIC HEALTH; WATER POLLUTION.

RESEARCH REPORT

POLYCHLORINATED BIPHENYL FOOD LEVELS AFFECT PREGNANCIES IN MONKEYS

After six months of a diet containing lower levels of *polychlorinated biphenyls* (PCBs) than are allowed in some human foods, the ability of female monkeys to achieve and maintain a pregnancy is greatly reduced, according to NATIONAL INSTITUTES OF HEALTH studies.

PCBs are stable chemicals widely used in industry for the past 40 years. They are present in the industrial wastes that pollute the air and water, and eventually are found in varying amounts in such foods as fish and poultry. The FOOD AND DRUG ADMINISTRATION considers these foods to be safe for human consumption if they contain less than five parts per million of PCB.

In experiments conducted at the WISCONSIN REGIONAL PRIMATE RESEARCH CENTER, half this level (2.5 ppm PCB) was contained in the diet given to eight adult female rhesus monkeys. After six months on the diet and following three matings with normal male monkeys, only three of the eight females became pregnant. In the other group of eight females on a diet containing 5 ppm PCBs, only one became pregnant. In a group of females on an untreated diet, nine out of ten became pregnant after three normal matings.

Because female rhesus monkeys have a 27-day menstrual cycle and share many other characteristics with human females, they are considered ideal models for studies of human reproduction. In this study, the PCB diet lengthened the period of menstrual flow, increased menstrual bleeding, and increased the metabolism of steroid hormones in the subjects. These altered hormone levels may have caused the reduced rate of successful pregnancies.

Male reproductive capability was apparently unaffected by the PCB diet. Those male monkeys who for one year received the diet containing

5 ppm PCB continued to sire off-spring by normal females at the usual rate.

Previous investigations at the Primate Center in which higher level PCB diets (25 to 300 ppm) were used reported that the monkeys showed pathological symptoms of hair loss, acne and enlarged livers. The present study is the first indication of the consequences of nonhuman consumption of levels of PCBs permissible in human food.   NIH515

POLYCYSTIC OVARIES, ovaries affected with multiple *cysts* (sacs filled with fluid or gelatinous material). Such cysts are not a threat to life, although they may cause trouble when they grow to huge size. The condition is characterized by associated symptoms of absent menstruation, abnormal uterine bleeding, hairiness of the face, and occasionally obesity and retarded breast development. *See also* CYST; OVARIES.

POLYCYTHEMIA, a chronic disease of the blood characterized by overgrowth of the bone marrow and increased production of the red blood cells—many of them nucleated—and also of hemoglobin and white blood cells. The normal red blood cell count is about 5,000,000 per cubic millimeter for men and 4,500,000 for women, the corpuscles being non-nucleated, and about 8,000 white blood cells. In polycythemia the red blood cell count rises up to 7,000,000–10,000,000 and the white cell count to 10,000–25,000. The blood is thickened by its high cellular content. The incidence of the disease is high in Jews and low in blacks, and more common in men than in women. The cause is unknown.

The most common symptoms are severe headache, a feeling of fullness in the head, ruddy complexion, dizziness, fainting spells, ringing in the ears, numbness and tingling in the hands and feet, distended veins, occasional spells of memory loss, quick tiring, disorders of vision, enlarged spleen, and hemorrhages in the skin or mucous membranes. Blood clots in the veins, bleeding from the bowel or stomach, and cirrhosis of the liver are the most common complications. Treatment includes *radioactive phosphorus* either intravenously or by mouth. *See also* BLOOD CONDITIONS; ERYTHREMIA; RED BLOOD CELLS, DISEASES OF.

POLYMYOSITIS, a form of the disease *dermatomyositis* in which the muscles are affected, but not the skin. It strikes women more often than men, usually in the 30–50 age group. The victim experiences extreme weakness in the muscles of the neck, throat, shoulders, trunk and hips. Though there is no cure for this disease, drugs and physiotherapy help to stem its progress. *See also* COLLAGEN; DERMATOMYOSITIS.

POLYNEURITIS, *multiple neuritis,* inflammation of many nerves, causing paralysis and loss of sensation in the affected areas. The most common causes are alcoholism, diabetes, vitamin B deficiency, infection, and various poisons including barbiturates, lead and other heavy metals. *See also* NERVOUS SYSTEM *and* **medigraph** NEURITIS.

POLYP, a benign growth that hangs by a *pedicle* (stalk) from the surface of a body cavity, varying widely in nature and structure depending on its origin. A *sessile polyp* is attached by a broad base. A *nasal polyp* contains a soft overgrowth of mucous membrane tissue from the nose and generally indicates a chronic infection of the underlying bone. A *rectal or bladder polyp*—arising from these organs and having a tendency to bleed—is originally benign but in some cases potentially malignant. A *uterine polyp* is one of the causes of spotting or bleeding between menstrual periods. It requires close watching because of the danger of malignancy. A *placental polyp* contains proliferating fragments of the afterbirth. An *adenocarcinomatous polyp* is one that has progressed to malignancy.

The most common treatment for polyps is surgical removal. Smaller polyps may be destroyed by electrolysis or application of chemical *escharotics* to convert the polyp into a scar. *See also* CANCER; CERVIX; NOSE; TUMOR *and* **medigraphs** DEVIATED SEPTUM; HAY FEVER; SINUSITIS.

POLYPHAGIA, excessive eating. Since this is one of the symptoms of diabetes, it is wise to investigate an abnormal increase in appetite. *See also* APPETITE.

PORES, small openings on the skin for the sweat and sebaceous (oil) glands.

Enlarged (*dilated*) pores are common in acne. The pores become clogged with hardened skin oil (*comedones*) and form blackheads when the surface collects dirt. The usual home treatment for dilated pores and blackheads is with steam and thorough washing with soapsuds and warm water followed by vigorous drying with a Turkish towel. Candy, chocolate, fatty foods, face creams, powder and cosmetics should be avoided, as they tend to aggravate the condition. *See also* COMEDONES; SKIN *and* **medigraph** ACNE.

PORPHYRIA, a hereditary metabolic disorder characterized by considerably increased formation and excretion of porphyrin and related substances, showing dark discoloration of the urine and other symptoms. *See also* BIRTH DEFECT; GENETIC COUNSELING.

PORTUGUESE MAN-OF-WAR, a large floating tubelike jellyfish, having a large bladderlike sac and a saillike structure on top, abounding in the tropical waters of the Gulf of Mexico and sometimes carried northward as far as Miami Beach. Its sting is poisonous. *See also* JELLYFISH DERMATITIS.

PORT-WINE STAIN, a birthmark derived from the primitive blood vessels appearing as a flat discoloration of a skin area. It is harmless except for the disfigurement when located on the face, which may be concealed by a covering cosmetic available in various shades to match the complexion. *See also* BIRTHMARK; HEMANGIOMA.

POSTMORTEM EXAMINATION. *See* AUTOPSY.

POSTNATAL CARE of the mother. Childbirth is an ordeal for many women, and rest and relaxation are required for recuperation. The mother should rest in a reclining position for several hours every day and lie on her abdomen for about 15 minutes. During the first week, visitors and telephone conversations should be limited. All persons with colds and other infections must be kept out.

The diet of the nursing mother is important as it also feeds the infant. It should contain milk, eggs, butter, green vegetables, and fresh fruit including tomatoes and oranges for vitamin C. A vitamin supplement supplying the recommended daily allowances of vitamins A and D is also recommended. Coffee, tea and laxative salts should be avoided as they eliminate water and thus reduce the quantity of milk. The nipples should be washed gently after each nursing and lubricated with oil if they become dry or chapped.

Systematic mild exercises, especially those that strengthen the weak abdominal muscles, are advisable. Strenuous exercises and social functions that involve travel away from home are not permitted. Television and games such as bridge and backgammon help to pass the time of this difficult period. The mother should visit the doctor—after six weeks have passed—for a physical examination which will include a pelvic ex-

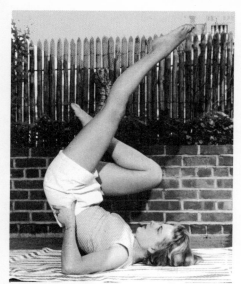

Postnatal Care—Weakened abdominal muscles need attention after a woman has given birth. Usually her physician will recommend exercises that are not too strenuous, such as the "bicycle ride" shown here. It not only tightens abdominal muscles, it slims and aids blood circulation in legs which may have received insufficient exercise in the last months of pregnancy.

amination (to be certain the reproductive organs have returned to their normal position). Under ordinary circumstances there is nothing to fear. *See also* CHILD-BIRTH; FEMININE HYGIENE; LOCHIA.

POSTPARTUM, the period following childbirth. *See* POSTNATAL CARE OF THE MOTHER.

POSTURAL DRAINAGE, a form of therapy, prescribed by doctors, for improved breathing in which gravity is used to drain out fluid that has accumulated deep in the tubes of the lungs. It is especially helpful to victims of asthma, chronic bronchitis, bronchiectasis and emphysema.

By lying in a series of different positions for short periods of time, mucus can be dislodged from the lung's *bron-*

chioles and moved along to the *bronchi* eventually reaching the *trachea* from where it can be coughed up more easily. The exercises of postural drainage are best done when the stomach is empty— for instance, before breakfast, late in the afternoon, and at bedtime—to avoid nausea or possible regurgitation. The whole process takes no more than 20–30 minutes each time.

A preliminary procedure that can be done while seated is the tapping of the chest from the bottom of the ribs to the shoulders, front and back, with the fingertips of one's cupped hands, but not excessively vigorously. This helps shake loose bronchial secretions and mucus plugs in distant parts of the lungs.

First exercise for postural drainage, to be done on a bed or carpeted floor:

1. Lie flat on the back without a pillow, arms at the sides, for 30 seconds.
2. Lie face down, inserting a firm pillow or books wrapped in a towel— for a thickness of 4–6 inches— under the lower abdomen, for 30 seconds.

Second exercise, to be done on a bed or carpeted floor:

1. Lie on left side, arms straight down, a pillow under the head; hold for 30 seconds.
2. Swing the right shoulder and torso forward, pivoting on the left shoulder; hold for 30 seconds.
3. Repeat as above while lying on the right side—30 seconds on the side; then swing the left shoulder and torso forward, pivoting on the right shoulder, and hold for 30 seconds.

Third exercise to be performed on a bed or board with the foot raised about 14 inches higher than the head:

1. Lying on the back, place small cushion or substitute under the buttocks; draw knees up as far as is comfortable with feet flat on the bed. Hold for 30 seconds.

Exercises for Postural Drainage

(Each Position held for 30 Seconds)

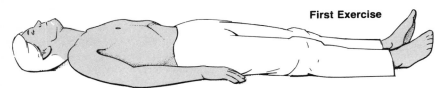

First Exercise

Lie flat on the Back, without a Pillow, Arms at the Sides

Lie Face down, with a Pillow under Abdomen

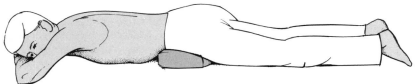

Second Exercise

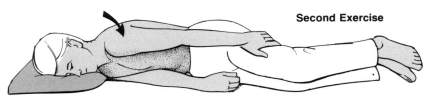

First lie on right Side, Pillow under Head, then
swing the left Shoulder and Torso forward

Third Exercise

Lying on the Back, Cushion under
Buttocks, Knees drawn up and
Feet flat on Bed

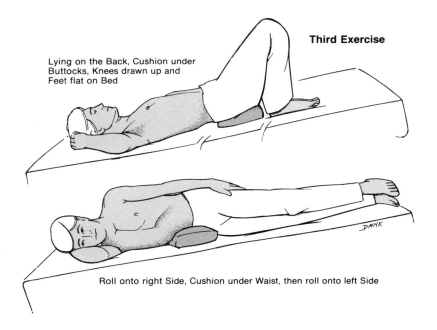

Roll onto right Side, Cushion under Waist, then roll onto left Side

2. Roll onto the left side, the cushion between the hip and bottom rib; hold for 30 seconds.
3. Roll onto the right side, and repeat as above; hold 30 seconds.

The final position is to empty the mucus the previous positionings have raised to the upper part of the bronchial tubes; it is done with the bed in its normal position. Lie across the bed face down, with hips and legs on the bed, head and torso hanging over the edge, forearms resting on the floor, and hands supporting the forehead. The neck should be in a straight line with the back to form a 45-degree angle with the floor. Place a bowl nearby for the sputum that will drain into the mouth. Sputum may not be produced at the first performance of postural drainage exercises, but fluids will be worked loose and may be coughed up later.

Personal physicians should be consulted by individuals for recommendations regarding additional or different exercises and their frequency. *See also* ASTHMA; LUNGS *and* **medigraphs** BRONCHIAL ASTHMA; BRONCHIECTASIS; BRONCHITIS; EMPHYSEMA.

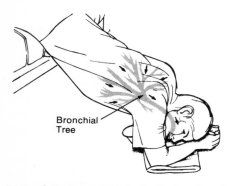

Postural Drainage—This is the final position in postural drainage. A series of reclining exercises have dislodged clogging mucus from the deep smaller tubes of the lungs and into the larger branches of the bronchial tree. The upper torso hanging at an angle from a bed, as illustrated, allows gravity to complete the process—the mucus drains into the mouth for expectoration.

POSTURE, the carriage of the body in walking, standing or sitting. Women in some cultures maintain an erect posture by carrying a basket of laundry on the head, and in the western world, fashion models are taught to do so by walking with a book on the head.

Modern men and women are inclined to slump and thus assume an unhealthy and unattractive posture. Certain abnormal postures are mostly the result of faulty habits of standing, walking and sitting. The *lordotic posture* appears as a forward curvature of the spine in the loin region; the *kyphotic posture,* as a backward curvature. Lordosis is largely the result of carelessness and can be corrected by learning to stand and sit erect in military fashion. Kyphosis results from tuberculosis of the spine, osteoarthritis or rheumatoid arthritis, and is aggravated by bad posture. Lordosis and kyphosis are not only unsightly but also tend to displace the abdominal organs and interfere with their physiological functions.

Good posture includes the sitting and resting position as well as the standing. In standing, the ideal posture is erect with the abdomen and chin drawn in and the shoulders square and high. In sitting, the body is erect and the head is poised over the location of the hip bones. A constant bent or droopy posture while at work or rest results in stretching and loosening of the ligaments and permanent sagging of the organs.

Good posture should be practiced regularly before a mirror. As one grows older, assuming bad posture is easy. A few simple exercises daily can help to correct these bad postural habits and thus avoid the backache which often results from them.

Schoolchildren may develop postural defects when they are seated at a desk which is too high or too low. Wearing high-heeled shoes is often responsible for backaches and may contribute to postural defects of the spine. The principal offenders are the three- and four-inch-high platform shoes worn by some people today. *See also* BACKACHE; KYPHOSIS; LORDOSIS; SPINAL CURVATURE.

POULTICE, an old home remedy for localized pains, consisting of linseed, flour or clay mush applied to the skin to provide heat and moisture.

PRECOCITY, early development of maturity, either mental or physical. *Mental precocity* is apparent in schoolchildren when they show superior intelligence to their classmates and the measured intelligence quotient is correspondingly higher. *Physical precocity* appears in such conditions as *pineal disease,* where the sexual organs of boys develop at an earlier age than usual. *See also* GENIUS; INTELLIGENCE; PINEAL GLAND; SEXUAL PRECOCITY.

PREECLAMPSIA, toxemia of late pregnancy. *See also* **medigraph** ECLAMPSIA AND PREECLAMPSIA.

PREFRONTAL LOBOTOMY. *See* PSYCHOSURGERY.

PREGNANCY, the period of childbearing, usually about 280 days, beginning with conception and ending with childbirth. To estimate the date of confinement, take the first day of the last menstrual period, count back three months, and add one year and seven days.

The signs of pregnancy become apparent soon after a woman's expected menstrual period does not take place. The earliest signs are in the breasts, which enlarge, feel heavy and show visible veins through the skin. The nipples darken, are surrounded by a darkened circle (*areola*), and are studded with little protuberances known as *Montgomery's tubercles.* The nipple discharges a whitish opaque secretion called *colostrum.*

The skin in certain areas becomes darker, especially around the nipples and in a straight line down the middle of the abdomen. Sometimes tender itching pinkish stripes are seen about the abdomen, breasts and thighs. Later they become white and disappear. Dark blotches may appear on the face, hands or elsewhere, called "the mask of pregnancy" when located on the face; there is a temporary growth of downy hair (*lanugo*) of the same type as that which covers the fetus about the fifth month.

Morning sickness with nausea and vomiting occurs in almost 50 percent of pregnant women at about the fifth or sixth week and usually clears up in 1–3 weeks. When the trouble persists and becomes more severe, it is called *pernicious vomiting of pregnancy* and requires medical attention.

With morning sickness, the diet should consist of frequent small meals including milk, broth, orange juice, ginger ale, and a multivitamin supplement. The woman should eat a cracker before getting up in the morning and limit her fluid intake.

In examinations using a finger inserted into the vagina, the physician perceives a progressive enlargement of the womb and also a softening of the tip. Through the speculum, the examiner notes that the mucous membrane of the vagina is darkened.

The lower abdomen begins to show a slight bulge around the third or fourth month of pregnancy, becoming progressively larger each month and rising higher in the abdomen. *Quickening* is an early symptom observed by the mother when she feels the fetal movements inside her abdomen. With a finger inside the vagina, the physician can detect the fetal movements and also outline the contour of the fetal body. The fetal heartbeat can be heard through a stethoscope—160 beats per minute during early pregnancy.

Complications of pregnancy include *ectopic gestation* (pregnancy in the Fallopian tube), *preeclampsia* and *eclampsia* (toxemia), *malposition of the fetus, uterine bleeding, anemia, high blood pressure, kidney disease, diabetes, miscarriage, twisting of the umbilical cord, death of the fetus,* and *premature* or *delayed labor. See also* AMNIOCENTESIS; AMNION; ANTENATAL; ANTEPARTUM; AREOLA; BAG OF WATERS; BIRTH DEFECT; CESAREAN SECTION; CHILDBIRTH; CONCEPTION; DETECTING TWINS; FALLOPIAN TUBES; FALSE PREGNANCY; FEMININE HYGIENE; GENETIC COUNSELING; MISCARRIAGE; MORNING SICKNESS; POSTNATAL CARE OF THE MOTHER; PREGNANCY TESTS; PRENATAL CARE; PRENATAL DEVELOPMENT; PRENATAL MEDICINE; REPRODUCTIVE SYSTEM; TOXEMIA; UTERUS *and* **medigraphs** ECLAMPSIA AND PREECLAMPSIA; ECTOPIC PREGNANCY; GERMAN MEASLES; TOXOPLASMOSIS.

PREGNANCY TESTS. There are a number of laboratory tests for pregnancy, the most reliable of which is the *Aschheim-Zondek.* A positive diagnosis is indicated when a sample of the woman's urine—injected into an immature female mouse or rabbit—induces swelling and congestion of the ovaries and enlargement of the follicles.

There are many variations of this test. In *Brown's test,* blood serum is used instead of urine. In the *Bercovitz test,* 5–6 drops of the woman's blood diluted with 1 drop of normal saline solution—instilled into the woman's eye—are supposed to indicate pregnancy when dilation or contraction of the pupil follows. The *Dienst test* is based on the increased antithrombin in the serum and urine of pregnant women; the *Fall's test,* on the reaction to a dilute suspension of colostrum injected into the forearm. The *Guterman test* depends on a chemical reaction to addition of sulfuric acid to a specimen of urine. A positive chemical reaction to *histidine* contained in pregnant urine is another procedure.

The many chemical and biological tests for pregnancy provide a means of confirming the diagnosis with considerable accuracy. *See also* ASCHHEIM-ZONDEK TEST; GENETIC COUNSELING; PREGNANCY; TESTS.

PREMARITAL CHECKUP. Both partners should be examined by a physician before they take the marriage vow. They must be in good health and, in particular, free from syphilis—as determined by blood tests—gonorrhea and tuberculosis. If they plan to have children, their ancestral history is most important, as many serious diseases are hereditary. Any person in poor health should not assume the responsibility of marriage. It could lead to serious consequences for both parties and particularly for any future children. *See also* GENETIC COUNSELING; KAHN TEST; PLANNED PARENTHOOD: WASSERMANN TEST.

PREMATURE AGING. A man is as old as his arteries, said the famous physician Sir William Osler. The age of 65 is usually set as the time when old age begins and retirement is advised. Many younger men are prematurely senile because of heredity, bad living habits, or intercurrent illnesses. The complications of premature aging include degenerative heart disease, hardened arteries, strokes, angina pectoris, cataracts, glaucoma, enlarged prostate, emphysema, chronic arthritis, senile warts and habitual constipation. As a general rule, men age earlier and have shorter lives than women. *See also* AGING.

PREMATURE BIRTHS, babies born before the full term of pregnancy (280 days) or weighing less than 5-1/2 pounds (2494.75 grams). According to statistics, five percent of all babies are born prematurely. Those born before the end of 28 weeks or weighing less than 2-1/5 pounds rarely survive, although exceptions have been recorded. In one case, an infant weighing only 1.6 pounds at birth weighed 17 pounds and 5 ounces at one year of age. Premature birth, the major cause of infantile mortality, is due mainly to an abnormality in the fetus or impaired health of the mother during pregnancy. By the time most premature infants are six months to a year old, they attain the normal weight for their age.

The premature baby is frail, feeble, and peevish, and its head is disproportionately large. It looks like an old person with prominent facial bones and flabby soft parts. Its principal handicaps are inability to regulate the body heat, delicate digestion, and susceptibility to infection.

A dangerous complication is the formation of *pulmonary hyaline membranes* which interfere with breathing and may cause suffocation within one to three days if not absorbed by the action of the white blood cells or removed surgically.

Regulation of the body heat in an incubator is the first step in the care of premature infants. The *isolette* is one type of automatic incubator. Another incubator, designed at the National Institute for Medical Research in London, features a ripple mattress which registers movement of the baby by monitoring the flow of air in the ripples. If the baby stops breathing, the air stops flowing and an electrical device sounds an alarm. Portable incubators have been developed for births taking place at home, so that the baby can be put into the device almost immediately after birth and then taken to the hospital.

Breast milk in large quantities is the best food for premature babies, using a wet-nurse if necessary. Since high caloric

Premature Births—The birth weights of these five premature infants total just over nine and a half pounds. The baby at extreme left was born weighing one and a quarter pounds and is not fully developed. At the right, the baby has more than doubled her weight in 68 days. But at four pounds, five ounces she is still below the five-and-a-half-pound minimum for normal birth weight.

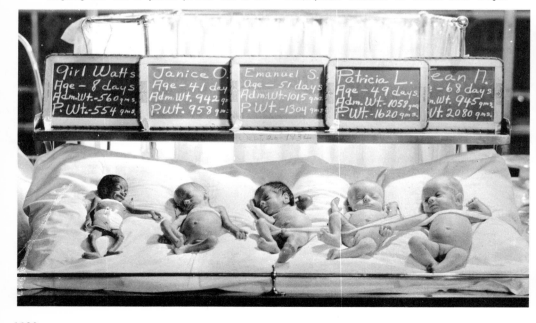

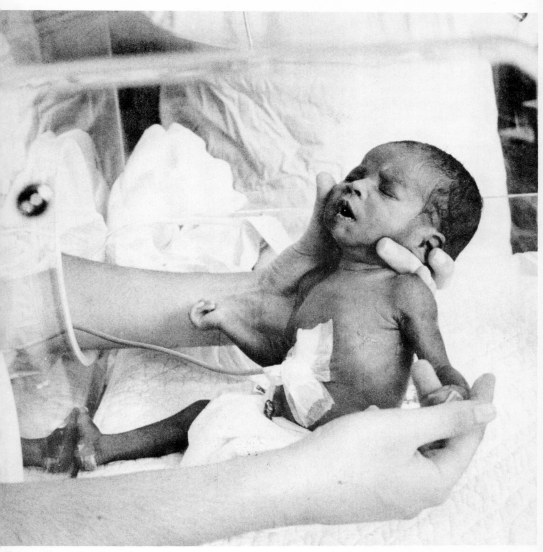

Premature infants present a special problem for physicians. Because of the precarious condition of such babies, incubators have assumed an indispensable role in their care. Modern incubators are very sophisticated. Besides regulating the temperature and humidity of the infant's environment, supplying its oxygen at whatever optimum concentrations, and filtering out its exhaled carbon dioxide and moisture, the contemporary incubator records the temperature, heartbeat, and breathing of the baby and stores these data on magnetic tape for instant reference by doctors and nurses. An added safeguard is an alarm system which goes off when the baby's condition deviates seriously from normal, giving attendants immediate alert of the emergency. The incubator, made of transparent plastic, is equipped with side portholes fitted with flexible plastic curtains through which attendants can put their arms to perform essential functions without disturbing the controlled atmospheric environment inside.

Premature babies are often afflicted with respiratory distress associated with acidosis (abnormal acidity of blood and tissues). To analyze the blood, a catheter is inserted into an umbilical artery or vein (above). It can monitor the oxygen content of the blood.

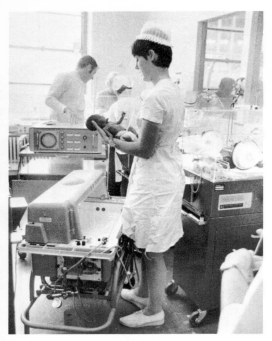

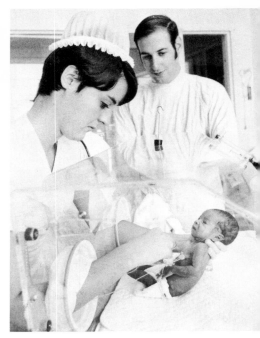

Through the umbilical catheter *(below)*, solutions of sodium bicarbonate may be given to maintain normal acid-base balance of the blood and tissues and thus enhance respiratory mechanisms. Scrupulous maintenance of temperature within the incubator also helps maintain proper chemical balance. Oxygen and humidity may be increased as required. Above right, the infant's heartbeat is monitored. Most essential tests can be performed without removing the baby from its environment. Left, arrival from delivery room.

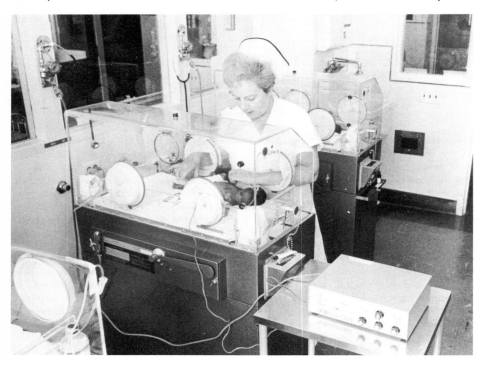

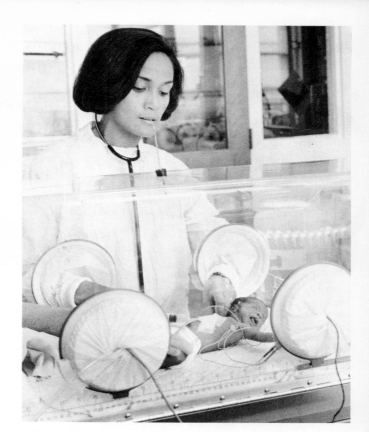

The intensive care incubator shown here is called an isolette. This ingenious invention has been responsible for saving many lives.

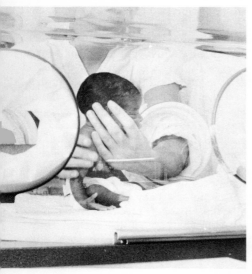

This premature infant (top) is given a battery of tests—all of which will assist his chances for survival. The multi-purpose umbilical catheter is in place, the heartbeat is being monitored, and he will undergo an electroencephalogram to determine if any brain damage has occurred during birth. Left, a nurse inserts her arms through the flexible apertures. Below, the baby is fed through a tube. Note the elaborate controls.

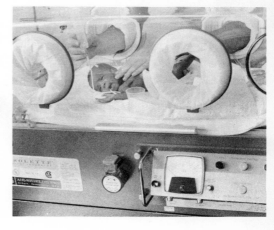

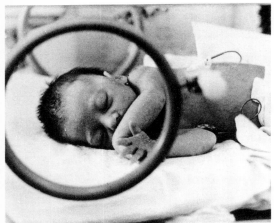

Courtesy, National Institutes of Health

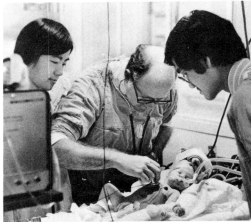

Courtesy, National Institutes of Health

Premature Births—Electronic monitors keep a constant watch as this three-and-a-half-pound baby sleeps in a premature infants research center. Respiratory distress is the most common problem of premature babies. Research has developed therapy to improve their survival rate.

Premature Births—Medical students observe a physician checking a baby on a respirator. Difficulty in breathing affects 20–25 percent of premature infants in the United States. Often these immature babies are also unable to regulate body heat and must be placed in incubators.

Premature Births—A mother learns to feed and care for her premature baby during daily hospital visits. The infant began life weighing just one pound and a half. Thanks to modern techniques in treating the many complications of prematurity, more such tiny infants are surviving and progressing to normal development.

Courtesy, National Institutes of Health

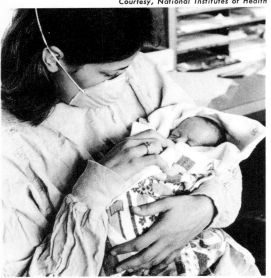

feeding is required to enable the baby to catch up on weight, daytime intervals of two hours and nighttime of three hours are recommended. Later, as weight and strength are attained, standard infant milk formulas may be substituted, with careful precaution that they not be fed in excessive amounts that may upset the delicate digestion and cause vomiting. Cod liver oil or other sources of vitamin D—not to exceed a daily potency of 400 U.S.P. units—is recommended for prevention of rickets. As a source of vitamin C, tomato or grapefruit juice is preferred to orange juice, since the latter sometimes upsets digestion.

Due to the baby's low resistance to infection, special precautions must be taken in the care of the premature infant to protect it from contact with those who may transmit colds, influenza, or pneumonia.

Just as the premature baby catches up on its weight during the first year, it likewise advances mentally. In the early months, coordination is poor and the baby learns slowly. But as it grows up, the infant has every prospect of equaling other children in mental capacity. *See also* BIRTH DEFECT; GENETIC COUNSELING; HYALINE MEMBRANE DISEASE; INFANT DEATHS; OXYGEN; RETROLENTAL FIBROPLASIA.

Rᴇsᴇᴀʀᴄʜ ᴇᴘᴏʀᴛ *follows* HYALINE MEMBRANE DISEASE.

PREMATURE EJACULATION, occurrence of the male sexual climax within less than a minute after the penis enters the vagina, usually leaving the woman sexually aroused without satisfaction. It is estimated that approximately 25 percent of married couples fail to reach the climax at the same time. The problem may be due to hypersensitivity of the head of the penis, irritation of the trigger mechanism of the ejaculation reflex, or a psychoneurosis related to the sex life. Application of a numbing ointment containing *benzocaine* or *dibucaine* to the head of the penis before intercourse helps to delay the climax. *See also* EJACULATION; EJACULATORY SYSTEM; SEXUAL ABNORMALITIES.

PREMENSTRUAL TENSION, symptoms of emotional irritability, headache, enlargement of the breasts, and weight gain of 3–10 pounds appearing during the week preceding the expected menstrual date. Authorities estimate that it affects about 60 percent of women and is due mainly to retained water in the system, caused by disordered secretion of *progesterone* and *adrenocortical hormone*. Some women become so nervous that they quarrel with others and even commit acts of violence. The generally accepted treatment is a dehydration regimen beginning 12–14 days before the expected menstrual date and implemented by limitation of the fluid intake to a quart daily, a salt-free diet, and administration of a diuretic. *See also* MENSTRUATION.

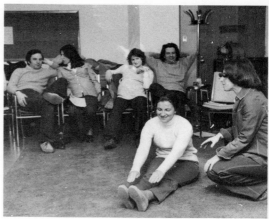

Courtesy, March of Dimes

Prenatal Care—Parents-to-be watch a prenatal exercise being demonstrated. Prepared childbirth classes have become an important part of prenatal care by educating couples in all aspects of pregnancy and birth. In addition to information, there is emphasis on exercises to strengthen and better control women's muscles most involved during pregnancy and labor.

PRENATAL CARE. When a woman skips a menstrual period, she should suspect pregnancy and should visit her doctor. The doctor can determine by physical examination—or, if needed, by laboratory tests—whether or not she is pregnant.

If a woman is pregnant, she should try to make certain that her baby will be healthy. Thus, her own health during the nine months of pregnancy is important. All detrimental activities must be stopped: smoking, hard liquor, inadequate sleep and heavy work are proscribed.

A balanced diet providing the customary proportions of milk, meat, fish, green and yellow vegetables, and fruits is essential. Iron, calcium, and vitamins may be deficient, so a multivitamin-mineral supplement providing the recommended daily allowances of all essential vitamins and minerals is advisable. A prospective mother usually gains about 14 percent in weight during the nine months; a weight increase of more than 20 pounds is far too much.

At each examination, the doctor will measure the blood pressure and possibly take a specimen of urine. Any unusual symptoms—such as morning nausea, vomiting, headaches, swellings, sore breasts, and bleeding from the vagina—should be reported to the doctor immediately. *See also* BIRTH DEFECT; GENETIC COUNSELING; PREGNANCY; PRENATAL DEVELOPMENT; PRENATAL MEDICINE *and* **medigraphs** ECLAMPSIA AND PREECLAMPSIA; ECTOPIC PREGNANCY; GERMAN MEASLES; TOXOPLASMOSIS.

Rᴇsᴇᴀʀᴄʜ ᴘᴏʀᴛ *follows* TOXOPLASMOSIS.

PRENATAL DEVELOPMENT. Life begins with a single fertilized egg cell in the Fallopian tube, which is carried upward to be lodged in the uterus. Here it begins to develop by multiplication of its cells. Up to the third month of pregnancy it is known as the *embryo,* thereafter as the *fetus.*

Three primary layers of embryonic tissue develop: the *ectoderm* (outer layer) from which the skin, the nervous system, and the lining of the stomach and rectum form; the *mesoderm* (middle layer), which gives rise to the muscles, connective tissue and blood vessels; and the *entoderm* (inner layer), which forms the lining of the intestines and related glands. The *limb-buds,* from which the arms and legs are developed, and the rudimentary nose, eyes and ears appear in the fifth week, which is the time when they may be destroyed by a deforming drug such as *thalidomide.* The head enlarges greatly and is bent forward. In the third and fourth months, the fetus is suspended by a stalk from the inside of the uterus called the *allantois,* which later forms the placenta, through which the fetus is nourished. The development of the various organs from these rudiments constitutes the science of *embryology. See also* AMNION;

BIRTH DEFECT; CONCEPTION; EMBRYO; FETUS; PREGNANCY; PRENATAL CARE; PRENATAL MEDICINE; UTERUS.

PRENATAL MEDICINE, the application of scientific knowledge to the care of the unborn child. It begins before pregnancy with investigation of the heredity and health of the prospective parents. The mother-to-be should consult her physician once a month in the early pregnancy and every two weeks later on. The examination will evaluate the size of the pelvis to determine whether childbirth can take place naturally, the mother's health, and the size and growth of the fetus. The diet will be such as to permit a weight gain of 14 percent during the nine months, but a gain of 20 pounds must be controlled. The mother should drink plenty of milk to supply calcium and phosphorus for the infant's bones, and also balanced proportions of meat, fish and fresh fruits and vegetables. Doctors advise most pregnant women to take a dietary supplement containing the recommended daily allowances of all essential vitamins and minerals. Next to calcium, the most important mineral for pregnant women is iron. During pregnancy the physician takes the blood pressure routinely and also has specimens of urine and blood examined as possible indicators of complications. At each examination, the doctor will question the patient concerning her vision, headaches, bleeding, unusual swellings and will possibly conduct a physical examination accordingly. The principal danger signals are persistent nausea and vomiting, vaginal bleeding, headaches and blurred vision. Excitement, emotional disturbances, and sexual intercourse during the latter months of pregnancy must be avoided. Next to heredity, the most important means of giving birth to a healthy child is the observance of good hygiene during pregnancy. Therefore, smoking, heavy drinking and inadequate sleep are bad habits for which the child may have to pay a heavy price. *See also* BIRTH DEFECT; GENETIC COUNSELING; PREGNANCY; PRENATAL CARE; PRENATAL DEVELOPMENT.

PRESBYCUSIS, partial deafness in old age, usually affecting the *cochlea* (hearing organ of the internal ear embedded in the petrous portion of the temporal bone). The loss of hearing is greatest for the higher frequencies. The condition is progressive and usually permanent. The ordinary hearing aids are not effective in this type of deafness, but recently invented devices provide considerable improvement of hearing for some people. *See also* DEAFNESS; EAR; HEARING AIDS.

PRESBYOPIA, reduced acuity of vision and farsightedness due to inelasticity of the crystalline lens as people grow older, with consequent loss of power of accommodation to distance. As a result, the image focuses behind the retina and near vision is impaired, as evidenced by difficulty in reading small, closely-spaced print unless it is held at a distance.

The first sign of presbyopia is usually in the 40's and the condition becomes progressively worse with advancing years. For near vision, corrective convex lenses are required, adjusted to the subject's occupation with regard to the distance of the visual object from the eye. For ordinary readers, a distance of 12–16 inches from the eyes is customary. Musicians may require bifocal lenses, so they can see both the score and the conductor, as may radio and TV performers, who must see both the script and the director. Linotypists with presbyopia should be fitted with convex lenses which correct their vision at a distance of 12–13 inches. The eyes should be reexamined at least once a year to adjust the glasses to changes in the degree of presbyopia. *See* ACCOMMODATION; EYE; EYEGLASSES; LENS.

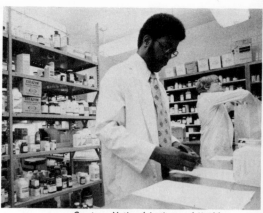

Courtesy, National Institutes of Health

Prescription—A prescription specifies a medication, the quantity to be dispensed and instructions for taking it. A pharmacist is responsible for accurately filling the prescription and must ascertain that it was indeed written by a physician. This pharmacist checks an order form for pharmaceuticals. Keeping his stock complete is important to sick people, too.

PRESCRIPTION, a written order signed by a licensed physician instructing a pharmacist to prepare the specified medication with instructions for its use. In former years, the prescription usually called for several ingredients, *polypharmacy,* but prescription of a single ingredient is now regarded as the wisest course because of the possibility of interaction of the various constituents.

Medications are of two classes: *Rx,* which can be dispensed only on prescriptions; and *OTC* (over the counter), which are available without a prescription. Only a month's supply of certain narcotic and dangerous drugs can be dispensed, and the patient's name and address must be written on the prescription. For such drugs, the physician in the United States must be licensed by the Drug Enforcement Agency of the Department of Justice, and certain narcotics require a special prescription form in triplicate. It is customary for the pharmacist to check the prescription with his reference books, so as to avoid possible error. In case of doubt, the pharmacist phones the doctor for verification. *See also* DOSAGE; PHARMACOLOGY.

PRESSURE POINTS, small areas on the skin of considerable sensibility to pressure. *See also* BEDSORES; FIRST AID; HEMORRHAGE.

PREVENTIVE MEDICINE, the application of hygienic and scientific measures to prevent the occurrence of diseases in the body. Typical examples are cessation of smoking cigarettes to obviate lung cancer, use of vitamin D to prevent rickets, use of vitamin C to prevent scurvy, use of the condom to obviate veneral diseases, vaccination to prevent smallpox, injections of triple typhoid vaccine to prevent typhoid and paratyphoid fevers, and various other forms of inoculation for prevention. *See also* CANCER PREVENTION; HYGIENE; IMMUNIZATION; NUTRITION; POLLUTION; PUBLIC HEALTH; QUARANTINE; VACCINATION.

PRIAPISM, abnormal erection and stiffness of the penis unrelated to sexual desire. It occurs in certain injuries and diseases of the spinal cord and also in cases of stone in the bladder. It is relieved by immersing the penis in cold water. *See also* PENIS.

PRICKLY HEAT, *heat rash, miliaria,* an acute inflammation of the sweat glands, common in children, characterized by intense itching and eruption of numerous tiny blisters and elevated pinkish spots. The most common sites are on the chest, back, waistline, and skin folds. The eruption subsides in a few days and may be followed by flaking of the skin. It occurs on exposure to intense heat, particularly moist heat, during the summer or in the tropics. The principal complications are chafing, par-

ticularly in obese persons, and infection of the skin due to scratching.

For persons who are subject to prickly heat, these precautionary measures are advised.

1. Wear light clothing during hot weather.
2. Bathe frequently and use a dusting powder after drying the skin.
3. Never use soap, which increases itching and may aggravate the inflammation.
4. Drink water and other liquids freely. Air conditioning may prevent the attack.

Cool clothing, dusting powders, and abundance of water or other liquids, with vitamins B_1 and C to replenish the loss in the sweat, are useful. The most commonly employed medications to relieve the itching include lotions of *menthol* or *camphor.* If infection occurs from itching, an antibiotic may be prescribed. Bathing twice daily for 10–20 minutes in a tubful of warm water containing oatmeal or starch is helpful.

PROBE, a slender flexible rod with a blunted end used to explore a cavity or wound or search for a stone in the bladder, or by military surgeons to locate a bullet. X-ray localization has taken the place of probing for bullets. *See also* MEDICAL INSTRUMENTATION.

PROCTITIS, inflammation of the anus or rectum, due most often to anal gonorrhea following anal intercourse or irritating treatments for hemorrhoids.

PROCTOLOGY, the study of diseases of the rectum and anus.

PROCTOSCOPE, an instrument for inspecting the anus and rectum. *See also* MEDICAL INSTRUMENTATION.

PROGESTERONE, the hormone secreted by the *corpus luteum* (yellow sub-

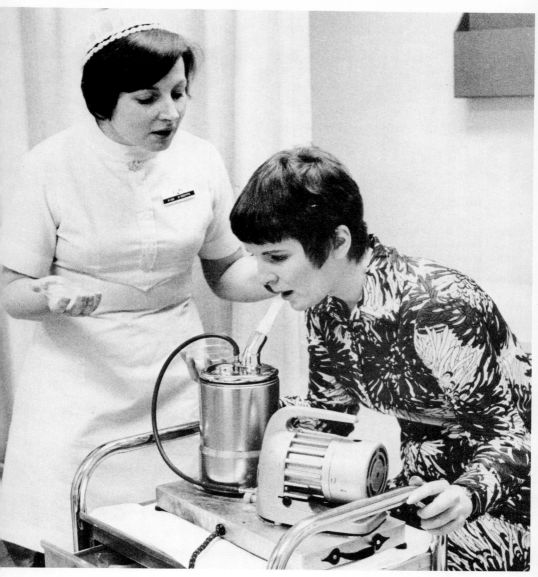

More and more attention is being paid to preventive medicine. It may be a cliché, but is still entirely valid, that "an ounce of prevention is worth a pound of cure." To nip any kind of bug in the bud is the best sort of remedy. Regular physical examinations cannot be too urgently advocated. Such periodic checkups can detect diseases and disorders in their early stages, when they are far easier to eradicate or control.

A general physical examination should include inspection of the skin, lymph nodes, eyes, ears, nose, mouth, throat, heart, thy-roid gland, lungs, breasts, stomach, intestines, rectum and reproductive organs, as well as tests of the blood, musculo-skeletal and neurological systems. Should the patient have a specific complaint, attention should focus on determining its source.

Modern medical science has developed numerous sophisticated techniques and devices in testing and diagnosis. Above, a patient's sputum is collected and washed by an aerosol machine preliminary to laboratory analysis. This test will reveal if cancer cells exist in the lungs or respiratory tract.

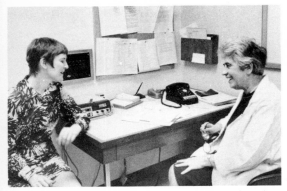
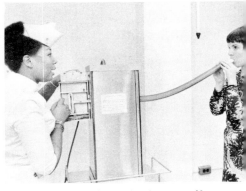

The first step in any medical examination is assembling the patient's prior medical history *(above left)*. The specific tests can then commence. Above right, a patient is examined for possible bronchial problems. The machine can identify cases of emphysema. A graph on the "auto-analyzer" *(center left)* records the results of a blood analysis. The physician *(center right)* points out a detail of importance in the patient's x-ray. X-rays are a standard and indispensable diagnostic tool. Bottom left, a "biotronic tonometer" measures intraocular (inner eye) pressure in a test for possible glaucoma. Many cases of blindness can be prevented if the conditions giving rise to glaucoma are located in time. Bottom right, slides of blood samples are stored in these "staining dishes."

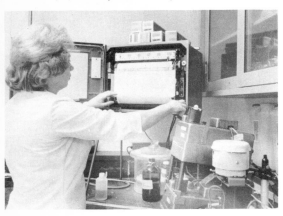
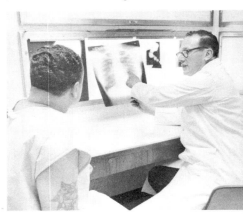
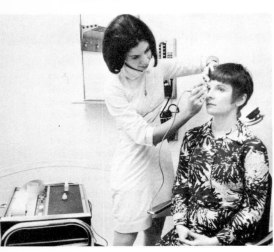
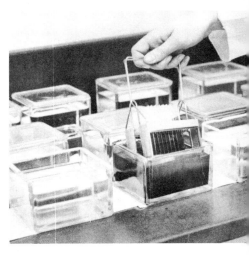

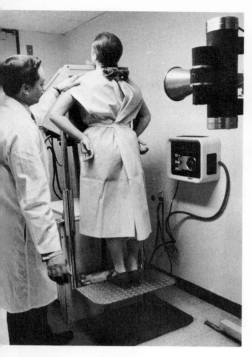

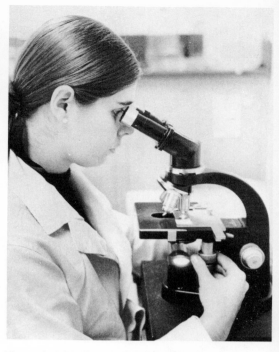

The elaborate equipment above (top left), called a photoroentgen machine, takes chest x-rays. The platform on which the patient is standing can be raised or lowered to accommodate height. The examiner here guides the patient into the best stance.

The technician (top right) examines a slide under a binocular microscope. Medical technicians perform many of the more routine chores connected with physical examinations. Below, a nurse takes a patient's blood pressure. At right, standard medical utensils.

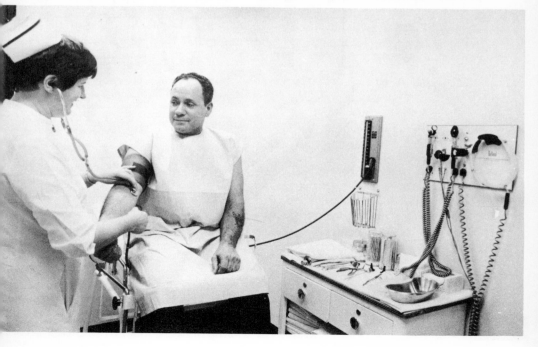

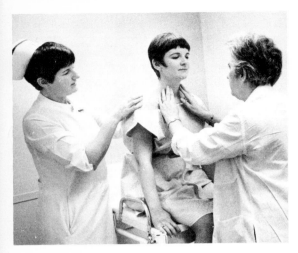

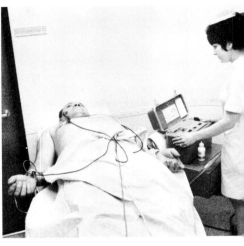

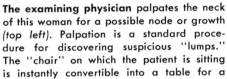

The examining physician palpates the neck of this woman for a possible node or growth *(top left)*. Palpation is a standard procedure for discovering suspicious "lumps." The "chair" on which the patient is sitting is instantly convertible into a table for a prone or supine examination. Above right, a nurse takes an electrocardiogram. The physician will interpret the information from this machine and can usually tell if there is any heart malfunction. Below, a wide-area x-ray examination.

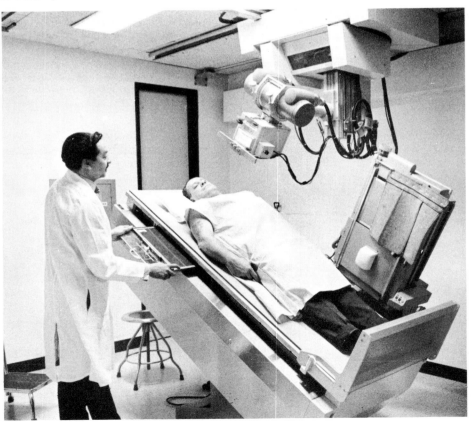

stance) of the ovary whose function is to prepare the uterus for reception and development of the *fertilized ovum* (female sex egg) by growth of its lining membrane. Progesterone is administered by injection or absorption from the mouth in the treatment of certain menstrual disorders and is also a constituent of oral contraceptives. *See also* ADRENAL GLAND; FEMALE SEX HORMONES; HORMONES; MENSTRUATION; ORAL CONTRACEPTIVES; OVARIES; PITUITARY. RESEARCH REPORT *follows* CANCER.

PROGNOSIS, prediction of the outcome of an illness based on the person's condition and on scientific knowledge concerning the usual course and result in such illnesses, together with the presence of certain symptoms and signs that indicate the expected outcome. Prognosis is the most uncertain branch of medicine. *See also* DIAGNOSIS.

PROLAPSE, the falling down or sinking of an organ from its normal position. The organs most generally affected are the uterus, hemorrhoids from the rectum, the umbilical cord, and the iris (circular colored disc of the eye) through a wound in the front of the eyeball.

Prolapse of the uterus results from a stretching of its ligaments during labor. The uterus falls downward and the cervix is pushed through the vagina, sometimes protruding. The prolapse may cause backache and other discomforts, interferes with sexual intercourse, and exposes the cervix to irritation and infection. After the physician has replaced the uterus manually, it may be held in place with a *pessary* (a device used to support the uterus in its normal position). Sometimes an operation is performed by which the uterus is stitched onto an abdominal ligament. *See also* HERNIA; INTUSSUSCEPTION; PESSARY; *and* **medigraphs** HIATUS HERNIA; INGUINAL HERNIA; INTESTINAL OBSTRUCTION.

PROPHYLACTIC, a remedy or procedure that aims to prevent certain diseases. *Venereal prophylaxis* utilized mercurial ointment to prevent syphilis and silver salt injection to prevent gonorrhea. Public health authorities seldom recommend such prophylactics any more because they are thought to be inadequate. *Dental prophylaxis* provides periodical dental examination and care for treatment of cavities, accumulated tartar, inflamed gums, and other oral diseases. *See also* CONDOM; ORTHODONTIA *and* **medigraphs** GONORRHEA; SYPHILIS.

PROSTAGLANDINS, unsaturated fatty acids which affect a multitude of actions in the body, such as the role of endocrines and reproduction, the mobility of the gastrointestinal system and its secretions and the functions of the blood vessels and the kidneys. They are involved in inflammation and in the passage of water and electrolytes through membranes of the body. Some 16 prostaglandins have been identified. Such drugs as aspirin and indomethacin inhibit the formation of prostaglandins.

Scientists have established the relationships of secretions from the kidney in blood pressure control. When these prostaglandins are given to people with high blood pressure, they decrease the blood pressure, increase the flow of blood through the kidneys and the body of water and sodium in the urine. Thus these prostaglandins have hormonal effects in regulating blood pressure. They are known as PGA and PGE. Eventually PGA may become the ideal hypertensive agent. Prostaglandins may also act to stimulate gonadotropin secretion by the pituitary gland. The prostaglandins are involved in the action of the ovaries in secreting hormones. They can also stimulate the uterus to contract and therefore are sometimes used to induce abortion.

One prostaglandin acts in the formation of red blood cells and may be important in controlling circulation of the blood through the capillary blood vessels. This prostaglandin is believed to induce sickling in red blood cells and to be involved in causing the platelets to stick together in coagulation of the blood.

The prostaglandins also participate in inflammation; they are particularly significant in the development and treatment of asthma. The "E" prostaglandins dilate the bronchial tubes, and the "F" prostaglandins constrict the bronchial tubes.

Prostaglandins act on the gastrointestinal tract, both stimulating and inhibiting movement of the intestines, secretion of gastric juices in the stomach and the use of sugar in the chemistry of the liver. Many of these substances are now being tested in laboratories to determine the limits of their action.

The nervous system can develop prostaglandins and use them in its functions. Some prostaglandins have been found in the spinal fluid. Studies in progress have shown effects on behavior, hunger, the temperature of the body, and regulation of the action of the heart.

The body also contains substances that inhibit actions of the prostaglandins, so that they are called *antagonists*. Because of this, the antagonists are being studied; if they can be isolated and prepared for use in the body, they may be used in the treatment of spontaneous abortion, diarrhea, spasm of the blood vessels, fever, sickle cell anemia, obstructive lung diseases, inflammation and in the eye, uveitis and glaucoma.

RESEARCH REPORT *follows* PERIODONTAL DISEASE.

RESEARCH REPORT

○   HIGH BLOOD PRESSURE MAY   ○
        RESULT FROM DEFICIENCY
○   OF PROSTAGLANDINS   ○

○   A deficiency in the kidneys of hor-
        mone-like substances known as *pros-*   ○
○   *taglandins* may be the underlying

cause of the development of *hypertension* (high blood pressure), according to researchers at the STATE UNIVERSITY OF NEW YORK in Buffalo. Injections of prostaglandins into hypertensive patients resulted in the restoration of normal blood pressure, normal blood flow in the kidneys, and normal salt and water excretion. These findings support the theory that hypertension may be a *deficiency* disease which can be remedied by replacement therapy.   NIH216

PROSTATE, a male sexual organ located at the neck of the bladder below the junction of the two pubic bones and in front of the rectum, through which it can be felt by the examiner's finger. It is conical in shape, about the size of a chestnut, and composed of muscular and glandular tissues. The function of the prostate is to secrete a fluid in which the sperm cells can live after ejaculation of the semen. The prostate surrounds the deeper part of the urethra, the tube through which urine and semen are ejected. When enlarged, it blocks urination by compressing the urethra.

Acute and chronic *prostatitis* may result from gonorrhea and other infections. These diseases can be treated effectively with suitable antibiotics.

In men over 50, *benign prostatic hypertrophy* (enlargement of the prostate) is a common trouble. It is benign in about 80 percent of cases and malignant in 20 percent. The presence of cancer of the prostate is suggested by occasional drops of blood in the urine, and the urologist can feel hard lumps on the prostate by rectal examination. Benign enlargement is slowly progressive with difficulty in urination, delay in starting and finishing it, a constant urge without result, and *residual urine* (the amount that can be removed by a catheter after the person has tried to empty his bladder). The recommended treatment is surgical removal of the prostate by either of two standard operations: *transurethral resection* (through the urethra) or the *two-stage suprapubic operation* (through the abdominal wall just above the junction of the two pubic bones). The latter operation does not cause impotence. *Electrical dissection* of the prostate can be performed through a tube passed into the prostatic area. In place of surgery some men prefer repeated catheterization, though it ultimately and usually leads to infection of the bladder.

In cancer of the prostate, surgical removal offers the only hope of prolonging life. If metastasis to the bones and vital organs occurs, removal of the testicles and injection of the estrogenic female sex hormone delay the inevitable fatal outcome and relieve the pain. *See also* BLADDER DISEASES; EJACULATORY DUCTS; EJACULATORY SYSTEM; GLANDS; PROSTATECTOMY; PROSTATISM; PROSTATITIS; REPRODUCTIVE SYSTEM *and* **medigraphs** PROSTATE GLAND ENLARGEMENT; URINARY TRACT PROBLEMS.

PROSTATECTOMY, surgical removal of the prostate for benign or malignant hypertrophy. *See also* PROSTATE *and* **medigraph** PROSTATE GLAND ENLARGEMENT.

PROSTATE GLAND ENLARGEMENT

T HE PROSTATE GLAND is an accessory organ of the male reproductive system. It surrounds the urethra at the base of the bladder and the alkaline fluid that it constantly secretes is thought to nourish and lubricate the sperm cells. The chief disorder that affects the prostate is the condition known as *benign enlargement*. About half the male population over the age of 50 suffers from prostate enlargement regardless of sexual circumstances.

Cancer of the prostate accounts for 10 percent of all male cancer deaths in the United States. It rarely occurs before age 60 and if diagnosed early enough can be treated with considerable success.

causes
The specific cause of benign prostatic enlargement is unknown. It is thought to be the hormonal changes that accompany aging. The condition is not inflammatory, nor is it related to cancer of the prostate for which the cause is also unknown.

symptoms
Since swelling of the prostate interferes with bladder function, the earliest symptoms are increasing difficulty in beginning to urinate and a feeling that the bladder is never emptied. The need to urinate becomes more frequent, and a burning sensation may accompany the passing of urine, due in part to the onset of infection.

Cancer of the prostate may produce no symptoms in its early stages, or it may cause the same discomforts as benign enlargement.

complications
A consequence of prostate enlargement can be a kidney disorder known as *hydronephrosis* that results from the spread of infection originating in the bladder because of urine retention. Complete obstruction of the bladder by the swelling of the gland may make urination impossible and require hospitalization so that the victim can be catheterized.

Undetected and untreated cancer of the prostate will eventually travel (*metastasize*), especially to the bones and the lungs.

treatment
The preferred treatment for an enlarged prostate is removal of the entire gland by an open operation through the abdominal wall. This procedure is known as

Prostate Gland Enlargement

Cancer of the Prostate

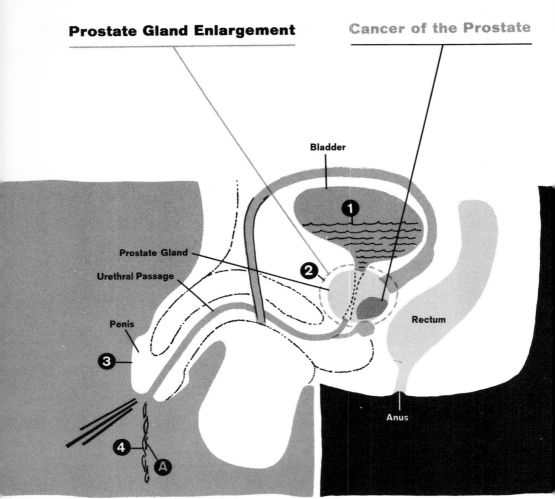

Bladder

Prostate Gland

Urethral Passage

Penis

Rectum

Anus

Enlargement

1. Difficulty clearing bladder of urine

2. Swelling of Prostate Gland constricts urethral passage through it

3. Difficulty starting urination

4. Lessening of force and quantity of urine

Cancer

Symptoms similar to Prostate Gland Enlargement plus

A. Occasional drops of blood in urine

B. Pain in pelvis and thigh bones as cancer spreads

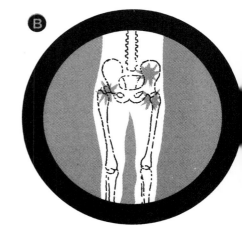

1208

a complete *prostatectomy* and is always preceded by a bilateral vasectomy which results in sterility but not in impotence.

Cancer of the prostate may be effectively treated in its early stages with the administration of female hormones. Removal of the entire gland may be preferred treatment. If the cancer has metastasized, combination therapy may slow down the progress of the disease over a long period.

prevention

At present there is no known way of preventing prostatic enlargement. The ravages of cancer of the prostate can be halted by early detection which is accomplished only by having a rectal examination once a year after the age of 40.

PROSTATISM, a condition of urinary obstruction without enlargement of the prostate, in which prostatic symptoms are present but the cause is located elsewhere. The causes include stricture of the *urethra* (the exit tube from the bladder); a stone in the bladder, with irritation; an enlarged lobe inside the bladder, causing obstruction; an enlarged *colliculus seminalis* (*verumontanum*) which lies close to the deep urethra, the *ejaculatory ducts* that discharge semen during intercourse, and the prostate; narrowing of the ejaculatory ducts with back pressure on the *seminal vesicles* (semen reservoirs); and *hydronephrosis* (distention of the pelvis of the kidney with urine due to an obstruction to its outflow). Congestion of the colliculus seminalis— sometimes due to prolonged masturbation or to the practice of withdrawal of the penis before sexual intercourse is completed—often causes symptoms which have been called *sexual neurasthenia.*

The physician can establish the diagnosis of prostatism by inserting a finger into the rectum, feeling the prostate in front, and finding that it is not enlarged.

The treatment varies according to the specific cause of the prostatism. *See also* PROSTATE *and* **medigraph** PROSTATE GLAND ENLARGEMENT.

PROSTATITIS, acute or chronic inflammation of the prostate due to infection, often as a complication of *gonorrhea.* The symptoms include discomfort in the perineal region deep between the thighs, itching around the end of the penis, and burning urination. On rectal examination, the prostate is found to be enlarged and tender and exudes pus into the urethra on pressure. A smear of the discharge identifies the responsible germ and a suitable antibiotic is administered. *See also* PROSTATE *and* **medigraphs** GONORRHEA; PROSTATE GLAND ENLARGEMENT.

PROSTHESES, artificial appliances used to replace lost natural structures. The most common prostheses are dental bridges and plates, artificial legs and arms, and glass eyes. *See also* ARTIFICIAL BODY PARTS; DENTURES.

PROTEIN, the basic material of which tissues and blood are composed, a nitrogenous compound of carbon, oxygen, hydrogen, nitrogen, and sometimes sulfur and phosphorus. The protein molecule combines 22 amino acids, ten of which are indispensable. Protein is the chief food required to build and restore human blood and tissues.

Complete proteins are those that contain the indispensable amino acids in large amounts. They include meat, eggs, fish, milk and cheese. *Incomplete proteins* are those that contain large amounts of dispensable amino acids, derived mostly from plants, cereals, and gelatin. For adequate nutrition, a diet rich in complete proteins is needed. When digested, protein is broken down into its constituent amino acids, which are absorbed into the bloodstream and reconstituted to make human tissue. For that reason, the essential amino acids have been called the "building stones" of the body. The two main types of complete protein are *albumins* and *globulins.* The purest albumin is egg white. The globulins include *fibrinogen,* needed for blood clotting; *musculin,* present in muscle tissue; *crystallin,* present in the lens of the eye; *edestin,* obtained from the seeds of hemp; *antibodies* to combat infections; and other proteins. The recommended daily intake of protein for a man weighing 150 pounds is about 100 grams, equivalent to about 12 ounces of cooked lean meat. Protein has great dynamic value and has no harmful effects on normal persons There are, however, certain illnesses in which the amount of meat in the diet must be restricted.

Protein deficiency may cause some metabolic disorders including cirrhosis of the liver and kwashiorkor. A diet high in starch and sugar but low in pro-

Protein—The building and functioning of body tissue requires proteins. What can happen with insufficient protein intake is illustrated here by two rats of the same age. The stunted growth of the smaller one is attributed solely to protein deficiency. This deficiency in pregnant and milk-producing rats also increases susceptibility to dental cavities in their offspring.

Courtesy, National Institutes of Health

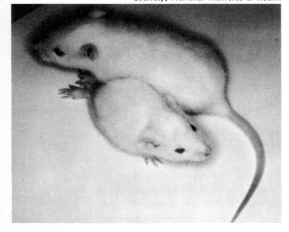

tein fails to supply the body with needed amino acids and may result in edema, a common complication of protein deficiency. *See also* ALBUMIN; AMINO ACIDS; DIGESTION; FIBRIN; FIBRINOGEN DEFICIENCY; FISH; KWASHIORKOR; MEAT; ANIMAL; MILK; NUTRITION *and* **medigraphs** BERIBERI; CELIAC DISEASE; PELLAGRA.

PROTOZOA, the simplest form of animal life, comprising single-celled organisms that multiply by fission—that is by splitting into two halves. *Bacteria,* on the other hand, are low forms of vegetable life.

The *ameba,* a primitive protozoon, grows in stagnant water and has been seen under the microscope by students in their courses of zoology. Most varieties of protozoa are harmless but some are parasitic and cause specific diseases. Among the pathogenic or harmful species of protozoa are the different types of *malarial plasmodia,* which are carried by mosquitoes to cause malaria; the *Endameba histolytica,* causing *amebic dysentery;* the varieties of *trypanosomes,* causing *African sleeping sickness* and *Chagas' disease; Leishmania donovani,* causing *kala-azar;* and others. *See also* INFECTION; INFECTIOUS DISEASES.

PROXIMAL, nearest to any point of reference as opposed to *distal,* which is farthest from such point. Thus the four bones of the fingers which are located next to the corresponding hand bones are proximal, while the four bones at the ends of the fingers are distal. The same applies to the bones of the toes. *See also* DISTAL.

PRURIGO, a chronic skin disease beginning in infancy or childhood, manifested by persistent and intense itching and spotty raised eruptions on the backs of the arms and forearms and over the calves. The cause is unknown and the disease is twice as common in males.

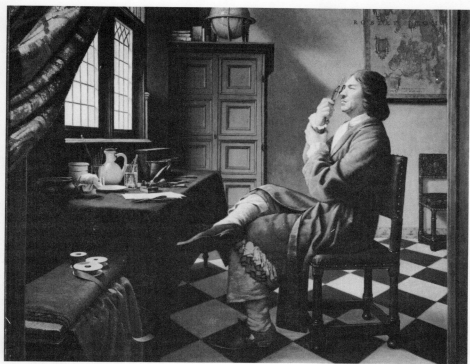

Protozoa—The first person to report having seen "animalcules"—now known as protozoa and bacteria—was this 17th century Dutch merchant, Antony van Leeuwenhoek. He studied the microscopic world through tiny lenses he ground and mounted himself. His discoveries eventually led to modern medicine's century-long onslaught against diseases caused by microorganisms.

Secondary infection and boils may result from scratching. There is no known cure but certain drugs reportedly relieve the itching.

PRURITUS. *See* ITCHING.

PSEUDOHYPOPARATHYROIDISM, a condition in which there is a physiological resistance to the parathyroid hormone. This disease resembles *hypoparathyroidism* in that the bodily abnormalities noted in chemical and clinical tests are similar. But in pseudohypoparathyroidism, the hormone—while actually sufficient in the body—cannot be utilized. The parathyroid tissue itself is normal; but for some reason the system is incapable of transmitting the hormone throughout the body.

The origin of pseudohypoparathyroidism is not known although some doctors believe it is due to a lack of end organ response. This disease afflicts few people. Those who do have pseudohypoparathyroidism are characteristically short, thick-bodied, with round faces and are often mentally retarded and inclined to cataracts. The disease affects bone growth so that metatarsal (foot) and metacarpal (hand) bones become shortened. This is evident when the patient makes a clenched fist and dimples rather than knuckles appear at the joints.

Pseudohypoparathyroidism can be diagnosed by the Ellsworth-Howard test in which a fasting patient is given some parathyroid extract intravenously. Following the injection, the person's urine is checked at intervals of several hours to measure the phosphate content. If the person fails to produce phosphate in the urine at all or in insufficient amounts, the test is considered positive. A person with a normal parathyroid might show an increase of five or six times the amount of phosphate usually found in his urine, if given such an injection, while a person suffering from hypoparathyroidism might produce ten times as much phosphate in the urine under such circumstances. However, someone with pseudohypoparathyroidism would show a maximum of twice his average phosphate content in the Ellsworth-Howard test. Because such people may often have convulsions as a symptom, the Ellsworth-Howard test is important in differentiating the disease from epilepsy.

The treatment for pseudohypoparathyroidism is the same as that for chronic hypoparathyroidism. The person is put on a high-calcium diet and given additional amounts of vitamin D, which aid in raising the calcium level in the body. *See also* PARATHYROID GLANDS.

PSEUDOPREGNANCY, *pseudocyesis,* is a condition in which many of the symptoms of pregnancy exist, but there is actually no fetus. Young women who greatly desire children and menopausal women account for most cases of pseudocyesis, commonly called *false pregnancy.*

Symptoms of pseudocyesis—like those of genuine pregnancy—are: increase in weight, increase in the size of the abdomen, enlarged breasts, irregular menstrual periods, and morning sickness. The causes of these symptoms are the depositing of fat in the abdominal area or the accumulation of abdominal fluid, endocrine disturbances of the ovaries, and disturbances of the adrenal and pi-

tuitary glands which account for the change in pigmentation of the breasts and the apparent mammary secretions.

The doctor may also detect what seem to be fetal movements but are in fact contractions of intestinal or abdominal wall muscles. The absence of a fetus can be determined by a bimanual examination, and by x-ray of the uterus. The doctor examines the area of the uterus with his hands in order to detect any signs of a fetus. In cases of pseudocyesis, the doctor must persuade the patient that she is not pregnant. *See also* HYPOCHONDRIASIS; PREGNANCY TESTS.

PSITTACOSIS, sometimes called *parrot fever,* is a disease contracted by humans usually from psittacene birds such as parrots, parakeets, or lovebirds but which can be transmitted by pigeons, domestic fowl, such as poultry, or by canaries and some other birds.

It had been thought for a long time that psittacosis was caused by a virus but doctors now believe that it is caused by a type of microorganism similar to rickettsiae. Humans can acquire the disease when they clean cages by inhaling the dust from excreta left by sick birds or by inhaling the dust from feathers of a diseased bird or from the bite of an infected bird. Psittacosis can also be transmitted from one person to another by inhaling the cough droplets or sputum of an infected person.

The incubation period for psittacosis is approximately two weeks or from 1–3 weeks. It is followed by symptoms ranging from a mild respiratory infection to severe atypical pneumonia. Psittacosis often appears with a dry cough, elevated temperature, sore throat, and a persistent headache. In severe cases rose-colored spots may appear. If the disease goes untreated, it may become chronic or even fatal.

In order to distinguish psittacosis from other forms of atypical pneumonia or infectious diseases, it is necessary to test the blood or sputum under carefully controlled conditions so that the disease will not be spread farther.

Treatment with antibiotics is most effective and recovery is aided by bed rest. The person with psittacosis is usually well in about 10–14 days. Because the disease is contagious, care must be used in treating the infected person and his contact with others should be restricted while he is ill.

PSORIASIS

PSORIASIS IS A CHRONIC SKIN disease that disfigures the faces and bodies of millions with recurrent red scaly patches. Psoriasis is neither dangerous nor contagious and affects men and women alike. It may appear for the first time during adolescence, coming and going throughout a lifetime.

causes

The cause of psoriasis is an inherited fault in the body's antigen-antibody re-

sponse to foreign organisms. It has recently been discovered that the *human leukocyte antigen* (HLA) *genes* are a decisive factor in resistance to particular diseases, including psoriasis. Whatever the organism that attempts to invade the body and cause this disorder, if the person's system lacks the HLA genes for producing antibodies against it, it cannot resist the disease. This genetic disability explains why psoriasis is one of the diseases that runs in families.

Psoriasis—A massive psoriasis patch covers this man's back. The scaliness, redness and itching are caused by excessive production of cells of the outermost layers of the skin. Though it may appear to be so, this chronic skin disease that runs in families is not contagious.

Courtesy, Gunderson Clinic, Ltd.

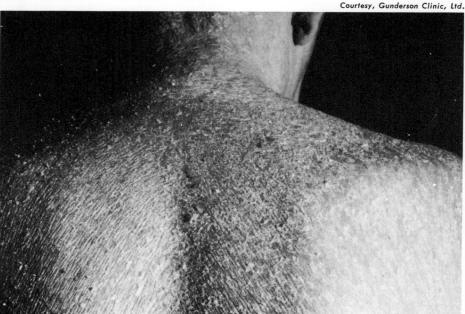

Psoriasis

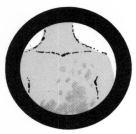

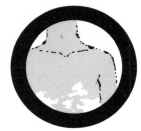

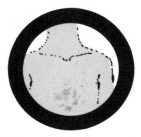

1. Starts as small red patches which enlarge and join together

2. Patches usually become covered with silvery-white, scaly skin

3. If scales fall off or are removed, red pinpoint area revealed underneath

Where Psoriasis Strikes

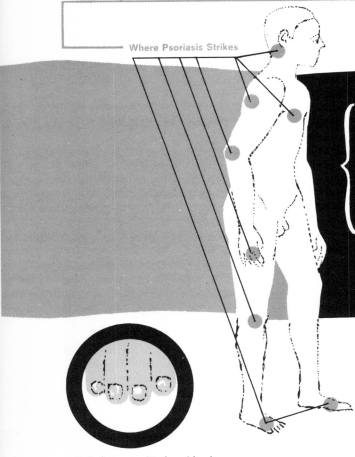

- Flares up with emotional stress
- Runs in family
- Children develop after strep infection
- Sometimes appears at site of skin injury
- Worsens in winter
- Little or no itching
- Not infectious

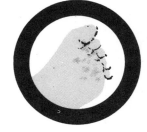

Nails become pitted or ridged with yellow spots — Soles of feet (and sometimes palms) may develop infection

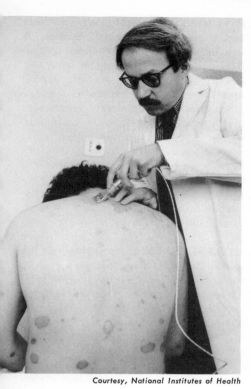

Psoriasis—The physician is using a special instrument to remove a thin sample of tissue from a psoriasis lesion. It will be preserved in liquid nitrogen and later analyzed as part of a research program. Possible abnormalities in cyclic nucleotides—substances that exert control over skin cell growth and convey cell messages—are being investigated as a cause of psoriasis.

symptoms

The symptomatic red and itchy psoriasis patches are produced when the skin cells multiply about ten times faster than they should. The parts of the body most frequently affected are the scalp, knees, elbows, chest, abdomen, palms and soles of the feet. Dot-shaped red marks may also appear under the fingernails.

treatment

People who suffer from psoriasis in its mild or acute form should not expect to be cured by any of the well-advertised patent medicines or special preparations, or by quacks who promise quick and easy cures. Such "cures" are at best worthless and at worst, harmful.

The conventional ultraviolet radiation therapy following the application of crude coal tar necessitates an inconvenient two weeks of hospitalization. More recently, the anticancer drug *methotrexate* has been administered as a way of slowing down skin cell reproduction by interfering with the genetic material in the cells, but this treatment cannot be used on a long-term basis because of its potential danger to the liver. A treatment called *photochemotherapy* has been evolved at Massachusetts General Hospital and combines oral doses of the photoactive drug *methoxsalen* with exposure to a specially designed ultraviolet light system that delivers enough radiation to activate the drug, but at a wave length that will not burn the person's skin. Permanent disappearance of symptoms has been reported after one month of this treatment on an outpatient basis.

RESEARCH
REPORT

PHOTOCHEMOTHERAPY CLEARS
SKIN LESIONS OF PSORIASIS
PATIENTS

The skin lesions of a group of *psoriasis* patients have completely cleared up in response to a new combination therapy administered at MASSACHUSETTS GENERAL HOSPITAL. Treatment consisted of oral doses of the photoactive drug *methoxsalen* and exposure to a recently developed *high-intensity long-wave ultraviolet light system*. Although the successful results are considered preliminary and will in most cases require maintenance therapy, they could lead to a safe and effective method of dealing with psoriasis on an outpatient basis. Up to now, some success has been achieved with the use of methotrexate, but this drug may be associated with severe liver toxicity. The conventional ultraviolet radiation treatment following

O application of crude coal tar requires hospitalization for up to two weeks.

O Reports indicate that the orally administered methoxsalen, which has been used for 20 years in treating the pigment disorder *vitiligo*, was well-tolerated by the psoriasis patients. The interaction of the long-wave ultraviolet light and the drug, termed "photochemotherapy," presumably retards the characteristic proliferation of psoriatic skin by inhibiting epidermal DNA synthesis.   NIH225

RESEARCH REPORT

PSORIASIS STUDIES ADVANCED BY SKIN-GRAFTED MICE

Mice that are successfully maintaining skin grafts from *psoriasis* patients are providing researchers with the first living models for the study of the development and possible treatment of this chronic skin disease. The transplantations were accomplished by scientists at the UNIVERSITY OF UTAH COLLEGE OF MEDICINE in Salt Lake City, using an inbred strain of laboratory rodents born without *thymuses* and thus unable to mount a thymus-dependent immune response that would result in rejection of the grafts.

Three psoriasis patients provided skin—both healthy and psoriatic samples—for the grafts that were received by 11 mice. Ten mice with successful grafts survived for four weeks, during which biopsies taken on two occasions indicated graft skin thickening that is typical of the disease.

Psoriasis research, which has previously been hampered by the lack of animal models, is now expected to accumulate new data leading to a possible means of preventing or effectively treating the disease. NIH1215

PSYCHEDELIC DRUGS, drugs that produce freedom from anxiety, mental relaxation, a dream-like state, and highly imaginative thought patterns bordering upon hallucinations. The most common psychedelic drugs are *LSD* and *mescaline. See also* PEYOTE *and* **medigraphs** LSD ABUSE; MESCALINE ABUSE.

PSYCHIATRY, the diagnosis, treatment and prevention of mental diseases. A *psychiatrist* is a physician who specializes in that field of medicine. *See also* APATHY; COMPULSION; DEFENSE MECHANISM; DELUSIONS; DEPRESSION; ELECTRIC SHOCK TREATMENT; EMOTIONAL DISTURBANCES; GENETIC COUNSELING; GROUP THERAPY; HYPNOSIS; HYSTERIA; INVOLUTIONAL MELANCHOLIA; MANIC-DEPRESSIVE PSYCHOSIS; MENTAL HEALTH; NEUROSIS; OBSESSIONS; PARANOIA; PERSONALITY; PHOBIAS; PSYCHOANALYSIS; PSYCHONEUROSIS; PSYCHOSIS; SCHIZOPHRENIA.

PSYCHOANALYSIS, exploration of the mind, Freud's method of delving into the subconscious mind to discover psychological patterns responsible for neuroses and psychoneuroses. His technique combined free association of ideas, dream analysis and hypnosis. *See also* DREAMS; HYPNOSIS; PSYCHIATRY.

PSYCHOLOGY, the science that studies the functions of the mind. A *psychologist* is a scientist who specializes in the study and practice of psychology. *See also* ANTISOCIAL BEHAVIOR; BEHAVIOR; EMOTION.

PSYCHONEUROSIS, an emotional disorder of the subconscious mind—apart from *psychosis* (insanity)—occurring in two forms: *hysteria* and *compulsion neurosis.*

Hysteria is manifested by great suggestibility and imitation of physical diseases such as paralysis and blindness. Compulsion neurosis—which usually stems from an obsession—is subconscious performance of acts contrary to conscious will. *See also* HYSTERIA; MENTAL HEALTH; NEUROSIS; PSYCHIATRY.

PSYCHOPATH, a person afflicted with a mental disease classified as a form of insanity. *See also* MENTAL HEALTH.

PSYCHOSIS, a mental disease involving disintegration of the personality or escape from reality. The most common psychoses are *schizophrenia* and *manic-depressive psychosis. See also* MANIC-DEPRESSIVE PSYCHOSIS; MENTAL HEALTH; PSYCHIATRY; SCHIZOPHRENIA.

PSYCHOSOMATIC DISORDERS, mind-body disturbances that originate in psychological distress and eventually produce a physical disorder. A typical example is provided by ulcer of the stomach or duodenum. Anxiety, for instance, can lead to disturbances of their functions and eventually ulceration due to the psychological stress and tension. Psychosomatic disturbances may take place in any of the involuntary organs of the body, including the digestive tract, the lungs, the heart, the blood vessels, the genitourinary system, the glands of internal secretion, and the skin. The emotional state may also aggravate existing physical disorders, as in the case of asthma, colitis, and benign prostatic enlargement. *See also* EMOTION; HYPO-CHONDRIASIS *and* **medigraphs** ULCERATIVE COLITIS; ULCERS OF THE DIGESTIVE TRACT.

PSYCHOSURGERY, an operation of last resort for violent and dangerous mental patients, in which the nerve fibers connected with the frontal lobes of the brain are severed. In some cases aggressive patients are rendered docile and safe by this operation.

PSYCHOTHERAPY, treatment of emotional and mental disorders by psychological means. Sometimes drugs are used to establish communication. *See also* ELECTRIC SHOCK TREATMENT; GROUP THERAPY; INSULIN SHOCK THERAPY; OCCUPATIONAL THERAPY; PSYCHOANALYSIS.

PSYCHOTROPICS, agents that affect the mind, such as antidepressants, tranquilizers and hallucinogens.

PTOMAINE POISONING. *See* FOOD POISONING.

PTOSIS, the sagging or dropping of an organ or structure, such as *gastroptosis* (dropped stomach), *nephroptosis* (fallen kidney); or drooping of the upper eyelid from paralysis of the third cranial nerve. Most ptoses result from stretched ligaments. *See also* GASTROPTOSIS.

PUBERTY, the age at which the sex organs begin to function and at which sexual features begin to appear. The average age in boys is from 13–16, in girls from 11–14. At comparable ages in school, girls are superior to boys, but this difference disappears in later years. It may explain the preference of girls for boys older than themselves, which often persists in later years. The period from puberty to maturity is *adolescence.*

In boys during puberty, the penis and testicles become enlarged, often the habit of masturbation begins, hair on the face begins to grow, and the voice deepens. In girls, the principal changes are enlargement of the breasts, broadening of the hips, and the beginning of menstruation. Both boys and girls rapidly grow taller during puberty under the influence of pituitary hormones, until the full height is attained, at which time further growth ceases. In both boys and girls, a prominent change is greater interest in the opposite sex. Parental guidance at this critical age is most important. Boys must be warned of the danger of contracting venereal diseases and girls of pregnancy as well as VD. The parent should explain that menstruation is a natural function, so that the young girl will not be terrified by the first sight of blood coming from her vagina. Boys take pride in their strength, not only of their muscles but also of their character —qualities which should be encouraged. At the age of 18, a boy is fully developed both physically and sexually.

Young people in some societies are greatly concerned about *acne,* which causes them embarrassment. Fortunately these blemishes are amenable to medical treatment, and usually recede in a few years. *See also* ADOLESCENCE; FEMININE HYGIENE; MALE PUBERTY; MASTURBATION; MENSTRUATION; NOCTURNAL EMISSION; SEX EDUCATION.

PUBIC, pertaining to the hairy region in front of the lower abdomen and just above the sexual organs, where the two pubic bones come together.

PUBLIC HEALTH, supervision of the health of a community by qualified public officials, covering all aspects of sanitation. In the United States, the Public Health Service, with branches in all large cities, has national supervision over community health problems, the control of biological drugs, and the dissemination of educational information. The Food and Drug Administration controls the sale of foods, drugs, cosmetics and appliances as to safety and effectiveness for their intended use. The states and cities also employ local public health officials and the federal Environmental Protection Agency is largely concerned with air, water and other environmental contamination. Both the Public Health Service and the Food and Drug Administration are branches of the Department of Health, Education, and Welfare. *See also* ENDEMIC; EPIDEMIC; EPIDEMIOLOGY; HYGIENE; POLLUTION; PREVENTIVE MEDICINE; QUARANTINE.

PUERPERAL FEVER, infection of the vagina and uterus around the time of childbirth. Two famous physicians at about the same time suggested and demonstrated that *puerperal sepsis* was carried to childbearing women by the unclean hands of physicians or medical students. They were Dr. Oliver Wendell Holmes of Boston and Dr. Ignaz Philipp Semmelweis of Hungary.

PUERPERIUM, the period from delivery of the infant to the time when the uterus regains its normal size, usually about six weeks. *See also* POSTNATAL CARE OF THE MOTHER.

PULMONARY DISEASES, diseases affecting the lungs, including among others *tuberculosis, lung cancer, pneumonia, pleurisy, lung abscess, empyema* (a collection of pus in the pleural cavity), *pulmonary edema, emphysema, bronchial asthma, bronchial degenerative dilatation, pneumothorax, pneumoconiosis* (inflammation of the lungs due to inhalation of dust, iron, marble, coal or asbestos), *psittacosis* (parrot fever), *lung cysts, lung cavities, lung gangrene, atelectasis* (collapse of all or part of a lung), *pneumonic plague,* and *Q fever* (resembling influenza). *See also* LUNGS *and* **medigraphs** ADENOMA, BRONCHIAL; ANTHRACOSIS AND ASBESTOSIS; BRONCHIAL ASTHMA; BRONCHIECTASIS; BRONCHITIS; EMPHYSEMA; LUNG ABSCESS; LUNG CANCER; PLEURISY; PNEUMONIA; SILICOSIS; TUBERCULOSIS.
RESEARCH REPORT *follows* ASBESTOSIS.

PULMONARY HEART DISEASE

PULMONARY HEART DISEASE is a coronary disorder related to various respiratory and lung diseases: chronic conditions such as *emphysema* or *bronchial asthma,* or pulmonary diseases that are occupational in origin and that result in scarring of the lungs. Pulmonary heart disease is always aggravated by smoking.

causes
When pulmonary abnormalities develop that interrupt or interfere with the flow

Pulmonary Heart Disease

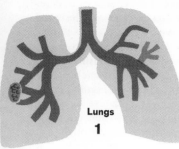

Lungs
1

1. . . . Serious Lung Disease . . .

Blood clot (embolus)

Bronchiectasis

Asthma, other chronic conditions

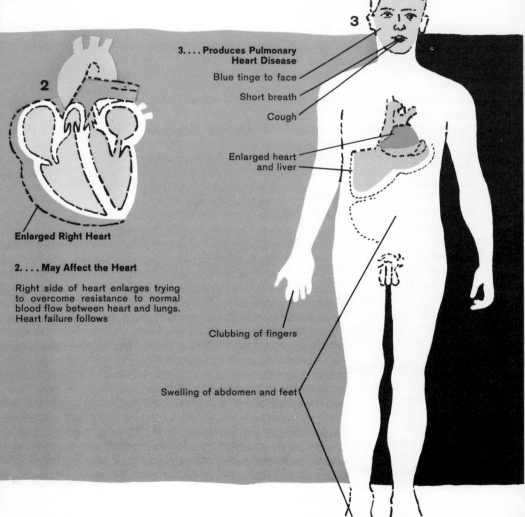

2

Enlarged Right Heart

2. . . . May Affect the Heart

Right side of heart enlarges trying to overcome resistance to normal blood flow between heart and lungs. Heart failure follows

3

3. . . . Produces Pulmonary Heart Disease

Blue tinge to face

Short breath

Cough

Enlarged heart and liver

Clubbing of fingers

Swelling of abdomen and feet

of blood between the heart and the lungs, extra pressure is placed on the right side of the heart, causing it to enlarge. In addition to the chronic diseases, other causes may be the formation of a pulmonary embolus (mass) that blocks circulation to the lungs or, less frequently, lung cancer.

symptoms

One of the most immediately observable signs of pulmonary heart disease is the slightly bluish cast to the skin caused by *cyanosis,* the condition in which circulatory disturbance results in inadequate reoxygenation of the blood in the lungs. Because of the underlying respiratory disorder, the victim usually has a chronic cough and is short of breath. Swelling of the extremities as well as enlargement of the liver and the *barrel chest* associated with emphysema are other symptoms.

complications

The most likely complication of untreated or advanced pulmonary heart disease is heart failure.

treatment

Irregular heart action resulting from a serious lung disease is best treated by dealing with that disease. In most cases, this means removal from the environmental conditions that are responsible for the bronchial or lung damage.

PULMONARY STENOSIS, an obstructive narrowing of the *semilunar pulmonary valves* located between the right ventricle of the heart and the pulmonary artery, which carries blue unoxygenated blood to the lungs. Most often the condition is a birth defect in children. The most common symptoms are *cyanosis* (blueness), shortness of breath, quick tiring, and a typical heart murmur. The diagnosis may be confirmed by an *electrocardiogram* and *fluoroscopic* examination. The treatment is surgical. Earlier

methods were to introduce a *valvulotome* (a special instrument designed to cut obstructive heart valves) at an optimal age of 4–12 years or to by-pass the obstructed valve by establishing an artificial detour of the circulation.

The present approved method employs open-heart surgery with use of an artificial heart-lung device. The surgeon inserts a miniature knife through a tiny slit in the heart wall and, working by a sense of touch, eliminates the obstruction in or near the pulmonary valve. *See also* HEART; HEART SURGERY.

PULSE, an intermittent change in the blood pressure within the arteries transmitted with the heartbeat (*systole*) and the following rest phase (*diastole*). People usually feel the pulse at the wrist over the flat lower front end of the radius bone. The experienced touch of the physician not only counts the pulse rate but also observes its regularity and roughly estimates the pressure within the artery. The procedure for taking the pulse is to place the index finger, not the thumb, lightly on the radial artery at the wrist and count the beats for a full minute. Usually the person whose pulse rate is being counted is at rest, seated or lying down. The pulse may also be felt over an artery located on the back of the foot (*dorsalis pedis*). The average normal rate of the pulse for men is 72, women 75, and infants 100–120.

A pulse rate above 90—the high normal—is called *tachycardia;* below 60—the low normal—*bradycardia.* Tachycardia occurs during exercise and excitement, in *exophthalmic goiter,* and in fevers, where the pulse rate increases about ten per minute for each degree of temperature elevation. In *paroxysmal tachycardia,* the pulse rate may increase up to 300 beats per minute and then suddenly snap back to normal. In *auricular fibrillation,* the pulse is very rapid and also absolutely irregular. Digitalis and quinidine slow and regulate a rapid and irregular pulse. Many long-distance runners have an exceedingly slow pulse rate, such as 40–65. In *heart block,* where the impulse to contract fails to pass from the atrium to the ventricle and the ventricle beats independently with its own rhythm, the pulse rate is persistently as low as 40–50 and other symptoms are present. The sympathetic nerves accelerate the pulse rate; the *vagus* (*pneumogastric*) *nerve* slows it down. *See also* BLOOD PRESSURE; BRADYCARDIA; HEART BLOCK; TACHYCARDIA.

PULSELESS DISEASE, a disease characterized by absence of the pulse from its usual location at the wrist, blackouts of consciousness, visual disturbances and cataracts, believed to be due to hardening of the large arteries located in the neck and below the collarbone. *See also* medigraph ARTERIOSCLEROSIS.

PUNCTURE WOUND. *See* WOUNDS.

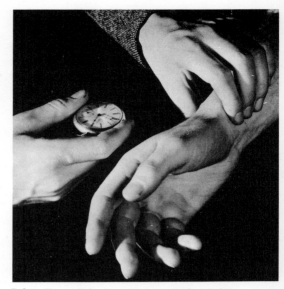

Pulse—The radial artery at the wrist just below the thumb is the most common place to feel a pulse beat with the fingers. The thumb is never used to take a pulse because it has a pulse of its own that would cause confusion.

P.U.O., *pyrexia* (fever) *of unknown origin.* Such fevers give great concern to patients and doctors. Often long and intensive study may be required to determine some cause when fever is apparently the only symptom. However, most of such fevers are ultimately found to be due to some common disease in which other symptoms are not prominent.

Scientifically, this is defined as an illness that lasts at least three weeks with fever at least $1\frac{1}{2}°F$ above the normal on several occasions and for which no cause can be found. Such fevers may occur in viral infections or common colds. Infections are found to be responsible for about 40 percent, tumors or cancers for about 20 percent, and collagen and blood diseases for about 15 percent, which leaves about 25 percent of cases in which unusual conditions are ultimately determined. For instance, fever may be a prominent symptom for

weeks or months before such conditions as rheumatoid arthritis or lupus erythematosus are diagnosed. In long-enduring instances of fever of uncommon cause, attempts are sometimes made by the administration of suitable drugs or even by exploratory operations to determine a specific cause. *See also* FEVER.

PUPIL, the circular opening in the colored iris in the front of the eyeball through which lights passes to the *retina.* It contracts in light and dilates in darkness and also contracts in accommodation when focusing on close-up objects. *Belladonna* and *atropine* dilate the pupils; *opium* and *heroin* contract them almost to a pinpoint. In *locomotor ataxia,* the typical *Argyll Robertson pupil* is one that responds to accommodation but does not contract to light. A hazy or milky colored pupil suggests the presence of a *cataract. See also* EYE.

PURGATIVES. *See* CATHARTICS.

PURPURA, a condition due to fragility and increased permeability of the blood capillaries characterized by numerous small round flat hemorrhagic red spots called *petechiae* which persist when pressed. Some people suffer more extensive hemorrhages under the skin or in the joints than others do. Many different forms of the disorder have been described.

There are three main types: *purpura simplex,* a familial disorder occurring mostly in females and not associated with well-defined defects of blood clotting; *purpura hemorrhagica,* with decreased

blood platelets and delayed coagulation, often fatal; and *symptomatic purpura,* with causative factors that include infections, certain drugs, anemia, leukemia, heart and kidney diseases, radiation, and allergies.

The treatments which have been employed include blood transfusions, steroids, vitamin K, and iron for hemoglobin replenishment. The results of such treatments other than transfusions have been indefinite, and numerous other agents have been tried without any benefit. Sometimes surgical removal of the spleen helped to stop the bleeding tendency. In one study, removal of the spleen combined with administration of the steroids proved successful in 92.3 percent of a group of 271 cases of *thrombocytopenic purpura* exhibiting a deficiency of the blood platelets and a prolonged bleeding time. Remissions of the disease following administration of the steroids are common, but side effects of prolonged use present a hazard. *See also* BLOOD CONDITIONS; COAGULATION; ECCHYMOSIS; PETECHIA; THROMBOCYTOPENIA *and* **medigraph** LEUKEMIA.

PUS, a thick creamy yellowish or greenish discharge or collection of waste composed of broken-down white blood cells and decomposed tissue formed as a natural defense against infection. *See also* ABSCESS; INFECTION; INFLAMMATION.

PYELITIS, an inflammation of the renal pelvis, the funnel-shaped sac of the kidney which transports the urine down the ureter connecting tube to the bladder. The usual cause is an infection carried to the kidney via the bloodstream and often affecting women in pregnancy. The symptoms are chills, fever, abdominal pain, backache and pus cells in the urine. *See also* KIDNEY; PYELONEPHRITIS *and* **medigraphs** NEPHRITIS; URINARY TRACT PROBLEMS.

Various Types of Purpura

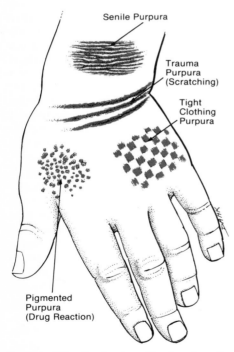

Senile Purpura

Trauma Purpura (Scratching)

Tight Clothing Purpura

Pigmented Purpura (Drug Reaction)

Purpura—This disorder is a bleeding from the capillaries into tissues, evidenced by small red patches and bruises on the skin. It can stem from low blood platelet count, certain drugs and diseases, or abnormally thin capillary walls.

PYELONEPHRITIS, combined infection of the kidney and its pelvis—the collecting funnel of urine. It is the most common type of kidney infection. The symptoms are similar to those of *pyelitis. See also* KIDNEY; PYELITIS *and* **medigraphs** NEPHRITIS; URINARY TRACT PROBLEMS.

PYEMIA, an infection of the blood with a pus-forming germ, which lodges in various organs and tissues to form abscesses. Depending on the identity of the infecting germ, a suitable antibiotic is available to stop the infection. *See also* BACTEREMIA.

PYLORUS, the connecting tube between the stomach and the *duodenum* (the first part of the small intestine). It is closed by the *pyloric valve,* which opens on signal from the hormone *secretin* to permit passage of partially digested food into the duodenum. Enlargement and spasm of the pyloric muscles, common in babies, causes an obstruction which results in vomiting and loss of weight, sometimes requiring surgery. The pylorus is the location of many *peptic ulcers. See also* STOMACH *and* **medigraph** ULCERS OF THE DIGESTIVE TRACT.

PYOGENIC, producing pus, a property of many harmful germs including the common *staphylococcus,* a dot-shaped organism growing in groups like a cluster of grapes. Most antibiotics destroy the pyogenic germs.

PYORRHEA, a discharge of pus from under the gums resulting from decay of the sockets that lodge the teeth and from *gingivitis* (gum infection). Accumulation of tartar around the necks and roots of the teeth is an important factor. Even-tually the affected teeth loosen and may be lost. An early warning sign is bleeding gums. The progress of pyorrhea can be delayed considerably by routine brushing of the teeth, a visit to the dentist every three months to scrape off accumulated tartar, and a low-sugar diet. *Vitamin C* and *calcium gluconate* are helpful. *See also* GINGIVITIS; GUMS; TEETH.

PYRIDOXINE, essential vitamin B_6, widely present in a variety of foods. The major functions of pyridoxine involve protein and amino acid metabolism. The symptoms and signs of *deficiency* include oily skin, chafing, inflammation of the skin, splitting and dry scaling of the lips and corners of the mouth, inflammation of the tongue and mouth, neuritis, and convulsions in infants. In addition to its corrective value for these deficiency symptoms, pyridoxine is useful for *peripheral neuritis* caused by certain drugs and in the prevention of the side effects of *L-dopa* (levodihydroxyphenylalanine) used in the treatment of *Parkinson's disease.* It was formerly employed in the treatment of nausea and vomiting of pregnancy but this use has been discredited. *See also* NUTRITION; VITAMIN DEFICIENCIES; VITAMINS.

PYROMANIA, an obsessive preoccupation with fires for the sake of the thrill or for other reasons. Pyromaniacs start many conflagrations and experience a morbid thrill at the sight of the flames and smoke. Arson is a serious crime and sometimes causes the death of innocent victims in addition to the loss of property. *See also* MANIA; MENTAL HEALTH.

PYROPHOBIA, a morbid dread of fire. *See also* PHOBIAS.

Q

Q FEVER, *nine-mile fever,* an infection resembling influenza and caused by a *rickettsia,* an organism that is intermediate in size between viruses and bacteria. The infection is spread by tick bites, inhalation of contaminated dust, or infected milk and dairy products. The disease was first recognized in an outbreak among slaughterhouse and dairy employees in Queensland, Australia, in 1937 and later by isolation of the rickettsia from ticks in Nine-Mile Creek, Montana. In 1940, 15 cases with lung complications and x-ray findings of atypical pneumonia occurred in the state of Washington.

The symptoms are similar to those of influenza—fever, chills, headache, muscular pains and severe weakness. The onset is usually 14–26 days after exposure to the rickettsia. Mild attacks last only a few days, but in severe cases the temperature may rise as high as 104° F. (40° C.) and may stay that high for two or three weeks. The disease usually ends in complete recovery. The death rate is low—less than one percent.

Complications include atypical viral pneumonia and inflammation of the lining membrane of the heart. The disease has been prevalent in Australia, Montana, California and Texas. A few cases have been reported in New York City and Boston. The principal carriers of the rickettsia are wood and cattle ticks, wild rodents, cattle and goats.

Some antibiotics are effective in combatting it. Therapy should be continued for approximately a week even though the temperature drops to normal in two days. *See also* INFECTIOUS DISEASES; RICKETTSIAL DISEASES.

QUACKERY, the practice of medicine by unlicensed persons or the application of treatments which are not generally recognized as appropriate by the profession. The quack promises to cure cancer and other incurable diseases and thereby swindles many desperately ill persons who have been told the unhappy truth about their health by qualified physicians. Before the passage in the United States of the Food and Drug Act in 1906, itinerant quacks roamed around the country lecturing about their so-called cures and selling their nostrums to the gullible public. There was a soothing syrup containing opium for crying babies, a sarsaparilla syrup for syphilis, and an alcoholic compound for epileptic fits. Testimonials were the main stock in trade of the quack. His portfolio contained letters from persons who wrote that the medicine had cured them of cancer, but in many cases the deception was exposed by the authorities in the form of a death certificate. The quack is really a salesman who advertises his wares by public lectures, radio or publicity. In the United States, fortunately, he is restrained by the Food and Drug Administration, the Federal Trade Commission, and in other nations, by various similar authorities. Some people who believe quacks are aware that some of the greatest medical discoveries were applied without having any real scientific foundation; for example, ether, digitalis, quinine, ephedrine and reserpine. But certain new drugs which were once credited with great healing properties have been shown by later scientific studies to be dangerous or ineffective. The secret remedy, once exploited by quacks, is no longer available because the Federal law requires disclosure of the active ingredients on the label. One of the most dangerous forms of quackery is the advertisement that tells the truth as far as it goes but which by artful devices misleads the reader or viewer into believing that the drug is a cure. The reader's unwarranted inferences are the cause of self-deception. *See also* PANACEA.

QUADRIPLEGIA, paralysis of both arms and both legs. The more common causes are poliomyelitis and *Landry's acute ascending paralysis*. The latter is a disorder that is due to an acute infection of the spinal cord, beginning in the lower limbs and ascending to paralyze the muscles of the upper limbs and other muscles. This disorder terminates with paralysis of the respiratory center in the *medulla oblongata* (the central and vital nerve center in the brain) and death. Other causes of quadriplegia are diphtheria and leprosy. *See also* PARALYSIS.

QUADRUPLETS, four children born in one labor. *See also* MULTIPLE BIRTH.

QUARANTINE, restrictions and detention placed on the entrance and exit of persons, animals and ships to localities where communicable infectious diseases are prevalent. The period of quarantine is usually 40 days, which was enforced during the Middle Ages to prevent the spread of plague. Quarantine may be enforced for the longest *incubation period* (time from the date of exposure to the outbreak of symptoms) of the disease.

Public health authorities in most countries are constantly on the alert to guard against the introduction of infectious diseases from foreign countries. As examples, the United States imposed quarantine on cattle and beef as a protection against foot-and-mouth disease and in Great Britain, dogs brought into the country are quarantined until after the incubation period has proved that they do not have *rabies* (*hydrophobia*). In 1918–19 a devastating epidemic of influenza with many deaths from pneumonia broke out in the United States following the arrival of people in Boston from a ship that had not passed through quarantine. *See also* INFECTIOUS DISEASES; ISOLATION; PUBLIC HEALTH.

QUICKENING, the first consciousness of pregnancy experienced by feeling the fetal movements of the unborn child, usually during the 16th–18th week of pregnancy. The physician confirms the diagnosis by listening to the fetal heartbeat with a stethoscope. *See also* PREGNANCY; PRENATAL DEVELOPMENT.

QUININE, the most active alkaloid of *cinchona bark,* specific for the prevention and cure of malaria. Cinchona bark —which had long been known by the Incas in Peru—was introduced into Europe by the Jesuits in 1632. The United States Pharmacopeia recognizes quinine officially as *quinine sulfate*. In addition to malaria, quinine is used for relief of leg cramps, headache, muscular pains, neuralgia, and as a bitter tonic to the appetite. During World War II, when quinine was in short supply, *quinicrine*

(*Atabrine*) was introduced as a substitute. Both quinine and quinicrine have unwanted side effects and are limited to prescription use. *See also* ALKALOIDS; ANTIMALARIAL DRUGS; ATABRINE *and* **medigraph** MALARIA.

QUINSY, a common name for *septic sore throat* with an abscess surrounding one of the tonsils. The symptoms are pain on one side of the throat, difficulty in swallowing and talking, unpleasant breath, coated tongue, disturbed taste and smell, and fever. Usually an antibiotic is prescribed, and incision of the abscess may be necesary to drain off the pus. *See also* **medigraph** TONSILLITIS.

QUINTUPLETS, five infants born at one labor. *See also* MULTIPLE BIRTH.

R

RABBIT FEVER, *tularemia,* a disease of rabbits and other rodents that is caused by *Pasteurella tularensis.* It can be transmitted to man by contact with diseased animals or their hides, by eating infected wild game, or by the bite of an insect that has fed on an infected animal. *See also* TULAREMIA.

RABIES

RABIES IS AN ACUTE VIRAL disease of the central nervous system transmitted to humans and to healthy animals through the infected saliva of a rabid animal—especially a dog, bat, squirrel, raccoon, or fox. It is always fatal unless treatment is administered before the appearance of the final symptoms.

cause

The infection is spread when the saliva containing the rabies virus enters any opening of the skin, whether a deep wound or a bleeding scratch, usually occasioned by the animal's bite. The disease can also be transmitted if a rabid animal so much as licks an already existing wound, as might be the case in a gunshot accident.

symptoms

Symptoms are most easily observed in a dog than in an animal in the wild: the dog becomes irritable, snappish, and has a high-pitched continuous bark. Within a few days, paralysis sets in and the muscles of the pharynx (throat) go into spasms that prevent swallowing (hence the term *hydrophobia*) so that there is either drooling, frothing, or choking on saliva. Total paralysis and death occur within ten days. The fatal effect of untreated rabies on humans occurs more rapidly the closer the bite is to the brain. Thus, a face bite from a rabid animal produces symptoms more rapidly than a bite on the body.

treatment

Emergency treatment for a bite from any animal consists of washing the wound thoroughly with strong soap and water and covering it with a sterile dressing until a doctor can be consulted about immunization. If possible, the animal should be kept alive in the custody of a veterinarian or a public health authority for observation. This precaution is obviously unnecessary if the dog is wearing a tag indicating rabies immunization. If

Rabies
Virus disease transmitted to man through saliva of rabid animals—particularly dogs and vampire bats

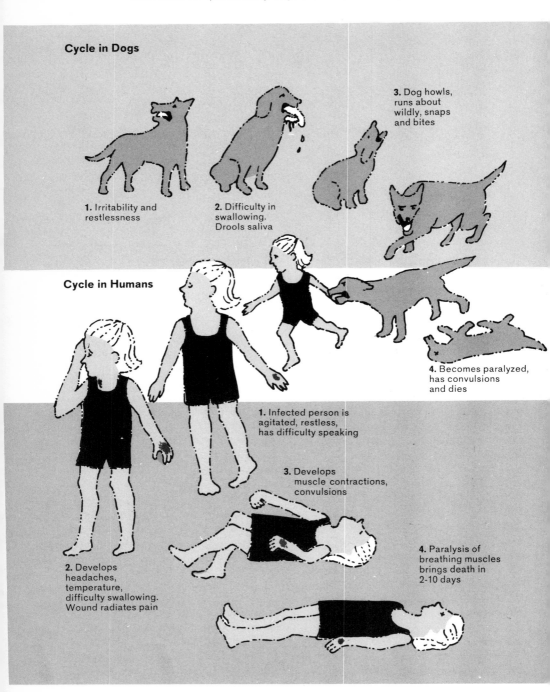

Cycle in Dogs

1. Irritability and restlessness

2. Difficulty in swallowing. Drools saliva

3. Dog howls, runs about wildly, snaps and bites

4. Becomes paralyzed, has convulsions and dies

Cycle in Humans

1. Infected person is agitated, restless, has difficulty speaking

2. Develops headaches, temperature, difficulty swallowing. Wound radiates pain

3. Develops muscle contractions, convulsions

4. Paralysis of breathing muscles brings death in 2-10 days

the bite occurs in the woods and the animal escapes, health authorities usually recommend that anti-rabies vaccine injections be undertaken immediately and continued over the necessary two-week period.

prevention
In most parts of the United States all dog-owners are required by law to have their pets immunized against rabies on a regular schedule, thus reducing the risk of transmitting the disease inside the city. The current carriers of rabies are bats that infect each other and creatures in the woods such as squirrels, foxes, raccoons, field mice, and so on. Children who spend time camping in the woods or adults on hiking trips should wear protective clothing, and if they receive a bite or scratch, should seek prompt medical attention.

RADIATION. *See* IRRADIATION.

RADIATION INJURIES. Most of what medical scientists now know about the effects of atomic (nuclear) and hydrogen (thermonuclear) bombs on human populations was derived from several major studies at Hiroshima and Nagasaki in Japan.

The three most lethal effects on human life are those attributable to *radioactive particles* (radiation fallout), *intense heat* and *blast shock* waves.

The first effect of an atomic bomb or hydrogen bomb is the blast effect. The second effect is that of intense heat which sets widespread fires and generates huge fire storms by sucking up all the available oxygen. Thus, even if a person succeeded in avoiding burns he might die of suffocation in a fire storm. The heat radiation of a 20-megaton bomb can cause third-degree burns to a person 45 miles from ground zero (the point directly under the detonation).

Victims of burn and blast do not present new problems to the medical scientist because the effects are quite similar to those of ordinary explosives. However, the blast and heat burns of atomic bombs are likely to be more painful than those of chemical explosions. After an exploding atomic bomb, *nitric acid* burns will be discovered in great numbers, because nitric acid is formed in the blast's first few seconds from nitrogen and oxygen (it is estimated that a one-megaton bomb generates about 5000 tons of nitric acid). Nitric acid is suffocating, caustic and highly corrosive. Its vapor is extremely damaging to the lungs, and treatment is that for nitrous gas poisoning.

The third effect is the most lethal and is one with which mankind had had little familiarity—the effect of *radiation fallout* on the human body. Some of the radiation from an atomic bomb explosion appears in the form of light, but most is in the form of invisible radiation fallout which includes x-rays, gamma rays, and radioactive particles of many varieties—about 200 in all. Some of the particles are intensely active but very short-lived, yet some will go on spewing out x-rays, gamma rays or other radiation for thousands of years. The high-speed particles—which are simply free electrons—produce ulcers on the outside of the human body, but inside they can cause other more serious injury. Fallout which is damaging to the skeleton includes the following *radioactive isotopes: calcium-45, strontium-89* and *strontium-90, yttrium-91, barium-140, lanthanum-140,* and all *uranium isotopes.* Those that affect the thyroid gland include all the several radioactive *iodine isotopes.* The liver is damaged by *manganese-56, cobalt-60, cerium-141* and *144, praseodymium-143* and *144* and *neodymium-147.* The particles *cesium-137* and *carbon-14* adversely effect the entire body.

Once a radioactive isotope enters the body, the amount of damage it does depends entirely upon the isotope's *physi-*

cal half-life—that is, its rate of decay, and upon its biological half-life—which is the average length of time the substance will remain in the body. Some radioisotopes have a rapid rate of exchange in metabolism and are soon excreted. For example, carbon-14 is eliminated within six months. On the other hand, strontium-90 displaces bone calcium, and where the rate of mineral exchange is very slow (as in an adult human), the isotope may remain in the bone marrow throughout the lifetime of the victim.

Radioisotopes do their damage through an ability to mimic close chemical relatives that are not radioactive. For example, strontium-90 masquerades as calcium, and iodine 131 or 132 is absorbed as stable iodine. In the latter case, the body captures iodine and concentrates it in the thyroid gland. Thus, a radioactive isotope may be focused upon a single organ. Strontium-90, a radioactive isotope of the element strontium, is the most feared of all the by-products of an atomic bomb explosion because it enters the body via milk and other food and emits beta particles from inside. Beta particles are highly damaging to many types of protein molecules and to bone cells. Strontium-90 produces anemias, leukemias and bone cancer. The latter requires a high dose of radiation.

Radiation sickness and leukemia are the most common effects of an atomic bomb explosion. Radiation sickness symptoms include nausea, diarrhea, internal bleeding, and a severe reduction in the white blood corpuscle count. If absorption of fallout has been heavy, symptoms appear in a few hours, but there is really no way to know if one has been subjected to excessive radiation fallout. Over a period of two days, a dose of 200 roentgens would make some persons ill, but it would probably take a dose in excess of 700 roentgens to cause death.

Treatment depends on length of exposure or severity of burns. For those who have radiation sickness, it is fairly certain that blood damage has occurred, and thus daily transfusions of blood may be needed. Large doses of antibiotic drugs will be needed to control infection, especially where many white blood corpuscles are destroyed. In the latter cases, the body loses its ability to fight infection. Severe burns are treated in the usual manner, but the physician may often be forced to treat compound injuries such as burns, radiation sickness and shock, all in one person. Since victims are apprehensive, mentally disturbed or frightened, sedatives will be needed. Heat blasts burns are extremely painful and pain-killing drugs will find heavy use. See also IRRADIATION; RADIATION SICKNESS.

RADIATION SICKNESS, an illness due to overexposure to x-rays, radium, cobalt, or a source of radiation such as an atomic bomb. The ill effects of excessive exposure to x-rays have long been known and operators were taught to protect themselves by wearing lead aprons and other nonabsorptive devices. Over a period of two days, a dosage of 700r (roentgen units) would normally cause death, 300r would make most people sick and kill some, and 200r would make some people sick but cause no deaths. However, even if radiation is absorbed in considerable amount, it is not always fatal. Various panels of experts are revising safety standards and air purity standards to protect the air from industrial radiation contamination.

The acute symptoms of radiation sickness are burns, loss of appetite, mild to severe nausea, fatigue, diarrhea, falling hair, transient sterility in women, internal bleeding, and aplastic anemia in the form of gradual loss of white blood cells and platelets and inability to form new ones. The degree of exposure to radiation can be determined by photographic film and instruments such as the Geiger counter. Pamphlets on radiotherapy and radiation protection in the event of atomic warfare are available from government agencies such as the National Council on Radiation Protection and Measure in the United States.

Modern scientific research indicates that an ominous effect of radiation is on the sex chromosomes, thus threatening the continued propagation of the human race. *See also* IRRADIATION; RADIATION INJURIES; RADIATION THERAPY.

RADIATION THERAPY, the therapeutic use of x-rays or radioactive substances such as radium and radioactive cobalt-60 isotope in the treatment of disease, primarily of a malignant nature. Radiation therapy is now widely used and radioactive isotopes are employed for specific purposes.

An *isotope* is an element which has the same atomic number as another element but a different atomic weight. A

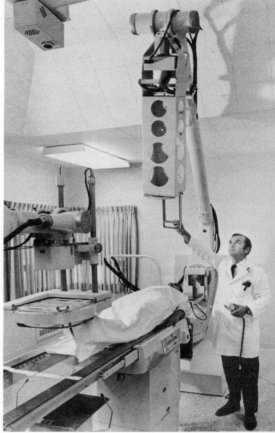

Courtesy, City of Hope

Radiation Therapy—An advanced multiple x-ray complex helps plan radiation treatment for a cancer victim. Radiation destroys malignant cells, which are usually young and thus more vulnerable. It also alters them so they are incapable of reproduction. Radiation dosages given are sufficient to treat the malignancy but not enough to permanently injure normal tissue.

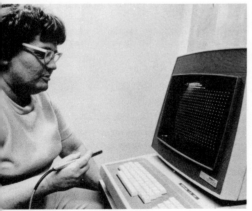

Courtesy, National Institutes of Health

Radiation Therapy—Understanding the mechanisms of the body's cellular system is a key to successful planning and application of radiation therapy. Here a scientist works with a mathematical computer model with graphic display output. The device allows a therapist to observe simulated life cycles of both normal and malignant cells as the treatment progresses.

radioactive isotope is one that decomposes spontaneously, emitting certain rays. Usually, when fed or injected, its course and concentration can be traced and tagged by use of a special instrument, the *Geiger counter*. Scientists are seeking to develop specific radioactive isotopes for many diagnostic and therapeutic uses. Their value and the dangers

of many have not yet been determined.
See also IRRADIATION; ISOTOPE; NUCLEAR MEDICINE; RADIATION SICKNESS; RADIOACTIVITY.

R̲ESEARCH
E̲PORT *follows* EWING'S SARCOMA.

R̲ESEARCH
E̲PORT

LEUKEMIA SURVIVAL TIME DOUBLED BY TOTAL BODY IRRADIATION

Treatment with *total body irradiation* has doubled the average life expectancy for *chronic leukemia* patients, according to studies sponsored by the NATIONAL CANCER INSTITUTE. Researchers claim that experiments with this treatment extending over a ten-year period have achieved remissions of a degree sufficient to alter the natural history of the disease in a significant number of patients.

One group of patients received the traditional combination of local irradiation therapy and anticancer drugs. Their median survival time was 27 months. Another group received total body irradiation, resulting in the complete disappearance of all symptoms in one-third of the patients. The median survival time of the second group was 57 months. Two patients were alive and free of the disease after ten years.

The total body irradiation treatment involved dosages of either five rads per day five times a week or ten rads per day three times a week. (A rad is the standard unit for measuring radiation dosage.) The differing dosages had no apparent effect on remission rates or survival times.

Scientists conducting the study point out that the total dosages which were administered are only one-tenth of the localized dosages used in conventional cancer therapy.   NIH615

R̲ESEARCH
E̲PORT

SALIVARY GLAND DAMAGE IS SIDE EFFECT OF HEAD/NECK RADIATION THERAPY

Patients undergoing radiation therapy in sufficiently high doses to treat cancer of the head and neck should be carefully guarded against tooth decay and also be guided in changing their eating habits. These recommendations for counteracting the discomfort and potentially damaging effects of *"dry mouth"* are the result of studies conducted at the UNIVERSITY OF TEXAS DENTAL SCIENCE INSTITUTE.

These studies indicate that a side effect of this category of radiation therapy causes permanent impairment of the salivary glands, thus definitely reducing the amount of saliva and lowering the level of its bacteria-fighting *bicarbonate* component.

The patients studied all had reasonably good teeth, and none had had previous treatment for cancer. Over a six-week course of radiation therapy, saliva and blood samples were analyzed. Blood levels of essential chemicals, including protein, remained the same before, during and following radiation. The flow of saliva over the same period was reduced over 80 percent. Most salivary salts became more concentrated, but there was a significant decrease in the bicarbonates which enable saliva to neutralize the bacterial acids that cause tooth decay.

During radiotherapy and for several months thereafter, the patients were given smaller, softer and more frequent meals to diminish the discomfort of "dry-mouth" eating. The change in eating patterns prevented serious weight loss and obviated need for stomach-tube feeding.   NIH815

R̲ESEARCH
E̲PORT

NEW DIET COUNTERACTS RADIATION ENTERITIS

A STANFORD UNIVERSITY scientist on a visiting fellowship at the INSTITUT GUSTAVE-ROUSSY in France has developed a specific *diet* that may overcome the severe *intestinal complications* resulting from *radiation treatment* of children with abdominal cancer. Among the 44 French children undergoing whole abdominal radiation therapy for control of malignancy, it was determined that subsequent *enteritis* and *bowel obstruction* were caused not by tumor recurrence, but by the radiation itself. Thus, although the cancer was arrested in many cases, the consequences of the therapy were also life-threatening.

As a countermeasure, a "diet by omission" was devised that eliminated all foods affecting the enteritis. It consists of a liquid blend of substances that can be taken through a tube if the patient is too sick to eat or drink it. It contains no proteins derived from wheat and other grains or from cow's milk and lactose, and it is low in fat and residue.

A dramatic reversal in the children's inflammatory condition followed the initiation of the diet. Roughage, gluten, milk, and fats were gradually added when x-rays and small bowel biopsies showed continuing improvement. The special diet, which was continued for two years in some cases, was gradually replaced by a normal one.

Follow-up studies of 14 of the long-term survivors of cancer, which were conducted for 19 months to seven years, indicate no deaths attributable to radiation enteritis, nor has there been any evidence of recurrent intestinal obstruction.

The diet is now under study at Stanford University.   NIH325

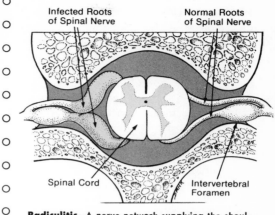

Radiculitis
Horizontal cross-section of Vertebral Column

Infected Roots of Spinal Nerve

Normal Roots of Spinal Nerve

Spinal Cord

Intervertebral Foramen

Radiculitis—A nerve network supplying the shoulder and arms originates from the branches of the upper spinal nerves. Inflammation of the nerves' roots causes acute shoulder pain.

RADICULITIS, inflammation of a nerve root, usually as it emerges from the spine. An example is *acute brachial radiculitis,* which produces the *shoulder girdle syndrome,* evidenced by atrophy (wasting away) of the shoulder girdle muscles and accompanied by sudden onset of acute pain in the shoulder which may radiate to the arm or neck.

The condition, which is disabling as well as painful, is usually the result of a recent or an old injury—most suffered in automobile accidents, others in sports or from blows or falls. Less frequently, infections, growths or metabolic disorders may cause the nerve root inflammation. In addition to analgesics and muscle relaxants, ultrasound, diathermy or moist heat may be used to relieve muscle spasm and pain. Surgery is rarely necessary.

RADIOACTIVE CONTAMINATION, the rendering of certain substances dangerous to health by causing them to emit alpha or beta particles or gamma rays in concentrations beyond safe levels. The most common sources of contamination are x-rays, radium, radioactive isotopes and atomic energy plants. Air and water are naturally radioactive to a certain degree and many of the non-marketed mineral spring waters in the United States have higher concentrations of radioactivity. The safe permissible limits of radioactivity have been published in the United States by the National Bureau of Standards. Extremely high levels of radioactivity can cause cancer, and animal experiments have shown that they may induce leukemia, malignant lymphoma and various other tumors. A high rate of lung cancer has been reported among European mine workers, presumably due to inhalation of radioactive dust. *See also* RADIATION SICKNESS.

RADIOACTIVE GOLD, a radioactive isotope of gold. Medically, it is implanted in tumors to restrain their growth. *See also* GOLD; ISOTOPE; NUCLEAR MEDICINE; RADIOACTIVITY.

RADIOACTIVE IODINE, sodium iodide isotope I-131, administered orally or intravenously, emits gamma radiation and reduces the physiological activity of the thyroid gland. It is used in the treatment of hyperthyroidism, exophthalmic goiter, angina pectoris, congestive heart failure, and thyroid carcinoma. As a result of its use, rapid heartbeats are slowed and the work load of the heart is reduced. Eighty-six percent of 231 persons suffering from hyperthyroidism and treated with radioactive iodine made excellent or good progress toward recovery. *See also* IODINE; ISOTOPE; NUCLEAR MEDICINE; RADIOACTIVITY *and* **medigraphs** HYPERTHYROIDISM; THYROID HEART DISEASE.

RADIOACTIVE ISOTOPES. *See* RADIOACTIVITY.

RADIOACTIVITY, the property of certain chemical isotopes of emitting alpha or beta particles or gamma rays through the disintegration of their atomic nuclei. These rays are traceable in the body by the Geiger counter. More than 150 *radioactive isotopes* are used experimentally in the treatment of various diseases. They include among many others *radioactive iodine* (sodium iodide I-131), used in the treatment of hyperthyroidism, exophthalmic goiter, angina pectoris, congestive heart failure and thyroid carcinoma; *radioactive gold* (gold-198) implanted in tumors to restrain their growth; *radioactive phosphorus* (sodium phosphate P-32) used in the treatment of chronic granulocytic and myelogenous

Radioactivity—The young woman at the rear left attended by a technician *(standing)* is undergoing tests that utilize radioactivity. The physician at the computer *(foreground)* reads the results. As an injected radioisotope passes through her body, the computer records what happens. The resulting changing picture permits physicians to observe the entire process. The computer tape of the tests can be stored for comparison with later scans to be made following treatment.

Courtesy, National Institutes of Health

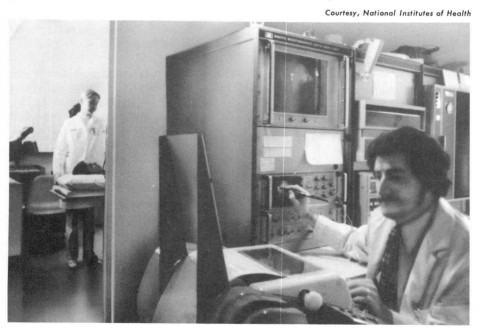

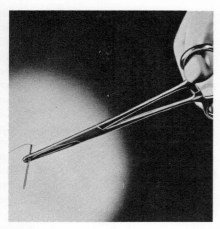

Radioactivity—A radioactive cobalt-60 needle is about to be implanted near an internal malignancy. This method provides continuous destructive irradiation of cancer cells.

leukemia and to provide relief in *polycythemia* (increased red blood cells); and *radioactive iron,* used in the treatment of iron deficiency anemias. The therapeutic uses of—and damage caused by—the various isotopes are under continuous investigation. The high uptake of minerals in radioactive isotopes has a great potential for both therapeutic and toxic results.

Many isotopes are used experimentally to apply radiation for both external and internal treatment. A notable example is cobalt-60 for deep therapy of cancer in inoperable cases. The great energy of the radiations emitted by cobalt-60 is evidenced by the fact that its penetration of body tissues is approximately the same as the radiation from a two-million-volt x-ray machine. Proper doses of radioactive cobalt-60 beamed at the malignant area are believed to restrain the growth of cancerous tissue without affecting the healthy tissue. Cobalt is now supplied to hospitals for investigative use in cases of inoperable malignancy. A unique beam has been developed which provides energy capable of obliterating completely the pituitary gland of the rat. Iron and

other minerals are tagged by isotopes so that their uptake and fate in the body can be measured accurately. Radioactive iron has enabled researchers to determine that the average lifetime of a red corpuscle is about 120 days. With the aid of isotopes, scientists are learning more about metabolism (the body's mechanism), including the relationships between cholesterol and arteriosclerosis and between sugar and diabetes.

With tagged isotopes, the life cycle of mosquitoes that cause malaria and yellow fever can be determined, as can the fate of digitalis and other drugs in the body. In one test by this new sensitive technique, the survival of one milligram of digitalis over 35 days in a human subject was established. One of the great achievements of this method of basic radiology is the detection of defec-

Radioactivity—A container of radioactive cobalt is focused to irradiate a throat cancer. Cobalt-60 emits high-intensity radiation, making it valuable therapy for inoperable cancers as well as surgery follow-up. Bombardment with subatomic particles converts an element into radioactive form, called a radioisotope.

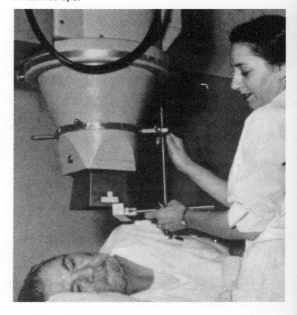

tive x-ray machines and films, a matter of great importance since authorities estimate that between one-third to one-half of all crucial medical decisions are made on the basis of x-ray information. *See also* ISOTOPE; NUCLEAR MEDICINE; RADIATION THERAPY; RADIOACTIVE GOLD; RADIOACTIVE IODINE.

RADIOGRAPHY, the diagnostic production, development, viewing and interpretation of x-ray films. A portable x-ray unit has been developed which employs *radioactive thulium* (a rare earth metal) as its source of radiation. A small amount of thulium encased in lead, which protects the operators, produces radiograms without the use of electricity, water or darkroom facilities. The unit—which weighs only 40 pounds—is simple to operate and produces a finished radiogram in 5–10 minutes. *See also* DIAGNOSIS; MEDICAL INSTRUMENTATION; RADIOLOGY; X-RAYS.

RADIOLOGY, the medical specialty which deals with x-ray diagnosis, and the therapeutic application of x-rays, radium, cobalt and other radioactive substances. A *radiologist* is a specialist in this branch of medicine. *See also* RADIATION THERAPY; RADIOACTIVITY; RADIOGRAPHY; X-RAYS.

RADIOTHERAPY, the use of x-rays, radium, cobalt and other radioactive substances in the treatment of the various conditions in which they are believed to be helpful, particularly inoperable cancer. *See also* RADIATION THERAPY.

RADIUM, a highly radioactive element found in *pitchblend* and other minerals in the earth's crust, identified by Pierre and Marie Curie in 1898. Its radioactive rays have an effect on the growth of human tissue. Radium is generally employed in the form of one of its salts, because they are more stable than the

element itself. Platinum or gold needles or tiny glass tubes called *seeds* filled with *radon* (a gaseous emanation of radium) are inserted into cancers and other tumors and in some cases allowed to remain permanently. The radium salts are used in the treatment of malignant tumors, especially inoperable cancer, as well as leukemia, polycythemia (increased red blood cells), and certain nonmalignant conditions. Inhalation or ingestion of radium, or body exposure to it may result in lung cancer, bone sarcoma, bony inflammation, blood disturbances, or burns. *See also* RADIOACTIVITY.

RAGWEED DERMATITIS, inflammation or allergy of the skin occurring mostly in adults during the pollinating season of July–September and recurring every year. The symptoms are redness, swelling and itching of the eyelids and inflammation of the exposed skin areas, especially the hands, wrists, ankles and face, which become worse following hunting, gardening or other contacts with the ragweed plant. The diagnosis is established by a patch skin test performed by an allergist. The best treatment is to avoid contact with ragweed during its season, including vacationing in an area where this plant does not grow. Certain drugs are useful in treating it, and sleeping in an air-conditioned room is a good preventive. *See also* ALLERGY *and* **medigraph** CONTACT DERMATITIS.

RALE, an abnormal sound produced in the lungs or bronchial tubes during breathing and heard by the doctor through a stethoscope. Various types of rales have been described but the most significant are these: *amphoric rales,* coarse tinkling sounds caused in lung cavities by fluid splashing inside; *crepitant rales,* fine dry crackling sounds heard during the first few deep inspirations, one of the early signs of lobar pneumonia; *cavernous rales,* hollow metallic sounds heard over cavities in late pulmonary tuberculosis which are produced by expansion and contraction of the cavity walls; *mucous rales,* sounding like a pipe blown through soapy water, heard in emphysema; and *sibilant rales,* high-pitched hissing or whistling sounds heard in bronchial spasm or asthma. Some doctors describe rales as coarse, medium, fine, moist and dry. *See also* AUSCULTATION.

RANULA, a retention cyst of a salivary gland located beneath the tongue, due to obstruction and retention of the secretion. It is usually treated by incision and drainage.

RASH. *See* EXANTHEM.

RAT-BITE FEVER, either of two similar bacterial diseases usually transmitted by the bite of an infected rat or other rodent. *Haverhill fever,* the most common of the two in the United States, is caused by the *Streptobacillus moniliformis; sodoku* is caused by the *Spirillum minus.* Rat-bite fever has been observed in practically every part of the world.

The symptoms begin 5–28 days after the bite of an infected animal with a sudden flare-up of the wound, fluctuating fever, chills, headache, weakness, enlargement of the lymph glands, and occasionally a skin rash. The relapsing type of fever is typical and may continue for weeks. The joints may be involved. The white blood cells are increased to more than twice the normal count. The diagnosis is confirmed by finding the responsible germ in the local eruption or regional lymph gland. The fatality rate without treatment is about 10 percent.

Most of the rat-bite wounds heal without treatment. If a wound persists or flares up, the bite should be cauterized and treated with a strong germicide. Penicillin injected into the muscles in large dosages is the most effective antibiotic, though some others are effective, too. The wound should also be checked to make certain that it does not contain the germs of rabies or plague. If the wound is of a deep-punctured nature, the precautions against tetanus should be employed. *See also* ANIMAL BITES AND WOUNDS; RAT CONTROL.

RAT CONTROL. The rat is one of the most dangerous enemies of humans. It transmits disease. It is the carrier of plague—which in epidemics decimated the human race—and also of typhus, rat-bite fever, hemorrhagic jaundice, tapeworm infestation, and food poisoning. It consumes food meant for humans. It feeds on and contaminates stored grain. These are reasons why one of the primary duties of public health officials is to kill the rat population.

Rats thrive on unsanitary conditions, especially uncovered garbage and offal. In poverty areas, the combination of inadequate disposal facilities and careless habits of some tenants accounts for the rapid multiplication of the rodents. Fumigation with hydrocyanic acid, carbon monoxide or sulfur dioxide gases is the acceptable method of destroying the rats. These gases are toxic to people, who must be kept out of the rooms where the gases are being used, and the doors and windows must be sealed to prevent the escape of the poisonous gas to adjoining apartments or dwellings. Ships coming from ports where rats are prevalent usually must be fumigated before landing, and usually this kills enormous numbers of the rodents.

The family cat or a rat-trap baited with cheese provides a household means of killing rats. Various rat poisons have been employed including red squill, strychnine, arsenic, warfarin, and ANTU. They are effective rodenticides but care must be taken to keep children and pet dogs and cats from eating them. One

Raynaud's Disease

Attacks precipitated by cold (low temperature) . . .

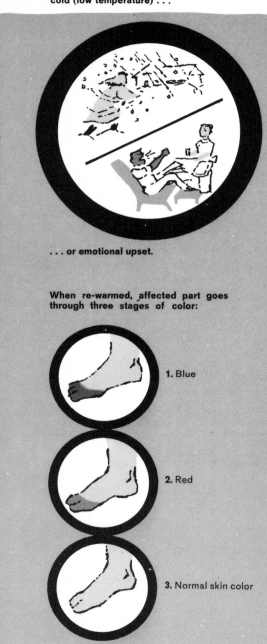

. . . or emotional upset.

When re-warmed, affected part goes through three stages of color:

1. Blue

2. Red

3. Normal skin color

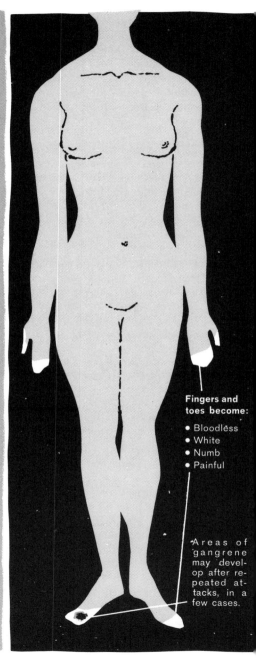

Fingers and toes become:

- Bloodless
- White
- Numb
- Painful

Areas of gangrene may develop after repeated attacks, in a few cases.

pound of ANTU is sufficient to kill 200,-000 rats. It is mixed with finely ground corn or wheat or cut-up vegetables, tomatoes or potatoes as bait. After the rat has eaten a small amount of this poison, its lungs fill up with body fluid and the animal dies of suffocation.

The best means of protection against rats is scrupulous sanitation in the home.

If there is no loose food or uncovered garbage in the home, the rats will either go elsewhere in search of food or starve to death. Also, sanitary facilities must be adequate if the home is to be protected against rats. *See also* BUBONIC PLAGUE; FLEAS; PLAGUE; PUBLIC HEALTH; RAT-BITE FEVER; TYPHUS *and* **medigraph** LEPTO-SPIROSIS.

RAYNAUD'S DISEASE

R AYNAUD'S DISEASE is a condition in which spasms in the superficial blood vessels of the extremities cause the fingers and toes to become *cyanotic* (bluish)—as occurs when tissues are deprived of oxygenated blood—and then to become numb and white. Attacks may last for minutes or hours, and eventually small and painful ulcers develop at the tips of the fingers. The condition is rarely seen in men and is most common in women of early middle age.

causes
Raynaud's disease may appear because of a disorder of the endocrine or nervous systems; because of sensitivity to substances such as tobacco or arsenic; it may be associated with a general circulatory disorder; it may be triggered by exposure to cold or by an emotional crisis.

symptoms
The chief symptom is the alteration in the appearance and sensitivity of the digits—more often the fingers than the toes —which turn blue, then white and numb, and then red. When the spasms of the blood vessels that bring these changes about are lasting, superficial ulceration develops and is quite painful.

complications
Only in rare cases does Raynaud's disease result in gangrene, and even then

tissue death is superficial and can be treated before too much damage is done.

treatment
If the disease can be traced to a glandular deficiency, hormone replacement therapy is effective. In most cases it is difficult to isolate the cause but for a considerable number of them, psychotherapy can be helpful. People vulnerable to the disorder are also advised to avoid severe cold, give up smoking, and protect their hands as much as possible. Where pain from ulceration is acute, sedatives are prescribed. Alcohol rubs sometimes help to prevent the vascular spasms. When the attacks seriously interfere with normal functioning, surgery may be recommended to remove the groups of nerve cells (*ganglia*) involved, thereby relieving the spasms.

REACTION, in medicine, the response of the body to a stimulus or drug. A very large number of *adverse reactions* to various new drugs occur, which are reported by physicians in medical journals and to government agencies. In some nations these are stored in a computer for the information of the medical profession. Other reactions, not caused by drugs, are described in medical texts. *See also* ALLERGEN; ALLERGY; CONVERSION REACTION *and* **medigraph** CONTACT DERMATITIS.

RECESSIVE, any physical characteristic that can be transmitted to future generations by the chromosomes. *See also* DOMINANT; GENETIC COUNSELING.

RECTOCELE, a bulge of the rectum into the vagina. *See also* HERNIA; VAGINA.

RECTUM, the last six inches of the colon (large intestine) beginning at the S-shaped *sigmoid* in the lower left side of the abdomen and ending at the anal opening. Its lower portion lies just behind the prostate in men and can be felt by a

The Rectum

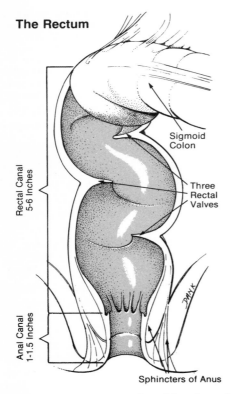

Rectal Canal
5-6 Inches

Sigmoid
Colon

Three
Rectal
Valves

Anal Canal
1-1.5 Inches

Sphincters of Anus

Rectum—The rectum stores the solid waste products of digestion before discharge through the anus. Crescent-shaped folds support the fecal matter as it descends from the large intestine. The muscular wall of the rectum is stronger than that of the colon, and that of the anal canal is thicker still. The internal and external sphincter muscles control the anus.

urologist by inserting a finger into the rectum (rectal palpation). The rectum is narrow at its beginning but dilates (becomes larger) below to form the *rectal ampulla.* It has two lateral curves, not being straight as its name might imply. The rectum is equipped with three or four folds know as *Houston's valves* that support the weight of the fecal matter and prevent its movement toward the anus, where its presence would excite a sensation demanding discharge. The rectum is further surrounded and supported by a dense tube of tough membrane and carries the *hemorrhoidal plexus* of veins, dilatation (expansion) of which produces the common disorder *hemorrhoids. See also* BOWEL; COLON; DIGESTION; INTESTINE *and* **medigraphs** CANCER OF THE COLON AND RECTUM; HEMORRHOIDS AND FISSURES; ULCERATIVE COLITIS.

RED BLOOD CELLS. *See* ERYTHROCYTES.

RED BLOOD CELLS, diseases of. The red blood cell does not have a nucleus. It is shaped like a disc with two concave sides. It measures about 7.5 microns in diameter and is two microns thick. (One inch is equivalent to about 25,000 microns in length.) There are about five million per cubic millimeter in the male and 4.5 million in the female. These cells are formed by the bone marrow, and the average span of life of a red blood cell is 120 days.

The red blood cells contain *hemoglobin,* a protein substance rich in iron that carries oxygen from the lungs to the tissues and removes carbon dioxide and waste products from the tissues.

Polycythemia is a disease in which there is an increase in the number and richness of the red blood cells. In this disease, both the red blood cell count and the hemoglobin percentages are above normal. People with polycythemia have a florid complexion and suffer from headaches and high blood pressure. The treatment is with drugs, special diets, and bleeding when needed to reduce the excessive amount of blood.

Pernicious anemia is a condition in which the red blood corpuscles are oversized but reduced in number. There is a lack of hydrochloric acid in the stomach and degenerative changes in the spinal cord, leading to paralysis in some cases. The treatment is by administration of liver extract, folic acid or vitamin B_{12}.

Iron deficiency anemia is very common in women. A daily supplement of up to 60 milligrams of iron is recommended for women as compared with a maximum of 27 milligrams for men. In children, iron deficiency anemia may be caused by a faulty diet; in men, it may indicate bleeding from the gastrointestinal tract, as from a gastric or duodenal ulcer or from hemorrhoids. The best treatment is a diet rich in liver and red meats and iron medication, best given during meals to avoid stomach upset.

Sickle cell anemia is a form of ane-

Red Blood Cells, Diseases of—There are millions of these disc-shaped red cells in each cubic millimeter of a person's blood. In polycythemia, the cells increase abnormally in number and richness causing high blood pressure, headaches and a florid complexion. Inadequate and abnormal formation of red cells, plus nonabsorption of vitamin B_{12}, occurs in pernicious anemia.

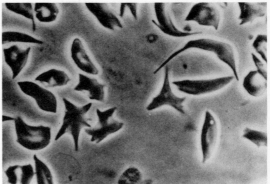

Courtesy, National Institutes of Health

Red Blood Cells, Diseases of—The red blood cells of sickle cell anemia show how the disease got its name. The cells are distorted from the normal disc shape by an inherited abnormal hemoglobin in the blood. The sickle shape increases blood thickness—retarding flow, blocking blood vessels, and causing cell death from lack of oxygen. There is also excessive red blood cell destruction, with recurring severe pain and eventual involvement of many organs.

mia that is inherited and occurs almost exclusively in blacks. It is characterized by sickle-shaped red blood corpuscles. The majority of its victims die during the first few years of life, and very few live beyond the age of 40. The onset of the illness is usually toward the end of the first year of life. The clinical course is that of a chronic severe blood-depleting disease, punctuated by periodic painful attacks of bone, joint, back and abdominal pain. There is no specific therapy as yet, and frequent blood transfusions may be necessary to sustain life.

Other diseases affecting the red blood cells include *secondary hemolytic anemias,* due to various causes such as lead poisoning, infections, and cancer and other malignant tumors; *aplastic anemia,* in which the bone marrow fails to form red and white blood cells normally; *leukemia,* in which the white blood cells multiply enormously at the expense of the red blood corpuscles; *Mediterranean anemia (familial thalassemia),* in which

Courtesy, National Institutes of Health

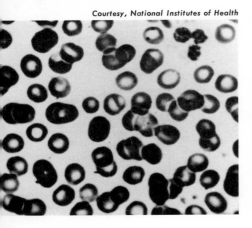

the production of hemoglobin and the red blood cells is impaired; and *hemolytic disease of the newborn,* in which the mother is Rh negative and the father Rh positive. The latter is a hereditary disorder which sometimes requires a complete exchange blood transfusion to save the infant's life. *See also* ANEMIA; APLASTIC ANEMIA; BIRTH DEFECT; BLOOD; BLOOD CONDITIONS; BLOOD TYPES; CHLOROSIS; ERYTHREMIA; ERYTHROCYTES; GENETIC COUNSELING; HEMOGLOBIN; IRON; MARROW; POLYCYTHEMIA; THALASSEMIA *and* **medigraphs** PERNICIOUS ANEMIA; SICKLE CELL ANEMIA.

REDUCING DIET. *See* DIET, REDUCING.

REFLEX, an involuntary response to a stimulus which passes through the lower spinal and nerve centers without conscious action by the brain. The most common automatic reflexes are *swallowing* chewed food, *laughing* in response to tickling, *jumping* out of the path of danger, *sneezing* when the nose is irritated, *coughing* on inhalation of tobacco smoke, *scratching* in response to itching; *erection* of the penis and *ejaculation* in sexual excitement and intercourse; and the *startle reflex* on hearing a sudden loud noise. Diagnostically, the most important reflex is the *knee jerk,* elicited by tapping the tendon immediately below the kneecap. The knee jerk is absent in paralysis of the lower spinal nerves, poliomyelitis, tabes dorsalis and general paresis; it is increased in diseases affecting higher nerve centers and in nervous individuals. *See also* BABINSKI REFLEX; BRAIN; KNEE JERK; NERVOUS SYSTEM.

REGENERATION, natural regrowth and repair of damaged or destroyed tissue. When the two fragments of a broken bone are brought together, they unite and cement the union with regenerated bone. If a nerve has been severed by a bullet or cut and the two ends are sewn together, the nerve will regenerate all the way to the end and eventually reestablish its full function. In the heart after a coronary thrombosis, the tributaries of the coronary artery regenerate cardiac tissue to repair the damage and reestablish the functions of circulation. Nature is provided with many regenerative devices to reestablish physiological action after it has been interrupted by injury or disease.

REGRESSION, a turning back of the mind in its adjustment to difficult and unpleasant situations, particularly in older persons, sometimes referred to as second childhood; a return to infantile behavior patterns. Many symptoms of inadequacy in senility result from a state of panic in the older person who feels

Reflex—An involuntary muscular action performed in response to a stimulation is a reflex. A tap of the doctor's hammer on the tendon below the kneecap tests for the knee-jerk reflex. Absence of the jerk or an excessive jerk indicates interference with the nerve pathways involved.

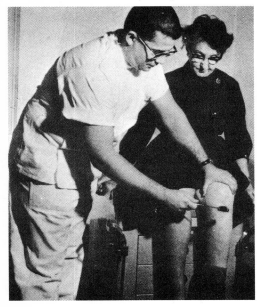

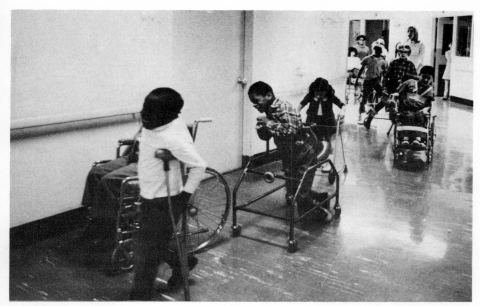

Rehabilitation—Wheelchairs, crutches, special "walkers" and braces are the mechanical means of rehabilitation for these crippled children. Just as important to their progress and ultimate ability to function is physical therapy. Skilled therapists guide them through exercises to develop maximum use of their limited muscular resources. In some cases, surgery is helpful.

rejected by society. Whether the feeling of neglect and isolation is real or imagined, the person reacts by building up tighter psychological defenses against the environment or by losing the usual defenses, thus regressing.

Early retirement has led many people to regress. Older people must constantly maintain their interest in life by keeping abreast of the times or developing hobbies or special interests. Extreme regression can make a person just as much an invalid as a stroke or other physical disease. It can be avoided by good psychological guidance. *See also* MEMORY; SENESCENCE; SENILITY.

REGURGITATION, a backflow of blood through a defective heart valve or the return of food from the stomach, gullet or duodenum (first portion of the small intestine) after eating, without vomiting. *Mitral regurgitation* is the return of blood from the left ventricle to the

left atrium during contraction due to imperfect closure of the mitral valve. *Aortic regurgitation* is the backflow of blood through the aortic opening during contraction because of an incompetent aortic valve. *Duodenal regurgitation* is the return of acid-digested food from the duodenum to the stomach.

REHABILITATION, the restoration of functions and useful activities to a disabled person by special devices, prescribed training, and many different methods employed by skilled workers in this field. A lame or crippled person can be rehabilitated by use of a cane to help him to walk, a paralytic by braces, supports and an ambulatory machine, and a mute person by an artificial voice box and speech therapy.

Formerly these victims were allowed to deteriorate in a bed or chair, suffering from *atrophy* (withering away) due to disuse of their muscles and enforced in-

validism. One important way to rehabili-
tate the invalid is to keep the person from
resting in bed excessively. Nowadays, patients are urged to stay out of bed soon
after an operation, sometimes even on
the first day. Much mental comfort and
encouragement are achieved by training
convalescents or invalids to perform their
usual activities as far as possible with
special training and devices. In the event
of paralysis or loss of the use of an arm
or a leg, active steps should be taken immediately to restore the function of the
defective limb, including providing the
person with an artificial limb if needed.
Some of the most useful citizens have
been restored to full activity after poliomyelitis and other debilitating diseases.
Early removal of casts and splints, massage, diathermy, and special exercises are
further aids to rehabilitation. Alcoholics
and narcotic addicts can often be rehabilitated by special training, will power,
and the use of nonaddictive drugs. *See
also* ARTIFICIAL BODY PARTS; OCCUPA-
TIONAL THERAPY; PHYSICAL THERAPY.

REITER'S SYNDROME, a combination
of *arthritis, conjunctivitis* (inflammation
of the membrane that lines the eye), and
urethritis (inflammation of the urethra),
all nongonorrheal.

RELAPSE, a return of the symptoms of
a disease after convalescence has begun.
Relapses are common in typhoid fever
and in rheumatoid arthritis on withdrawal of cortisone, but seldom occur in
pneumonia.

RELAPSING FEVER, any of a group
of specific infectious diseases caused by
spirochetes and transmitted to people by
lice, ticks, and sometimes bedbugs, characterized by a return of fever after the
beginning of convalescence. The symptoms are acute onset with chills, high
fever, backache, pains in the legs, enlargement of the spleen, delirium, and

sometimes convulsions. After a few days
the victim suddenly appears to recover
but suffers a relapse in about a week. The
death rate is about five percent or less.
Antibiotics are used for treatment. Aspirin and other salicylates are useful to
relieve pain and, with sponge baths, lower
high temperatures. *See also* BEDBUG; IN-
FECTIOUS DISEASES; TICKS *and* **medigraph**
LICE AND SCABIES.

RELAXANTS, agents that lessen tension. These include the barbiturates, the
tranquilizers, and the bromides. The most
effective muscle relaxants are *mephenesin*
and *meprobamate.* A hot tub bath is also
an excellent relaxant. *See also* TRANQUIL-
IZERS *and* **medigraph** BARBITURATE ABUSE.

REMISSION, an interval in the course
of a disease in which the symptoms subside or abate. Remissions occur naturally
in some cases of cancer and other malignant diseases and in rheumatoid arthritis.

RENIN, a substance secreted by the kidneys which causes the blood to liberate
angiotonin, a substance that causes the
arterioles to contract and thus raises the
blood pressure.

RENNIN. *See* DIGESTION.

REPRODUCTION, propagation of the
individual organism or species by producing other organisms or individuals of
the same species. In the ameba, a microscopic one-celled animal, reproduction is
by *fission*—that is, the single cell divides
into two equal halves. In flowering plants,
the pollen from the *stamen* (male organ)
is carried by the wind or insects to impregnate other plants of the same species.
In the human race, reproduction is accomplished by sexual union between a
man and a woman, the offspring inheriting the characteristics of both parents as
either dominant or recessive traits. *See
also* REPRODUCTIVE SYSTEM.

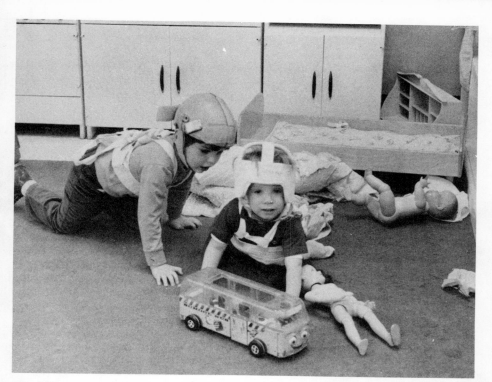

Disease is no discriminator with regard to age. It can and often does strike young children. When children have been disabled by disease or injury, they must be helped to return to normal living patterns as soon as possible. Sometimes this can best be accomplished in a children's rehabilitation hospital. Here, children with walking problems can be assisted by various therapeutic procedures. Some can have their disability corrected surgically. All can receive the moral support that is crucial to satisfactory recovery. Above, these young patients at one of the leading children's hospitals in the country suffer from difficulties with their balance. Since they are prone to fall down a lot, they are wearing protective helmets to protect their heads from injury. Right, this handicapped boy is working hard to overcome his disabilities.

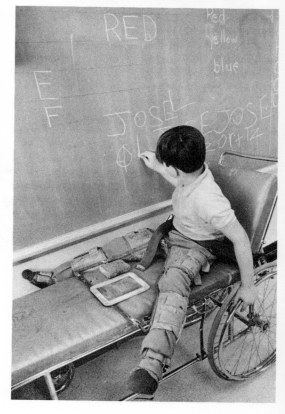

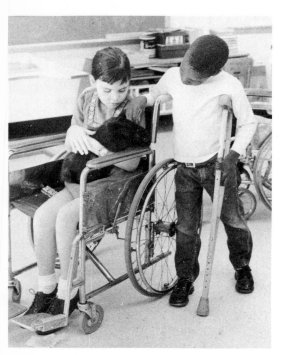

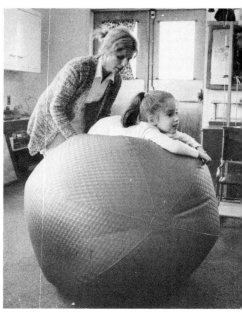

Two handicapped children take time away from their own problems to play with a rabbit *(left)*. A little girl *(above)* learns to climb and strengthen her muscles through the use of this big ball. A trained nurse helps. Below, despite their handicaps, these children can enjoy life in the pleasant atmosphere of this modern children's hospital.

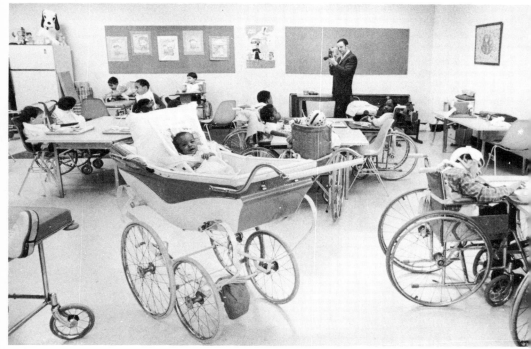

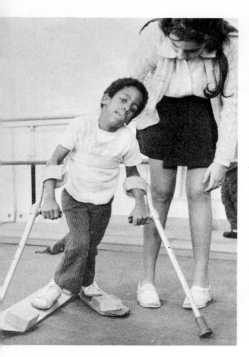

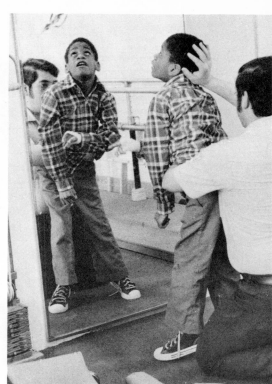

Children with walking problems are assisted with all kinds of therapy. Above, a boy takes some of his first steps in learning how to walk. The therapeutic ski-like shoes were especially designed for this purpose. Above right, this boy is learning proper head balance so he can begin to control his balance in walking. Right, walking in water is easier than on dry land; water is buoyant and thus helps support the body. This will help strengthen the weakened muscles of these young patients. The stainless steel swimming pool is also used for recreation.

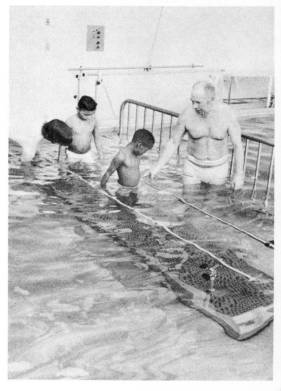

A variety of wheeled vehicles enable the patients to move from one class to another. No one studies or eats in bed. All are urged to move around independently.

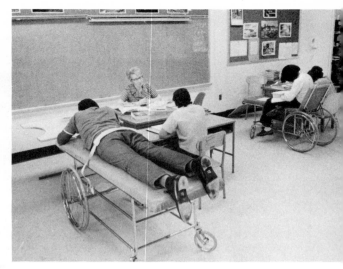

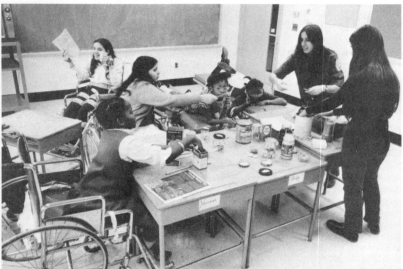

These girls work enthusiastically on a poster project. Keeping occupied is part of the therapy; the children don't brood when they are busy.

An attendant helps this boy put on a pair of ski-like therapeutic shoes (right).

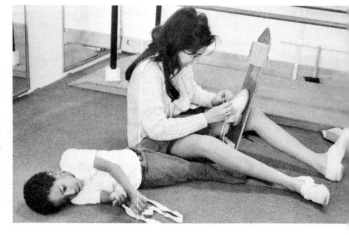

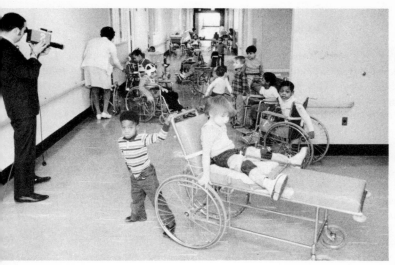

All the children help each other and learn to have patience for each other's defects *(above)*. In the therapy room *(right)*, a videotape is in use. Nurses and therapists can learn useful therapeutic techniques by rerunning the videotape for study. A record can be kept of the children's progress with the tape. Below left, the camera records a young patient's progress in the videotape studio of the hospital. Below right, tapes are stored for later study or comparison.

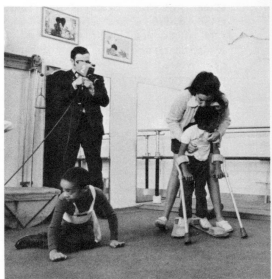

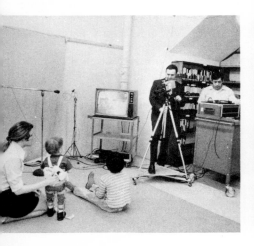

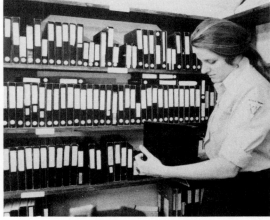

REPRODUCTIVE SYSTEM, those organs of the male and female involved in the regenerative process. This includes formation of reproductive cells, conception, sex determination and development, gestation, birth and patterns of inheritance. The differences in the female and male systems determine that the male is the instrument of fertilization, while the female nurtures and bears the new life.

The male sexual apparatus consists of the *penis, scrotum, testicles* and several internal glands such as the *prostate.*

The testicles—the *male gonads*—are the most crucial component of the male sexual system. These extraordinary glands determine and govern the maleness of the individual: the secondary sexual characteristics such as the beard, deep voice, heavy bones and narrow pelvis, and control his ability to procreate.

Deprived of the testicles, as in *castration,* the individual cannot procreate, and may lose some of the secondary characteristics—or fail to develop these characteristics at all if the castration occurs before puberty.

The testicles, which lie outside the body proper in a thin-skinned sac called the scrotum, consist of a large number of tubular structures called *seminiferous tubules,* and of cells between the tubules called *interstitial cells.* The seminiferous tubules, from puberty to senility, are constantly producing sperm cells (*spermatozoa*), the male reproductive cells. Production of these sperm cells is the primary purpose of the testicles, and their conveyance to the female reproductive tract is the primary purpose of the whole male sexual system.

The interstitial cells produce the male hormone *testosterone* which enters the blood stream and determines the male secondary sex characteristics. The seminiferous tubules all empty into the *epididymis,* a coiled tube partly covering the testicle which serves as a temporary storage area for the new sperm. The epididymis in turn empties into a long narrow duct called the *vas deferens (seminal duct),* through which the sperm cells pass to a larger storage area called the *seminal vesicle.* The seminal vesicles, in addition to serving as a storage area for sperm, also secrete a sticky viscous substance which aids in the preservation of the sperm and facilitates its further transport along the remainder of the seminal duct.

The seminal duct finally empties into the *urethra,* a channel which normally serves to convey urine from the bladder to the outside (hence the whole system is also called the *genitourinary tract*). At this point, the urethra is surrounded by the prostate gland, which secretes another sticky white substance into the seminal fluid containing the sperm. This further facilitates the transport and preservation of the sperm. This final combined fluid is called *semen.*

The urethra passes into the erectile organ called the penis. Two small glands called *Cowper's glands* or the *bulbourethral glands* occur in this area. When sexual activity takes place, these small glands secrete an alkaline fluid which neutralizes any traces of urine which might still remain in the urethra. The acid urine would otherwise be highly injurious to the sperm cells. During sexual activity, special muscles close off the urethra from the bladder, making it impossible for any fresh urine to enter the urethra while sexual activity lasts.

The penis, through which the urethra travels, serves as the organ of intromission into the female vagina for depositing the semen in the female reproductive tract. Under the impetus of sexual desire or excitement, the highly flexible tissues of the penis become engorged with blood, and the normally flaccid organ assumes a rigid, greatly enlarged position called an *erection.* The state of erection permits the penis to be inserted deeply into the

Reproductive System

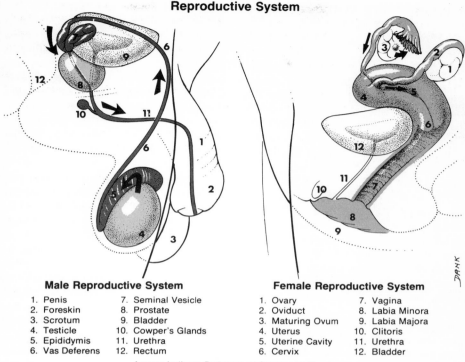

Male Reproductive System

1. Penis	7. Seminal Vesicle
2. Foreskin	8. Prostate
3. Scrotum	9. Bladder
4. Testicle	10. Cowper's Glands
5. Epididymis	11. Urethra
6. Vas Deferens	12. Rectum

Female Reproductive System

1. Ovary	7. Vagina
2. Oviduct	8. Labia Minora
3. Maturing Ovum	9. Labia Majora
4. Uterus	10. Clitoris
5. Uterine Cavity	11. Urethra
6. Cervix	12. Bladder

Arrows indicate Pathways of Sperm and Ovum

Reproductive System—*(Left)* Male sperm cells from the testicles pass into the urethra via the seminal ducts. Two white substances added along the way form the combined fluid called semen. The erect penis deposits semen deep into the female vagina. *(Right)* Monthly an ovary releases a mature female egg which enters a Fallopian tube. If the egg is fertilized by a male sperm cell, it passes into the uterus for development. Birth occurs through the vaginal canal.

vagina. The friction of the vaginal tissues against the penis—normally highly pleasurable to both partners—causes muscular spasms to occur in the penis and along the seminal tract, finally resulting in the *ejaculation* of the semen into the vagina, an event known as *orgasm* in which the pleasurable sensations are greatest. Following orgasm, the blood drains from the penis and it resumes its flaccid state. Every ejaculation contains several hundred million sperm cells; only one of these can fertilize the female egg cell, resulting in a new human being; the others die after a few days. Fertilization does not occur at all if no egg is present in the female tract.

The female sexual apparatus consists of the *ovaries, uterus, oviducts, vagina,* and several small associated organs. The ovaries—the *female gonads*—perform functions analogous to those of the testicles in the male: they germinate the female reproductive cells, and govern the female secondary sex characteristics such as the high-pitched voice, absence of a beard, development of the breasts, and wide pelvis.

The female reproductive cells, called eggs (*ova*) develop in the interior of the ovaries within fluid-filled sacs called *follicles*. As an ovum matures, it attaches itself to the wall of the follicle. When the ovum becomes fully mature, the wall of the follicle bursts and the ovum escapes with the liberated follicular fluid—a process called *ovulation*. It then passes into the oviduct where it may be fertilized by a male spermatozoon if sexual intercourse has taken place.

The ovaries produce the female hormones (*estrogens*). These include *estradiol*, which specifically determines the female secondary sex characteristics, and *progesterone*, which brings about physiological changes in the uterus to prepare it for the reception and nurture of a fertilized egg cell. Progesterone is secreted into the uterus for about a week each month following the release of the ovum or ova.

As in the male, the production of reproduction cells and the secretion of sex hormones begins at puberty—usually about the age of eleven or twelve in the

female. However, in the woman the sex glands cease these functions considerably earlier than in the male, usually between the ages of 45 and 50. This phenomenon is known as the *menopause*.

The uterus (*womb*), an organ capable of tremendous expansion, is where the fertilized egg develops into an embryo, a fetus, and finally a fully developed infant ready for birth. The vagina is the channel leading from the uterus to the outside of the body. It serves a twofold function: first, to admit the male penis into the female body so that semen may be deposited in the female reproductive tract, and—if conditions are propitious—an egg be fertilized; second, to serve as a channel for the birth of the developed infant, allowing it to emerge from the uterus into the outside world. Several small glands lubricate the vagina during sexual inter-

Reproductive System—The female reproductive cell (ovum) develops in and is released from an ovary. The much smaller male reproductive cell (sperm) is produced in the testicles. It is one of millions in the semen ejaculated into the vagina at the climax of intercourse. For conception to occur, one sperm must reach a female egg within a Fallopian tube. Attaching itself to the egg, the sperm head loses its tail and penetrates into the egg. Fusion of the egg's nucleus and the sperm head (fertilization) forms the first cell of a new human being.

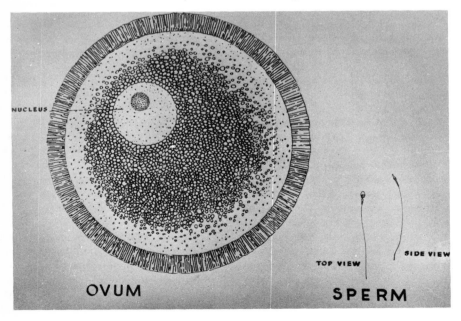

OVUM   SPERM

NUCLEUS

TOP VIEW   SIDE VIEW

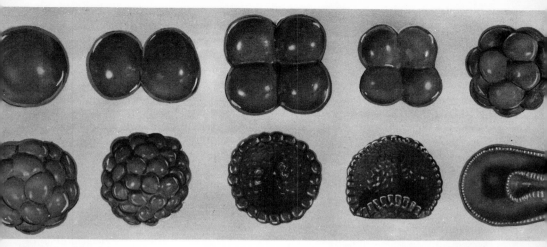

Reproductive System—With the formation of the first human cell by fertilization of an egg, mitosis begins. This is the complex process in which a cell splits into two new cells—each with the identical number and kind of genes and chromosomes as the parent cell. Repeated cell divisions finally form a solid mass of cells resembling a mulberry, the morula. Mitosis continues to the blastula stage—a fluid-filled ball of cells in a single layer. An indentation of the ball begins an alteration of shape into a hollow tube which eventually becomes the digestive tract.

course, facilitating the intromission of the penis and the passage of the semen. During intercourse, sensations of sexual pleasure occur in the vagina analogous to those the male experiences in the penis.

The entrance to the vagina resembles a small pair of vertical lips and is called the *labia minora*. Outside this is a larger pair of lips called the *labia majora* which encloses not only the entrance to the vagina but also the mouth of the urethra —through which urine is expelled—and, in front of that, the *clitoris*. The clitoris is a small fleshy projection which, in sexual excitement, may become erect, like a tiny penis. These external female sex organs are known as the *vulva*.

In young virgins, the opening of the vagina is covered by a thin membrane called the *hymen*. This disappears soon after intercourse is undertaken, and not infrequently even before.

Conception of a human being is an intricate event. In intercourse, the sperm cells are deposited near the mouth of the womb. These sperm cells may travel fur-ther, enter an oviduct, where one of them may meet with and fertilize one of the female egg cells. At once, by process of self-division, the fertilized egg cell—called a *zygote*—will begin to grow, feeding mainly on the food which it finds within itself.

Leaving the oviduct, this fertilized egg cell fastens itself to the inner wall of the womb. Soon, between the wall and the cell, the *placenta* develops. This is the channel of communication between mother and child, but the blood of the two never intermingles. Each, in the placenta, will have its own separate blood vessels. Other materials, however, such as fluids and gases, are passed from mother to child through the walls of these blood vessels, a process known as *osmosis*, which permits the mother to supply the child with such essentials as food, water and oxygen. The child may also use this channel to rid itself of waste.

The placenta, together with membranes developed during pregnancy, is eliminated after the birth of the child.

The new human being exists as soon as the sperm cell has fertilized the egg cell, at which time the sex is determined.

All females are composed of cells each of which contains *46 chromosomes*—the infinitesimal protoplasmic bodies which govern the chemical (genetic) make-up of the individual, and determine such factors as the color of the hair, eyes and skin, the features of the face, the intelligence, etc. Two of these chromosomes govern the sex of the female and are labeled for convenience as X chromosomes.

The cells of males normally also contain 46 chromosomes, two of which are specifically sex chromosomes. One of these—as in the female—is an X chromosome, but the other exhibits a distinct genetic composition and is labeled a Y chromosome.

Thus, females are said to possess an XX genetic make-up (because they have two X sex chromosomes in each of their cells), and males are said to possess an XY genetic make-up (because each of their cells contains one X sex chromosome and one Y sex chromosome).

However, the reproductive cells—the ova and the spermatozoa—contain only one sex chromosome each, sharply differentiating them from all other cells in the body. In the female—since all of her sex chromosomes are X chromosomes—the one sex chromosome in any given reproductive cell (ovum) will necessarily be an X chromosome. In the male, any given reproductive cell (spermatozoon) may on the other hand contain either an X chromosome or a Y chromosome. (The spermatozoa are produced by division of other, nonspecialized cells in the walls of the seminiferous tubules. Any one spermatozoon may thus be formed with either an X or a Y chromosome obtained probably by sheer chance from its parent cell, which contained both an X and a Y chromosome.)

If the ovum—carrying an X chromosome—should happen to be fertilized by a spermatozoon also carrying an X chromosome, the resultant individual will inherit only X chromosomes from both parents and will thus be an XX individual, or *female*. If, on the other hand, the ovum should happen to be fertilized by a spermatozoon carrying a Y chromosome, the resultant individual will inherit an X chromosome from the mother but a Y chromosome from the father, and will thus be an XY individual, or *male*. As can readily be seen, it is the genetic make-up of the father's fertilizing spermatozoon which determines the sex of the offspring.

There is no way of determining or ordaining which one of the several hundred million spermatozoa in an ejaculation will fertilize the ovum. Even if we could miraculously pick out one of these sperm cells from the many millions of other sperm cells around it, declare that this one would be the cell to fertilize the ovum, and then somehow see to it that it did in fact fertilize the conveniently available ovum, it would still be exceedingly difficult to ascertain with certainty whether this one given sperm cell were carrying an X or a Y chromosome. As it is, there is no conceivable way of performing any of these miracles. For better or worse, sex determination must remain in the field of chance.

It was discovered that certain males—notably some of those prone to antisocial or criminal activity—possess an extra Y chromosome in their cells. They are XYY instead of normal XY males. Certainly, not all criminals are thus genetically abnormal; nor are all XYY males necessarily doomed to a life of crime. But it has been estimated that one in 300 men may possess this genetic abnormality, caused by the inexplicable presence of two Y chromosomes in the father's fertilizing spermatozoon. Several studies among prison inmates in the United States and Great Britain revealed an incidence of as high as four percent of this genetic aberration. In addition to aggressive and violent tendencies, the XYY men tended to be tall, to have acne and to be of low intelligence.

It has also been determined that certain women have an analogous genetic abnormality in which their cells contain three X chromosomes instead of the usual two—in other words, they are XXX females. Sometimes, the possession of three X sex chromosomes in women is associated with another abnormal phenomenon known as *mosaicism,* in which the total number of all chromosomes in the cells—normally 46 in each cell—varies markedly in different cells. Thus, while all human beings normally have 46 chromosomes in each and every individual cell of his or her body (of which two are sex chromosomes), the victims of mosaicism may have as few as 45 chromosomes in some cells, or as many as 48 chromosomes in other cells. The extent of mosaicism in the general population has not been determined, but it has been noted that there is a high incidence of mosaicism among schizophrenics. The exact relationship between schizophrenia and mosaicism remains to be determined.

These discoveries opened up new areas of study in the fields of genetics, psychiatry and criminology. *See also* ACCESSORY SEX ORGANS; ADOLESCENCE; BIRTH CONTROL; BIRTH DEFECT; CERVIX; CHROMOSOMES; CLITORIS; CONCEPTION; COWPER'S GLANDS; EJACULATORY SYSTEM; FALLOPIAN TUBES; GENETIC COUNSELING; HORMONES; IMPOTENCE; MENSTRUATION; OVARIES; OVULATION; OVUM; PENIS; PROSTATE; REPRODUCTION; SEMEN; SEXUAL INTERCOURSE; SEXUAL LIFE; SPERM; SPERMATIC CORDS; TESTICLES; UTERUS; VAGINA; VAS DEFERENS; VULVA *and* **medigraphs** ECTOPIC PREGNANCY; MENOPAUSE; STERILITY.

RESCUE BREATHING. *See* RESUSCITATION.

RESECTION, the operation of cutting out and removing a section or complete segment of an organ. *See also* SURGERY.

RESERPINE, the active alkaloid of *Rauwolfia serpentina,* used as a tranquilizer in certain mental diseases, and also classified as an *antihypertensive* drug. Its efficacy was first questioned but is now generally accepted, and reserpine is used in many mental hospitals and also as a standard treatment for high blood pressure. The antihypertensive action develops slowly on oral treatment, but faster when injected. Reserpine is usually administered in conjunction with a diuretic.

Recent studies have shown that the value of reserpine in the treatment of mental disorders is limited but it is useful for reducing blood pressure. The most common side effects are mental depression and nasal congestion, and the drug should not be used if someone has a gastric or duodenal ulcer. *See also* ANTIHYPERTENSIVES; TRANQUILIZERS.

RESPIRATION. *See* BREATHING.

RESPIRATORY DISEASES, those that affect the lungs or other breathing apparatus. They include pneumonia, tuberculosis, influenza, pleurisy, emphysema, lung cancer, lung abscess, bronchitis, bronchiectasis, laryngitis, sore throat, and colds. *See also* BREATHING; COLD, COMMON; LUNGS; NOSE; RESPIRATORY SYSTEM *and* **medigraphs** ADENOMA, BRONCHIAL; ANTHRACOSIS AND ASBESTOSIS; BRONCHIAL ASTHMA; BRONCHIECTASIS; BRONCHITIS; DIPHTHERIA; EMPHYSEMA; HAY FEVER; HISTOPLASMOSIS; LUNG ABSCESS; LUNG CANCER; PLEURISY; PNEUMONIA; SILICOSIS; TUBERCULOSIS.

RESPIRATORY SYSTEM, the body's apparatus for breathing and inhaling oxygen and exhaling carbon dioxide and water vapor. It is composed mainly of the lungs and bronchial tubes, and its movements are activated by the midriff and the muscles between the ribs. By this mechanism, the lungs act like a pair of bellows. The apparatus begins in the nasal passages and is continued down the throat through the *larynx* (voice box). Breathing is automatically controlled by the respiratory center in the *medulla oblongata*—the nerve center in the brain. *See also* BODY; BREATHING; CARBON DIOXIDE; LARYNX; LUNGS; NOSE; OXYGEN; PHARYNX; RESPIRATORY DISEASES; TRACHEA.

REST, repose, cessation of labor and activity for the purpose of recuperating from a disease and for the proper functioning of the body. Rest may be obtained in bed, in an armchair, or simply by diverting one's mind from work to a game or hobby. *See also* HYGIENE; SLEEP.

RESUSCITATION, the revival of unconscious persons suffering from asphyxia or cessation of the heartbeat. Such injuries are commonly produced by drowning, inhalation of carbon monoxide, electric shock, surgical anesthetics, street accidents, or assaults.

Every adult should be taught how to administer first aid and perform artificial respiration, as their immediate application may save life. As a human being can live without air for only four minutes, time is of the essence. Most beaches and swimming pools are manned by lifeguards who can handle drowning and similar accidents efficiently. Policemen and firemen are also taught first aid and should be summoned if needed. Often, an ambulance doctor called in an emergency finds a police officer performing artificial respiration and thereby saving life.

In every case of asphyxia or heart stoppage, two persons are needed. One should perform artificial respiration and other emergency measures immediately; the other should use the telephone and summon outside help. A doctor should be called, but remember that most specialists are not expert in first aid and the victim may be dead before the doctor arrives. The victim should be carried immediately outdoors or to a room where there is plenty of oxygen. As soon as possible, the victim should be taken to the nearest hospital.

The person assigned to call outside help should consult the local telephone directory and dial the emergency numbers (police, ambulance, doctor, operator). The desk service of a hotel or large apartment house should be informed.

In the meantime, artificial respiration is being performed by the immediate first aid helper. That person should continue, even after the victim has stopped breathing, because every person is considered alive until pronounced dead by a doctor. Many a victim who appeared to have died has been revived by the persistent use of artificial respiration.

The standard procedure of artificial respiration is the Holger method, which has been adopted by the American Red Cross and approved by the American Medical Association. This method is lifesaving and should be taught by actual demonstrations to all persons who wish to qualify for first aid.

The Holger Method of Artificial Respiration. The lungs are controlled like a pair of bellows, with alternate expansion and contraction at the rate of 18 per minute to draw in air and then expel it.

The unconscious person is stretched out face downward and turned slightly to one side, with one hand on top of the other, the forehead resting on the hands and the elbows extended outward. The operator kneels on one or both knees in front of the victim's head, places the hands under the subject's arms above the elbows and rocks backward, drawing the victim's arms upward and toward himself. The arms are elevated until firm resistance is met, then replaced on the

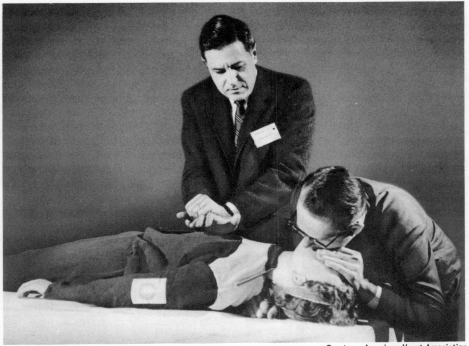

Resuscitation—Using a manikin, physicians demonstrate cardiopulmonary resuscitation (CPR)—a life-saving procedure in cases of cardiac arrest. One doctor uses external heart compression to stimulate blood circulation and heartbeat. The other gives artificial ventilation with mouth-to-mouth breathing. The latter is the most effective method of restoring breathing that an individual can use. The tilted-back position of the head is important when using this technique.

ground or floor. The operator then moves his hands to the victim's back, just below the shoulder blades, and rocks forward, exerting pressure on the back. The operator's arms are kept straight during both the lift and pressure phases, and the complete cycle is repeated up to 18 times per minute.

The hip lift back pressure performance of manual artificial respiration is another resuscitative procedure. This method combines alternate lifting of the hips with pressure on the middle of the back below the shoulder blades. With the victim in a prone position, the operator kneels on one knee near the victim's hip, straddles the person, and places the other foot near the opposite hip. He places his hands un-

der the hips, raises the pelvis vertically upward 4–6 inches, then replaces the hips on the ground and repeats the cycle. Lifting the hips produces active inspiration.

The ancient method of *mouth-to-mouth breathing* has been revived, particularly for newborn infants. The operator places his mouth over the child's mouth and nose, breathing into them at the rate of 20 per minute. If the infant's air passages are blocked, he is suspended by the ankles, bent over on the operator's arm, and given a few sharp pats between the shoulder blades. When the lungs have been inflated with the operator's breath, they are allowed to empty naturally and the procedure is repeated.

There are various physical apparatuses

for producing artificial respiration. In the *respirator,* the body (except for the head) is hermetically enclosed in a cabinet and respiratory movements are produced by introducing alternately pressure and suction. In the *Both respirator,* a wooden cabinet encloses the body (except for the head) with a rubber collar around the victim's neck. A small motor drives a bellows connected with the chamber by a flexible pipe. By means of a valve the bellows acts as a sucker, extracting and letting air in alternately. The *Drinker respirator* is a power-driven breathing apparatus similar in type to the Both respirator, the cabinet being of metal.

Asphyxia sometimes develops on the operating table because of a weak heart or administration of too much anesthetic. Anesthetists are in charge of this situation. They discontinue the anesthetic and administer oxygen. In depression of respiration due to *chloral hydrate* or *phenobarbital,* strong black coffee and amphetamines are useful.

Sometimes stimulants are needed to resuscitate the person from *syncope* (temporary heart failure). Manual compression or thumping of the heart through the second to the fifth spaces between the ribs on the left side of the chest and an injection of *epinephrine* (*Adrenalin*) are the measures usually employed. See also ACCIDENT PREVENTION; ASPHYXIA; DROWNING; FIRST AID.

RETARDATION, delay in physical or mental development. *See also* BIRTH DEFECT; GROWTH RETARDATION; MENTAL RETARDATION.

RETCHING, involuntary straining efforts to vomit, often without results, a common symptom of motion sickness.

RETENTION OF URINE, inability to urinate and accumulation of urine in the bladder, due most often to enlargement of the prostate and compression of the

first part of the urethra, which normally evacuates the urine. *See also* BLADDER DISEASES *and* **medigraphs** PROSTATE GLAND ENLARGEMENT; URINARY TRACT PROBLEMS.

RETINA, the innermost seeing membrane inside the eyeball which receives visual images and transmits them through the optic nerve to the brain and midbrain. The pictures are perceived and registered by the *occipital lobe* (back part) of the opposite side of the brain; sometimes, a reflex without consciousness is transmitted through the midbrain, as in the contraction of the pupils to light or accommodation. *See also* EYE; RETINITIS; RETINITIS PIGMENTOSA; RETINOBLASTOMA.

RETINITIS, inflammation of the *retina* (innermost seeing membrane of the eyeball) due to various causes including drinking wood alcohol, smoking tobacco, receiving excessive sunlight, or affliction with kidney disease, tuberculosis, diabetes, hardening of the arteries, syphillitic general paresis, or tabes dorsalis. *See also* EYE; RETINITIS PIGMENTOSA.

RETINITIS PIGMENTOSA, a hereditary disease of the *retina* (eye camera), usually transmitted by the unaffected mother to the male child and often skipping several generations (*recessive*). Authorities estimate that in the United States, for example, about 100,000 people have this disease.

The first symptoms appear in childhood or adolescence as night blindness and stumbling in the dark. The victims' range of vision is narrowed, so that they cannot see to the sides or above or below the visual object (*telescopic vision*). Eye specialists who examine the retina with an ophthalmoscope find areas of black coloring matter scattered throughout but mostly to the sides. The small retinal arteries and veins are gradually obliterated and replaced by scars. The principal complications are physical injuries due to poor vision.

There is no known effective treatment for retinitis pigmentosa, although vitamin A has proved helpful. The possibilities of research have been encouraging. One of the clues to the cause of this disease is *rhodopsin*—visual purple in the eye, composed of a protein and vitamin A. Human subjects who cannot absorb vitamin A lack rhodopsin and develop symptoms of retinitis pigmentosa. In the United States, the National Retinitis Pigmentosa Foundation has been established to find a cure for retinitis pigmentosa. *See also* EYE; GENETIC COUNSELING; RETINA; RETINITIS.

RETINOBLASTOMA, a malignant tumor of the retina occurring in early infancy, childhood, or at birth. It originates from the embryonic cells of the retina and may spread to distant organs in the same manner as *glioma*—a tumor of the nerve-supporting tissue. The eye and half of the visual field are destroyed by rapid growth of the malignant cells, which may spread to distant organs including the brain and the lungs. Both eyes are affected in about 25 percent of cases, and eventually the eyeballs can become perforated with extension of the malignant growth. There have been remarkable advances in the treatment of retinoblastoma in recent years. The tumor can be destroyed with

cryotherapy and radiation. *See also* CANCER; EYE; GLIOMA; RETINA.

RETIREMENT, withdrawal from one's customary occupation, often at the age of 65, ostensibly to provide vacancies for other employees. Unfortunately, many highly qualified persons with superior skill and experience are replaced by less qualified substitutes. However, private life still provides opportunities for gainful work apart from a full-time job. For many people, retirement leads to idleness, *hypochondriasis* (excessive concern with health) and alcoholism. In the United States, retiring boards for the Army, Navy and Air Force, composed of five or more commissioned officers, examine their personnel for their mental and physical fitness to continue military service or be retired. Social Security benefits and pensions help provide for financial security during retirement. *See also* AGING.

RETROLENTAL FIBROPLASIA, formation of scars behind the lens of the eye, detaching the retina and leading to blindness. The disease is most common in prematurely born babies raised in incubators with too much oxygen. These babies later develop the eye disease when the oxygen intake is reduced to the normal level. The disease can be prevented by avoiding an excessive amount of oxygen provided in incubators for prematurely born infants. *See also* EYE.

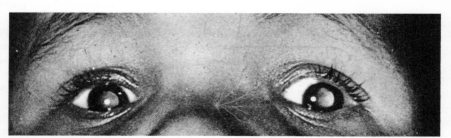

Retrolental Fibroplasia—These are the unseeing eyes of a victim of retrolental fibroplasia. The whitish pupils are caused by growth of an opaque membrane behind the lens of the eyes. As a premature infant, the child was confined to an incubator and given excessive oxygen. Until oxygen poisoning was discovered as the cause, the disease was common in premature babies.

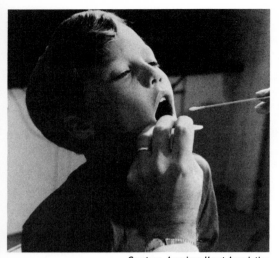

Courtesy, American Heart Association

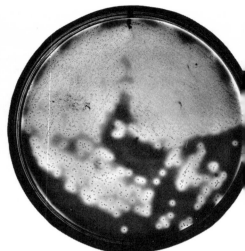

Courtesy, American Heart Association

Rheumatic Fever—A specimen is about to be swabbed from the boy's throat for laboratory testing. Prompt diagnosis and antibiotic treatment of a streptococcal infection is important in the prevention of rheumatic fever.

Rheumatic Fever—A culture of a "strep throat" specimen as seen through a microscope. Rheumatic fever can follow infection by streptococcal bacteria. This inflammatory joint disease may involve and permanently damage the heart.

RHEUMATIC FEVER

R HEUMATIC FEVER IS A BACTERIAL dis-
ease characterized by inflammation, swelling and soreness of the joints. It is always preceded by a strep throat or scarlet fever. In the past, it was called *growing pains* since it was and still is one of the diseases of childhood and adolescence. However, it can also strike young adults in the early twenties and the dangers are the same.

causes
In approximately one out of every hundred cases of throat infection by *Streptococcus* bacteria, the body's defense system against infection goes awry, so that the antibodies generated to fight the bacteria also attack the healthy tissue of the joints, tendons and heart valves. This happens because the bacteria contain substances (antigens) very similar in composition to components in the tissues that are attacked.

symptoms
Following an untreated sore throat or tonsillitis by a few weeks, either of which may have been so mild as to come and go without correct diagnosis, the victim suddenly develops a fever. The joints become inflamed, swollen and sore—not simultaneously, but one after the other. A skin rash appears and then disappears in one or two days. When inflammation of the brain tissue is involved, the patient develops *chorea* (St. Vitus dance) in which the arms and legs move jerkily and spasmodically. Inflammation of heart tissue becomes evident when lumpy nodules appear over the joints.

complications
In addition to the possibility of meningitis, the chief danger of rheumatic fever is its potential destructiveness to heart valve tissue. When the valves become inflamed, the formation of scar tissue is

Rheumatic Fever

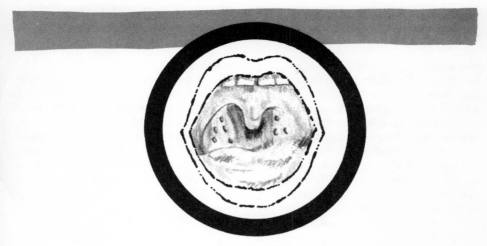

Usually preceded by tonsillitis or sore throat.

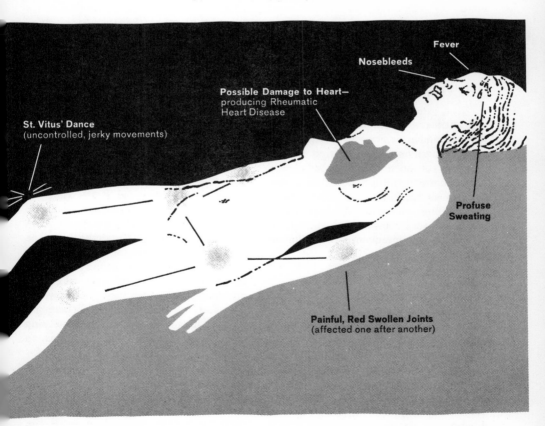

Fever

Nosebleeds

Possible Damage to Heart—
producing Rheumatic
Heart Disease

St. Vitus' Dance
(uncontrolled, jerky movements)

Profuse
Sweating

Painful, Red Swollen Joints
(affected one after another)

inevitable as they heal, leaving the victim with the condition known as rheumatic heart disease.

treatment

In all cases of rheumatic fever, the basic treatment consists of administration of antibiotics over a period long enough to eradicate any remaining streptococcal infection. Depending on the severity of the case and the acuteness of the symptoms, some bed rest may be essential, although the former practice of totally immobilizing the patient for several months is rarely necessary. Aspirin is prescribed to relieve joint inflammation and to control fever; hormones such as cortisone and ACTH may be part of therapy when there are signs of heart involvement. Continued supervision is mandatory, especially in the case of a growing child,

and any sign of recurrence of a strep infection must be called to the doctor's attention at once.

prevention

It is the considered opinion of specialists that if all cases of strep throat or strep tonsillitis were promptly and properly diagnosed by a laboratory test of a swab sample, and treated with antibiotics without delay, there would be no more cases of rheumatic fever. Unfortunately, it is still possible for a strep infection to be mild enough to escape detection and yet to be followed by rheumatic fever. The great advance in preventive medicine in this area has been treatment for this condition before significant damage has been done to the heart. And even such damage can now be repaired thanks to advances in cardiac surgery.

RHEUMATIC HEART DISEASE

R HEUMATIC HEART DISEASE is a condition in which the heart valves have been permanently scarred so that they do not open and close efficiently. More than one and a half million Americans of all ages suffer from this disability which may occur at any age, but most commonly starts between the ages of five and 19 as a consequence of rheumatic fever.

causes

In approximately one percent of all childhood and adolescent cases of streptococcal infections of the throat, tonsils, or ear, rheumatic fever is a complication. This disease causes an inflammation of the heart muscles and valves that leaves the affected tissues scarred, rigid and contracted. About half the adults diagnosed as having chronic rheumatic heart disease are unaware of having had a childhood attack of rheumatic fever.

symptoms

Because the edges of the damaged valves fail to close properly, or because the scarred tissue obstructs normal blood flow, the efficiency of the heart decreases, and in some cases the heart itself becomes enlarged to compensate for the leak. When a doctor listens to a rheumatic heart through a stethoscope, he can hear the characteristic *murmur* of the blood as it passes through the damaged valve. X-rays and other diagnostic procedures also detect the extent to which the heart has been damaged. There are many adults who have been suffering from heart disease with symptoms so mild as to be overlooked in daily life.

complications

It is extremely important for anyone with a *rheumatic heart* to be aware of the disability so that the necessary measures can be taken to ward off a recurrent attack

Rheumatic Heart Disease

Most rheumatic heart disease develops between ages of 5-20

Rheumatic fever predisposes toward development of rheumatic heart disease — but many cases develop without history of rheumatic fever

Palpitations or jumping sensation in chest are sometimes sign of rheumatic heart disease

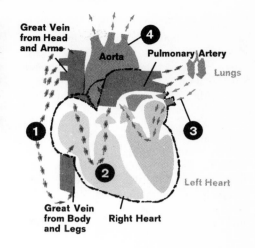

Great Vein from Head and Arms

Aorta

Pulmonary Artery

Lungs

4

1

3

2

Left Heart

Great Vein from Body and Legs

Right Heart

Normal Heart Action

1. Blood from body comes to heart through veins

2. Right heart pumps blood to lungs to get rid of carbon dioxide

3. Blood returns to heart after picking up oxygen supply in lungs

4. Freshened blood pumped out to body through Great Artery (aorta)

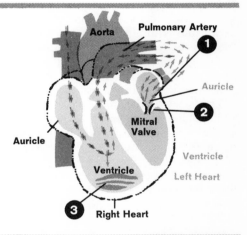

Aorta

Pulmonary Artery

1

Auricle

2

Mitral Valve

Auricle

Ventricle

Ventricle

Left Heart

3

Right Heart

Mitral Valve Affected

1. Scar tissue from Rheumatic Fever obstructs mitral valve or prevents it from closing properly

2. Blood backs up putting increased pressure on left auricle

3. Pressure feeds back through pulmonary veins and arteries to right ventricle. It may eventually become enlarged and fail

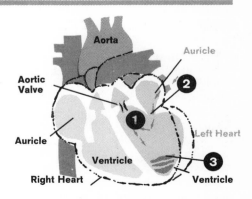

Aorta

Auricle

Aortic Valve

2

1

Auricle

Left Heart

Ventricle

3

Right Heart

Ventricle

Aortic Valve Affected

1. Scar tissue from Rheumatic Fever obstructs aortic valve or prevents it from closing properly

2. Instead of pumping through aorta to rest of body, blood backs up, putting increased strain on left ventricle

3. Left ventricle may eventually become enlarged and fail

of rheumatic fever. If such a recurrence is not immediately treated, it can further damage the heart to the point where heart failure is inevitable. An additional complication is the onset of *bacterial endocarditis* (inflammation of the inner lining of the heart).

treatment

Several new techniques have been developed in recent years for the surgical replacement of the damaged valves characteristic of rheumatic heart disease. The earliest replacement valve and the one still used in many hospitals is a mechanical contrivance made of plastic and metal. More recently, valves taken from human cadavers have been transplanted with considerable success and now successful use is also being made of heart valves taken from pigs. These transplants from pigs, which are in plentiful supply, have so far proved to be superior in every way to all other substitutes.

Treatment of rheumatic heart disease also requires continuing antibiotic therapy as a precaution. This is usually supervised by the victim's private physician. Also, many hospitals have *cardiac clinics* which operate on an outpatient basis for people with rheumatic heart disease, providing them with the necessary medications as a safeguard against the recurrence of rheumatic fever.

prevention

In most cases, rheumatic heart disease can be prevented only by being alert to the damaging effects of rheumatic fever. Since the accurate diagnosis of this disorder—once casually referred to as *growing pains*—involves laboratory tests, parents are advised to consult a doctor promptly about any acute sore throat accompanied by a fever.

RHEUMATISM, a general term commonly used to include various related diseases affecting the joints, muscles, tendons, bones and nerves, causing discomfort and disability. It is not a single disease but a conglomerate expression used for convenience in describing various twinges following exposure to cold, overexertion, and certain indefinite illnesses. The most common symptoms are pain and stiffness in the fingers, loss of manual dexterity, and difficulty in walking. Hot baths are helpful and the most useful drug for temporary relief is aspirin. The severe forms of rheumatism include *rheumatic fever, rheumatoid arthritis, spondylitis, sciatica, lumbago, bursitis, neuritis* and *myositis.*

RHEUMATOID ARTHRITIS

THIS FORM OF CHRONIC and crippling arthritis, which often attacks young adults and can persist into old age, affects the body joints and connective tissue with painful and disabling results. It is approximately three times as prevalent among women as among men and rarely occurs in childhood.

causes

Although no single cause for the disease has yet been isolated, current theory attributes rheumatoid arthritis to a fault in the body's autoimmune system, wherein disease-fighting antibodies are triggered by some circumstance into attacking not only abnormal cells or foreign or toxic invaders, but healthy cells as well, causing them to multiply. Normal human finger joints, for example, are lined with a *synovial membrane* one of whose functions is the secretion of a lubricating fluid. In rheumatoid arthritis, the multiplication of the synovial cells is so rapid

Rheumatoid Arthritis

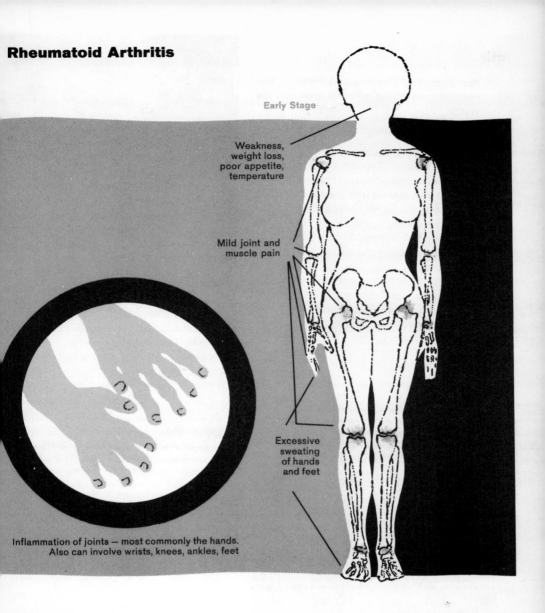

Early Stage

Weakness, weight loss, poor appetite, temperature

Mild joint and muscle pain

Excessive sweating of hands and feet

Inflammation of joints — most commonly the hands. Also can involve wrists, knees, ankles, feet

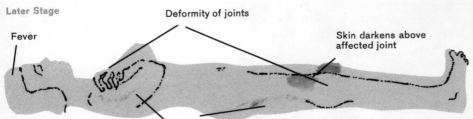

Later Stage

Fever

Deformity of joints

Skin darkens above affected joint

Muscles near inflamed joints develop spastic rigidity.　Fusion of joints, leading to progressive disability.

that unnatural swelling and eventual immobilization of the affected area are the result.

symptoms

Symptoms vary according to the severity of the disease. Typical early signs of rheumatoid arthritis are redness, swelling and soreness of the joints, especially of the fingers, wrists, knees, toes, or ankles. The shoulder, elbow and hip joints may also be affected. If the disease becomes acute, the person may suffer from fatigue, fever and severe immobilizing pain. Stiffness and soreness travel to other joints, and characteristic lumps or visible nodules develop at the sites of the bone prominences, resulting in deformity. In some cases, there may be a sudden remission of symptoms, or the symptoms may come and go for no apparent reason.

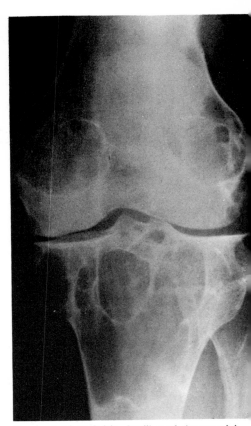

Rheumatoid Arthritis—Swelling of the synovial lining of a joint eventually erodes the cartilage that protects the bone ends from friction. This in turn leads to erosion of the bones. An x-ray film shows the extent of deterioration in a rheumatoid arthritic knee.

Rheumatoid Arthritis—Hands disabled by rheumatoid arthritis can still function with the aid of special equipment. This spoon handle with furrows will be less likely to slip out of distorted and stiffened fingers.

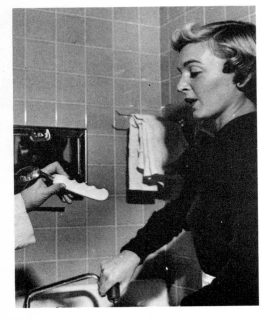

complications

If the rheumatoid disorder spreads to the muscles, or if the immobilization of the area makes muscle activity impossible, atrophy (wasting) of the muscles may lead to permanent disablement. In some cases, heart and lung tissue become scarred. During active phases of the disease, the spleen and lymph glands may swell.

treatment

No specific cure is yet known, but treatment is available to relieve symptoms. Periods of rest are recommended, usually alternated with exercise—such as swimming—designed to maintain muscle

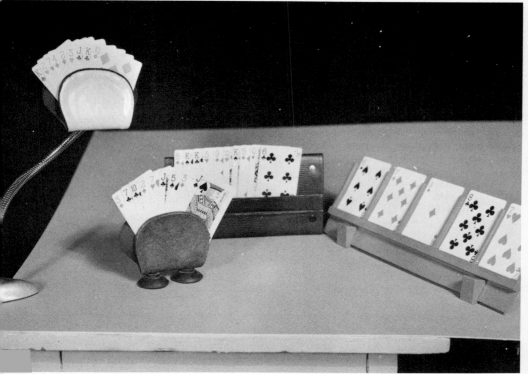

Persons afflicted with arthritis and other crippling diseases can now cope with many everyday activities more easily thanks to numerous self-help devices now available on the market. These inventions have helped to make life easier and more enjoyable for many thousands of people. Several of these implements are shown on these pages. Above, equipment for holding playing cards, especially designed to aid arthritis sufferers. The portable devices eliminate the need to hold or manipulate the cards by hand. Right, this gadget shuffles and dispenses the cards automatically. Arthritics can now play their favorite card games without undue discomfort or embarrassment.

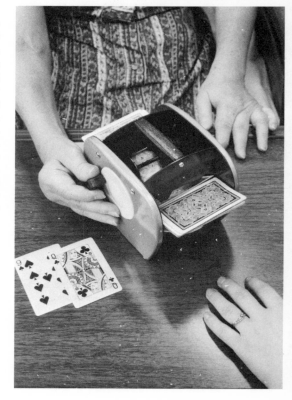

The self-help devices depicted in these photographs are all based on simple principles; but although they may seem obvious to us now, it still took the ingenuity of professional inventors to devise them.

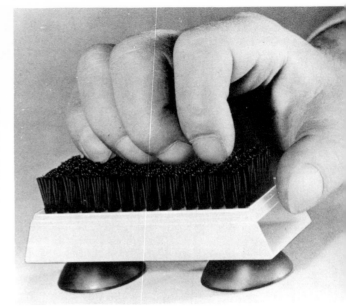

Sufferers from arthritis often have particular difficulty holding things. This vexing problem can now be circumvented by use of the many devices especially designed to assist such people. Above, this nailbrush can be attached at a comfortable height to a wall or sink by suction, eliminating the necessity for holding it by hand. It can be purchased in many department stores.

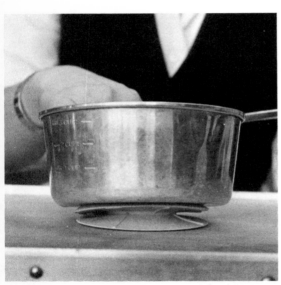

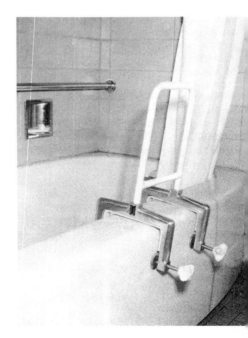

There are many uses for a two-sided rubber suction cup like the one above, which clings both to the counter and to whatever other utensil is being used. It holds pots to be scoured and bowls for mixing, and can be used to steady a dish to facilitate eating. Right, a device to assist a handicapped person in getting in and out of the bathtub. It attaches to the tub by suction. This implement can help to prevent accidents.

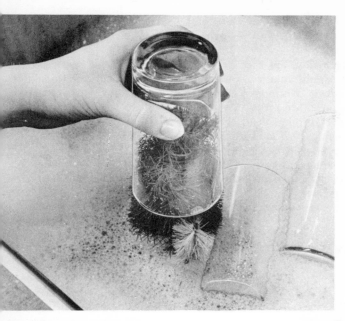

The brush *(above)* attaches to the sink by suction, and facilitates scouring, as with these glasses. Right, this can-opener can be operated with one hand and does not need to be held with the other as it is attached to the table surface by suction. Below, a device for removing the lids from sealed jars. Only one hand is needed to hold the jar.

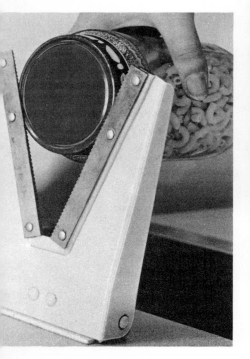

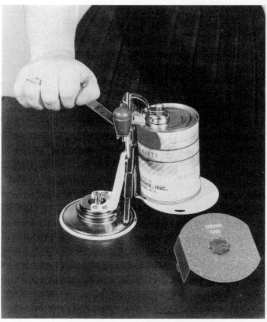

Self-help devices, such as those shown here, have proved a boon to the physically handicapped, freeing them from dependence on others for everyday routine chores, and promoting their psychological well-being.

function. Pain and inflammation are relieved by large doses of aspirin adjusted to avoid negative side effects. Hormone and cortisone injections are other forms of treatment. Medical supervision of diet and general health are also part of long-term therapy. Recent use of gold in the form of gold salts in solution given by injection appears to arrest bone and cartilage destruction in some cases.

R ESEARCH EPORT *follows* LUPUS ERYTHEMATOSUS.

R ESEARCH EPORT

○ **RHEUMATOID ARTHRITICS RESPOND WELL TO NEW COMBINATION THERAPY**

Rheumatoid arthritis patients are responding favorably to a new treatment that combines low-dose *cyclophosphamide* with *prednisone,* according to studies at the UNIVERSITY OF COLORADO sponsored by the NATIONAL INSTITUTE OF ARTHRITIS, METABOLISM AND DIGESTIVE DISEASES.

When cyclophosphamide alone was orally administered in high doses to a group of patients over a six-month period, inflammation of the joints progressively decreased and joint function improved, but the clinical improvement was accompanied by frequent toxic reactions.

In contrast, the group of patients treated with low-dose cyclophosphamide plus prednisone showed similar clinical improvement with fewer adverse side effects.

Continuing studies are attempting to determine whether long-term therapy with the new combination of drugs will produce undesirable side effects.   NIH925

RH FACTOR. *See* BLOOD TYPES.

RHINITIS, *head cold, coryza,* inflammation of the mucous membrane of the nose due to one of several specific viruses. It is one of the most common of all illnesses, with peaks of incidence in October and December. The prevalence of common colds is approximately 15 percent of persons per week during the winter months.

It accounts for half of all absences from work and a quarter of the total time lost. The disease is spread by personal contact with a cold sufferer or a healthy carrier or by the use of contaminated handkerchiefs, towels, spoons or glasses.

The symptoms are nasal congestion, dripping from the nose, headache, low fever and sneezing. The infection may spread downward to cause minor sore throat and through the Eustachian tubes to the middle ear to cause earache. Blowing the nose violently should be avoided, as it forces the discharge into the Eustachian tube leading to the middle ear.

The value of vaccines has not been established and no antibiotic is of value. Only when pneumonia complicates the cold is an antibiotic used. Nose drops are used to relieve nasal congestion, and gargles with antiseptic solutions are used to soothe the irritated throat. Aspirin may be taken to relieve headache or associated muscular pains. Usually, it is better to stay in bed for at least one day than to go about one's business.

Atrophic rhinitis (ozena) is a gradual destruction of the mucous membrane of the nose, with an offensive odor, fetid discharge, and formation of large foul-smelling crusts. The treatment includes frequent syringing of the nasal passages with alkaline and antiseptic solutions. *See also* COLD, COMMON; NOSE; OZENA.

RHINOLITHS, nasal stones or concretions formed from dried discharges. *See also* NOSE.

RHINOPHYMA, a large swelling of the nose with lumps due to acne and overactivity of the sebaceous glands, also called *toper's nose* or *whiskey nose.* The condition is disfiguring. The huge nose can be reconstructed by plastic surgery. *See also* NOSE.

RHINOPLASTY, plastic surgery on an oversized or deformed nose, commonly resorted to for cosmetic improvement. *See also* NOSE; PLASTIC SURGERY.

RHUBARB, a mild laxative drug which was formerly official for the treatment of occasional constipation. It consists of the dried root of the rhubarb plant. A mixture of rhubarb and soda is an old home remedy for irregularity of the bowels.

RHYTHM METHOD, a method of birth control which avoids the use of artificial contraceptives and depends upon abstention from sexual intercourse during the woman's fertile period. In women who menstruate regularly, ovulation—the fertile period—ordinarily occurs 12–16 days from the onset of the previous menstruation. Intercourse before or after this cycle cannot result in pregnancy. To insure success in this method, the woman must keep a record of her periods for 6–12 months, as variations may occur. The unfertilized ovum survives for only 24 hours after ovulation; therefore if intercourse is not performed during the fertile period, pregnancy cannot occur. As the temperature rises slightly during ovulation, the woman employing the rhythm method should also take her temperature every morning upon arising to determine her fertile period. Due to the burdensome details of the method and to variations in the menstrual cycle, the rhythm method often fails to avoid pregnancy. *See also* BIRTH CONTROL.

RIB CAGE, *thorax,* the bony case formed by the 24 ribs, the breastbone, and the 12 thoracic vertebrae. It lodges the heart, lungs, mediastinum, bronchial tubes, pleural cavity, the large blood vessels which flow to and from the heart, and the thoracic lymph glands. *See also* INTERCOSTAL.

RIBOFLAVIN, vitamin B_2. The foods rich in riboflavin include liver, egg white, milk, cheese, beef muscle, enriched cereals and greens.

The principal symptom of riboflavin deficiency is *cheilosis,* with pallor of the mucous membrane at the angles of the lips and softening and breaking down with cracks and fissures at the junction of the lips with the mouth, also soreness of the tip and margin of the tongue, greasiness and scaliness of the face, and cloudiness and inflammation of the cornea of the eye. *See also* CHEILOSIS; DEFICIENCY DISEASES; NUTRITION; VITAMINS.

RIBONUCLEIC ACID. *See* RNA.

RICKETS

RICKETS IS A DEFICIENCY DISEASE that affects the bones of infants and children. The name of the disease evolved from the Greek word for "spine."

causes
The cause of rickets is a lack of vitamin D in the diet, which in turn affects calcium and phosphorus metabolism. Since the action of sunlight on the skin produces vitamin D in the body, the absence of sunshine is a contributing cause of the disease. The children of the 19th century English industrial slums whose diet was poor and who were deprived of sunshine by smoke and fog (now known as smog) were especially vulnerable to rickets. Adults suffering from a vitamin D deficiency because of a metabolic defect or for other reasons develop a condition known as *osteomalacia* (softening of the bones).

symptoms
Rickets becomes apparent between six months and a year because the baby's growth is slower than normal and the bones are soft and bent where they

Rickets

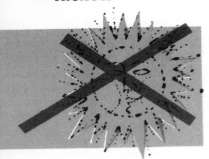

Develops in infants due to lack of Vitamin D

Sunlight prime source of Vitamin D, Mother's milk, egg yolk and cod liver oil can also supply infant's needs

Develops in Infants Between 3rd-18th Months

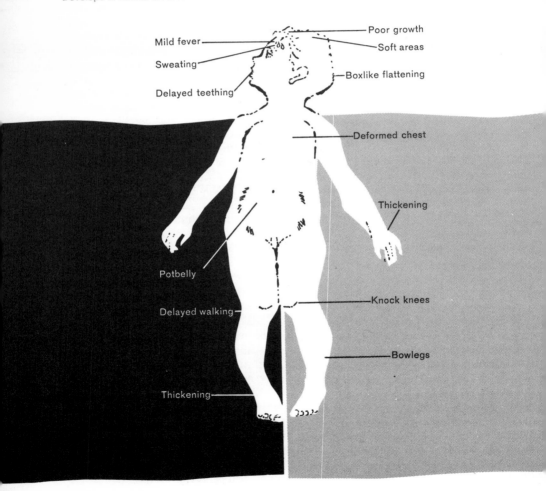

Mild fever

Sweating

Delayed teething

Poor growth

Soft areas

Boxlike flattening

Deformed chest

Thickening

Potbelly

Delayed walking

Knock knees

Bowlegs

Thickening

should be straight. Continuing decalcification produces such abnormalities as a misshapen skull and bandy legs that can scarcely support the body. The abdomen protrudes and diarrhea is chronic.

complications

If vitamin therapy is not undertaken at an early stage of the disease, the bones are permanently deformed and curvature of the spine is inevitable. Malformations of the permanent teeth occur before their eruption. Anemia is a likely complication and low resistance to infection is typical.

treatment

Rickets is now extremely rare in the United States thanks to the widespread use of milk fortified with vitamin D and the alertness of doctors and health station personnel to signs of deficiency diseases. Cod liver oil—at one time the preferred treatment for an active case of rickets—has been replaced by vitamin D in concentrated form. Where effectiveness of this therapy is limited by an inherited fault in calcium and phosphorus metabolism, the child is given massive doses of the vitamin and dietary supplements of calcium.

prevention

Rickets is now routinely prevented by the inclusion in the diet of milk enriched with "the sunshine vitamin." Vitamin D is also present in limited amounts in fish —especially cod, tuna, salmon and herring—and in eggs. Exposure to sunlight is another preventive measure, but overexposure, especially of an infant at the beach, should be strictly avoided.

RICKETTSIAL DISEASES, those caused by one of the rickettsial organisms, which are intermediate in size between the larger bacteria and the smaller viruses. Some rickettsiae are not visible under the ordinary microscope. Under the ultramicroscope, the rickettsiae have many different shapes but most of them resemble tiny rods. The rickettsiae are transmitted from the infected person to others by an intermediate host such as blood-sucking ticks, mites, lice, fleas and spiders.

The diseases caused by rickettsiae include *typhus fever, murine typhus, Rocky Mountain spotted fever, scrub typhus, Brill's disease, Q fever, trench fever, rickettsialpox,* and various epidemic diseases in the Mediterranean region and Australia. In general, the rickettsiae have four common features: they assume various different shapes; they multiply only within certain cells of susceptible animals; they occur in various parasites in nature; and they cause acute self-limited fevers in people, usually with a skin rash.

Usually the spread of rickettsial diseases can be prevented by mass delousing, the use of safe insecticides in areas where the infections are prevalent, and administration of protective vaccines to vast numbers of people. Certain antibiotics are also used. *See also* GERMS; INFECTION; INFECTIOUS DISEASES; PARASITES; Q FEVER; RICKETTSIALPOX; SCRUB TYPHUS; TRENCH FEVER; TYPHUS *and* **medigraph** ROCKY MOUNTAIN SPOTTED FEVER.

RICKETTSIALPOX, a disease that can afflict people living in impoverished areas. The infection is transmitted by small colorless mites infesting house mice and other small rodents. It affects adults as well as children.

About a week or two after the infective bite, a firm reddish blister appears at its site. This dries and forms a scab that drops off and leaves a small black ulcer. A skin rash resembling that of chickenpox appears elsewhere on the body, sometimes involving the mucous membrane of the mouth and disappearing in about a week. The systemic symptoms are fever, chills, sweats, headaches, muscular pains, and loss of appetite, lasting about a week.

The sanitary measure needed to eliminate rickettsialpox in poverty pockets is eradication of house mice by sanitation and fumigation. Protective vaccine may be used as may certain antibiotics. Aspirin is useful for relief of headache and muscular pains. *See also* RICKETTSIAL DISEASES.

RIGOR MORTIS, stiffness and rigidity of the muscles after death. It begins several hours after breathing stops as a result of the coagulation of the muscle protein. It is one of the signs observed by medical examiners in determining the approximate hour of the victim's death.

RINGING IN THE EARS, *tinnitus,* a sound which is perceived by the person who is troubled by it, but which does not originate outside his own body. Language may be inadequate to permit the person to describe it properly to the doctor, but the sounds have been verbally characterized as buzzing, ringing, hissing, blowing or roaring in the ears. These sounds must be differentiated from other sounds that people hear and that do not have any determinable source. Such sounds are auditory hallucinations that may include the sound of voices, music, bells ringing, or whatever the imagination may conjure and are symptoms associated with drug addiction, alcoholism, or psychiatric disturbances.

Most tinnitus is an annoyance difficult to diagnose and impossible to treat. Apparently some people have ringing in the ears because of the changes in the internal ear associated with *otosclerosis.* Even 25 percent of these people fail to improve after the operation for mobilization of the stapes (innermost of the three small bones of the middle ear). Some cases are associated with such serious conditions as damage to the tissues involved in hearing, changes in the blood supply, tumors which may occur in the middle ear, infections and inflammation

of the labyrinth, and sometimes toxic effects of drugs. If there are serious disturbances of the central nervous system —such as tumors, venereal infections, epilepsy, migraine or concussion—the approach to control of the underlying symptom of tinnitus is control of the underlying condition. In a few instances, tinnitus may be associated with hardened wax in the ear, inflammation of the external ear, or perforation of the tympanic membrane (eardrum). These conditions can be found on examination. Assuming, however, that no such physical changes can be detected, the physician will try to determine whether or not the ringing in the ears is constant or intermittent; whether the hissing or blowing sounds are associated with breathing or with a patent Eustachian tube. As with other symptoms, some victims find the ringing in the ears much more serious than do others—some even learn quickly to disregard the symptom. The otologist may make many specialized tests which go beyond the practice of the family physician. In some cases the patient may benefit from being told that the noise will be louder when he is nervous, tense or fatigued; or contrariwise when the environment is exceedingly quiet—as when he tries to go to sleep at night. Some of these people benefit by the prescription of mild tranquilizing drugs. The ringing in the ears may sometimes be masked or blocked by other sound—such as the music from a radio. Modern radios may be turned off by a timer at an established time.

In the course of the years, surgical operations have been suggested and tried in difficult cases ranging from cutting of the nerves to total removal of the labyrinth (inner ear) with which comes total hearing loss. However, in half of these cases, even such surgical procedures did not eliminate the tinnitus. Experimental use of ultrasound irradiation of the oval or round window areas has resulted in

80–90 percent improvement in tinnitus. *See also* ACOUSTIC NERVE; DEAFNESS; EAR; OTOSCLEROSIS *and* **medigraphs** BELL'S PALSY; BRAIN TUMORS; MÉNIÈRE'S DISEASE.

RINGWORM, the popular name for some fungus infections of the skin (*tinea corporis*). It is caused by parasites which invade various areas of the body, particularly in folds such as the crotch and armpit. The infection sometimes takes on a circular shape and the center seems to heal as it spreads outward. The area is sore and itchy.

Ringworm is highly contagious and can be spread from person to person and article to person. Animals can also spread the infection. Antifungal drugs are effective in treating the disease.

The best prevention of ringworm is cleanliness. Every day the entire body should be washed with soap and water, and dried thoroughly. Drying is very important since the fungi thrive where moisture is present. *See also* **medigraph** FUNGUS INFECTIONS OF THE SKIN.

RINNE TEST, a hearing test which compares the duration of bone conduction of sound with that of air conduction by use of measured tuning fork vibrations. Normally, air conduction lasts longer than bone conduction. Reversal of this relationship indicates a disease of the sound-conducting apparatus of the ear. *See also* DEAFNESS; EAR.

RIO GRANDE FEVER. *See* UNDULANT FEVER.

RNA, *ribonucleic acid,* an essential substance contained in all living matter. It is one of the components of the cytoplasm of cells, and in one of its chemical forms, it carries genetic information from the *DNA* (*deoxyribonucleic acid*) within the cell nucleus to the ribosomes where amino acids are synthesized into proteins. The stringing together of amino acids into proteins is the key step in the transmission of hereditary characteristics from one generation to another. *See also* DNA; GENETIC COUNSELING.

ROCKY MOUNTAIN SPOTTED FEVER

ROCKY MOUNTAIN SPOTTED FEVER is one group of diseases (including typhus fever, Q fever, and rickettsialpox) caused by microorganisms of the Rickettsia family and named after their discoverer, the American scientist Howard Ricketts. Rocky Mountain spotted fever is the most widespread of the rickettsial infections. It is also known as *tick fever, Eastern spotted fever* and *Cape Cod spotted fever.*

causes
Wild animals such as squirrels and chipmunks, as well as pet dogs, may carry the infectious organisms without themselves suffering any symptoms. Wood ticks feeding on the blood of the infected hosts pick up the vector (carrier) by which the disease is transmitted to humans. Rocky Mountain spotted fever cannot be transmitted from animal to animal, nor from animal to human, nor from human to human. It is transmitted through the bite of an infected tick or through its eggs.

symptoms
Major symptoms may become apparent at any time from one day to one week after a tick bite has occurred. Joint and muscle pains, chills and fever, nausea and vomiting, cramps, sensitivity to light, and sore throat may occur within a day of each other in any combination. In some cases, fever is high enough to cause delirium. The unique characteristic of Rocky Mountain spotted fever is the rash

Rocky Mountain Spotted Fever

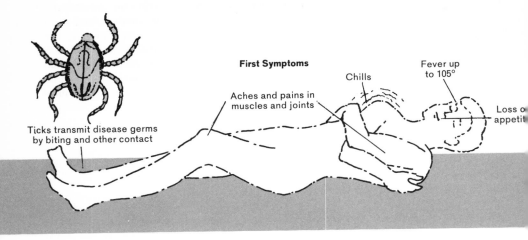

Ticks transmit disease germs
by biting and other contact

First Symptoms

Chills

Aches and pains in
muscles and joints

Fever up
to 105°

Loss of
appetite

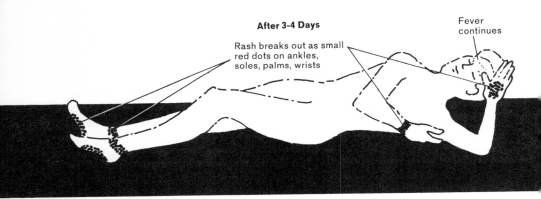

After 3-4 Days

Rash breaks out as small
red dots on ankles,
soles, palms, wrists

Fever
continues

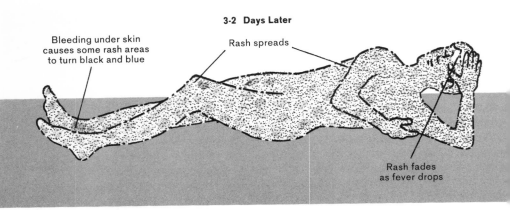

3-2 Days Later

Bleeding under skin
causes some rash areas
to turn black and blue

Rash spreads

Rash fades
as fever drops

that starts on the ankles and wrists, then spreads to the legs and torso, and sometimes involves the face.

complications
If not treated promptly, the disease can have fatal effects. Before antibiotics, it led to heart and kidney disablement as well as to bacterial infection—usually in the form of pneumonia.

treatment
Prompt administration of a combination of medicines that includes antibiotics usually effects a complete cure without any adverse aftereffects. Some mild cases may be self-limiting in about two weeks without any treatment.

prevention
People who live in areas where the disease is endemic usually concentrate on eliminating the ticks rather than in reducing their chance of infection by temporary immunization. This is especially the case since antibiotics afford completely effective treatment. Those who must frequent wooded areas or go through tall grass, or who are on hiking or camping trips are advised to wear protective clothing and to use suitable insect-repellent preparations. Summer vacationers in rural or beach areas should be alert to the warnings of public health authorities about tick infestation and should post such warnings where children and weekend guests can see them. Household pets should not be permitted to run loose in the country and should be inspected and treated regularly for ticks.

If a tick is visible under the skin of a person or a pet, it can be removed in the following way: a drop of alcohol or the application of a newly extinguished matchhead to the tick will cause its jaws to loosen their hold on the skin. It can then be removed with a pair of tweezers. Great care should be exercised in doing this, since crushing the tick while it is partially under the skin can also transfer the infection. Another method is to cover the tick with a "glob" of petroleum jelly; wait about 20 minutes (the tick will suffocate); then carefully remove the insect.

RORSCHACH TEST, a psychological test in which the person is shown a series of ten standard ink blots and immediately interprets them in terms of his own thinking. The responses disclose personality patterns, special interests, general intelligence, abnormal desires, and neurotic or psychotic tendencies.

ROSACEA, a skin condition resembling acne but including among its symptoms redness about the nose which may spread to the forehead and neck. Small dilated (expanded) blood vessels then appear and tiny pimples develop on the flushed areas. These pimples are more superficial than acne pimples and do not leave scars. The condition is sometimes called "whiskey nose," an unfair name because many people have rosacea who have never had

Rosacea—In this chronic disorder, facial skin is reddened by dilated blood vessels, with pimples in the flushed areas. It can also affect the eyelids and lead to superficial keratitis, a painful inflammation of the cornea which should be treated by an ophthalmologist.

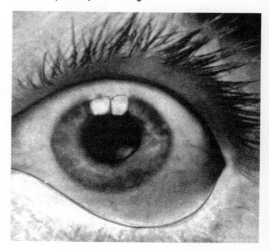

an alcoholic drink. The rush of blood to the affected area is a nervous reflex, stimulated often by alcohol and also by highly spiced foods. Washing the face with soap and cold water, or rubbing with ice, may reduce the flushed appearance of the skin. The most common medical treatment is through control of diet, including the elimination of alcohol, coffee, tea, nuts, eggs, extremely hot or cold foods, and highly seasoned and fried foods. The face should *not* be massaged. Rubbing irritates the inflamed skin and can spread infection. *See also* FACE.

ROSEOLA, a term applied to any rose-colored rash.

ROSEOLA INFANTUM, *exanthem subitum,* an acute disease of infants with high fever and a rash like that of measles after the fever falls. The disease, which strikes most often in the spring and fall, is believed to be communicable.

The onset of a 103–105°F. (39.4–40.5°C.) fever is sudden. It lasts for 3–4 days. Then the rash appears, mostly on the chest and stomach, and the temperature returns to normal.

The disease most often strikes children 1–3 years old. Aspirin and lukewarm water or alcohol sponge baths help keep the temperature below 103°F.

ROUGHAGE. *See* DIET, ROUGHAGE IN.

ROUNDWORM

A MONG THE WORMS RESPONSIBLE for parasitic intestinal infections are the *roundworms,* a general category that includes *hookworms, threadworms* and *pinworms.* However, the term "roundworm" is generally used for the giant intestinal roundworm scientifically known as *ascaris lumbricoides.* This infestation is more common in moist and warm climates than in cold and dry ones, and is endemic in parts of the world where public sanitation is primitive.

causes
Ascaris is the largest roundworm that infects humans. It resembles the earthworm and it is most often transmitted in contaminated human feces used as fertilizer. The eggs in the feces turn into larvae in the soil, and the larvae are carried into the digestive system when people eat the unwashed and uncooked produce containing them. The larvae travel from the intestines into the bloodstream, enter the lungs and the esophagus and finally return to the intestines where they reach maturity, achieving a length from 5–15

inches. The eggs are then excreted in the stool and the cycle is repeated.

symptoms
Sharp stomach pains and diarrhea are common. Children sometimes vomit the worms as they pass through the esophagus. Giant hives may erupt and the face may swell. Loss of appetite and conspicuous weight loss are other symptoms. In some cases, "wandering worms" may come through the skin near the groin or navel.

complications
If untreated, children may suffer from a loss of nutrients with signs of deficiency disease. The worms may also cause intestinal or pancreatic blockage, or they may obstruct the bronchial passages or the lungs, thus making the victim vulnerable to pneumonia. A severe infestation can be fatal to an infant.

treatment
Diagnosis is based on microscopic examination of a stool sample for the pres-

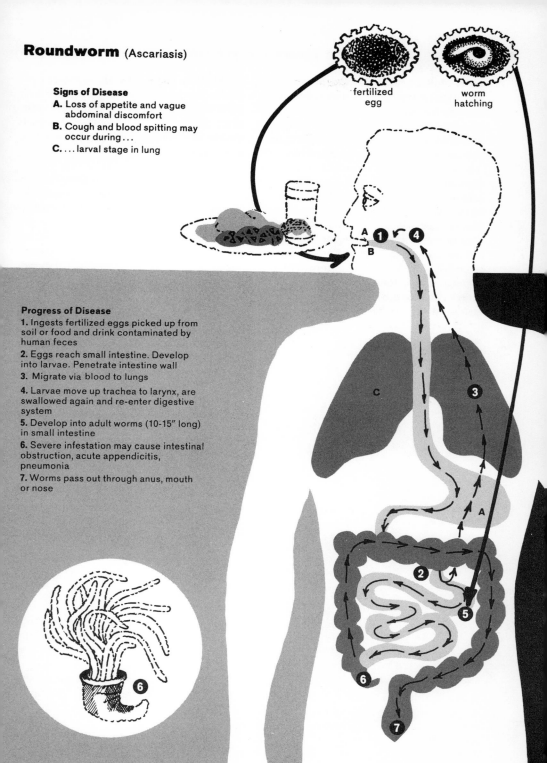

Roundworm (Ascariasis)

fertilized egg

worm hatching

Signs of Disease
A. Loss of appetite and vague abdominal discomfort
B. Cough and blood spitting may occur during...
C. ...larval stage in lung

Progress of Disease
1. Ingests fertilized eggs picked up from soil or food and drink contaminated by human feces
2. Eggs reach small intestine. Develop into larvae. Penetrate intestine wall
3. Migrate via blood to lungs
4. Larvae move up trachea to larynx, are swallowed again and re-enter digestive system
5. Develop into adult worms (10-15" long) in small intestine
6. Severe infestation may cause intestinal obstruction, acute appendicitis, pneumonia
7. Worms pass out through anus, mouth or nose

ence of the eggs. Treatment involves
medications that destroy the worms and
the eggs so that all vestiges of infection
are eliminated from the various parts of
the body. The destruction of the parasites is practically always complete.

prevention
Infection by roundworms can be prevented only by public health measures
that outlaw the use of human feces as
fertilizer and that educate the local population in self-protective habits of personal hygiene. Where these measures are
impossible to achieve, all foods should be
thoroughly cooked before they are eaten
and handwashing before meals should be
established as a ritual.

RUBELLA. *See* GERMAN MEASLES.

RUBEOLA. *See* MEASLES.

RUPTURE, a forcible tearing of a part
of the body, as for example rupture of
the uterus or a hernia. *See also* HERNIA;
RUPTURED DISC.

RUPTURED DISC, a forcible tearing or
breaking of one of the circular plates of
cartilage located between the adjacent
surfaces of the spinal vertebrae. A *herniated disc* is one that has been displaced
and protrudes through the surrounding
cartilage and fibrous tissue. A ruptured
disc causes severe backache and must be
repaired surgically. Other treatments are
under study. *See also* BACKACHE; LAMI-
NECTOMY; SPINAL INJURIES; SPINE *and*
medigraphs SLIPPED DISC; WHIPLASH IN-
JURY OF THE NECK.

S

SABIN VACCINE, a live vaccine taken by mouth for immunization against *poliomyelitis*. It is composed of three representative strains of weakened virus. A series of three adequately spaced doses of the vaccine produces an immune response in over 90 percent of the people who take it. It is recommended for infants and children and has been administered to millions of people. Experience indicates that widespread use of this vaccine —especially for children of preschool age—may come close to eradicating poliomyelitis. Vaccines are also available for each of the three virus types, and the trivalent vaccine combines them all. *See also* IMMUNIZATION *and* **medigraph** POLIOMYELITIS.

SACCHARIN, an artificial sweetener, 10 milligrams of which is equivalent in sweetening power to one teaspoonful of sugar. Saccharin is used as a substitute for sugar by diabetics, the obese and dieters, and also as a pharmaceutical aid to sweeten liquid medicines. *See also* ARTIFICIAL SWEETENERS.

SACROILIAC, the joint at the lower part of the spine connecting the *sacrum* (triangular-shaped bone at the base of the spine) with the *ilium* (expanded wing-shaped portion of the hip bone) which are bound and held together by ligaments. Looseness of this joint and *sacro-*

Sacrum and Sacroiliac

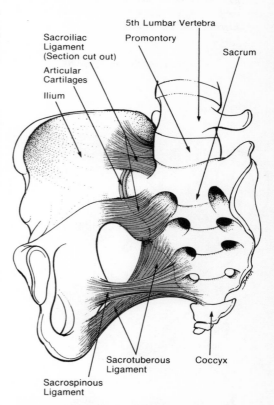

Sacrum and Sacroiliac—At the base of the spine and just above the coccyx, five fused vertebrae form the sacrum. The bone is wedged into the open section of the flaring upper hip bone (ilium). They are connected on each side of the spine by the sacroiliac.

iliac arthritis are common causes of low backache and sciatica. *See also* LOW BACK PAIN; VERTEBRA.

SACRUM, a large triangular bone in the lower part of the vertebral column and at the upper part of the pelvic cavity, where it is inserted like a wedge between the two hip bones. It is connected above with the fifth *lumbar vertebra* and below with the *coccyx*. The sacrum is formed by the five fused *sacral vertebrae*. (It was named as the "sacred bone" because the ancients believed it to be the seat of the soul.) Inflammation of the sacrum and sacroiliac joint are among the common causes of low backache and sciatica. *See also* SPINE; VERTEBRA.

The Salivary Glands

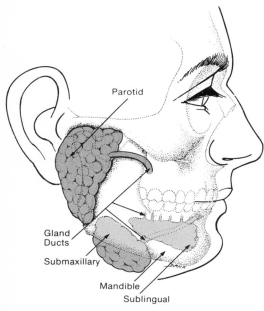

Salivary Glands—A drawing indicates the areas where the three major salivary glands supply saliva to the mouth. Saliva moistens food being chewed and starts to break it down as the beginning of digestion. The large parotid glands in front of the ears are those that become inflamed and swollen in mumps.

SADISM, a sexual perversion in which gratification is obtained by torturing others. It is named after the Marquis de Sade (1740–1814), a French nobleman who wrote two pornographic novels on the subject, spent much of his life in various prisons, and died in an insane asylum.

In addition to practicing sadism, many people suffer from fantastic sadistic concepts. Some women before marriage expect to be badly torn by the husband's penis. Freud remarked that to a certain extent surgery is a sublimated form of sadism serving a useful purpose. *See also* SEXUAL ABNORMALITIES.

ST. ANTHONY'S FIRE. *See* ERYSIPELAS.

ST. LOUIS ENCEPHALITIS. *See* ENCEPHALITIS.

ST. VITUS DANCE. *See* CHOREA.

SALICYLIC ACID, a chemical remover of corns and thickened skin tissue.

SALIVARY GLANDS, the three pairs of glands in the mouth region which secrete saliva: the *parotid glands*—the largest, lying below and in front of the ear; the *submaxillary glands*—the size of a walnut, situated mostly under the lower jawbone; and the *sublingual glands*—the smallest of the group, located in the floor of the mouth under the tongue.

Saliva contains the enzyme *ptyalin* to digest starch in the masticated (chewed) food. The saliva mixes with the food mass in the mouth to moisten and soften it, start the process of digestion, and prepare it to be swallowed. *See also* DIGESTION; GLANDS.

SALK VACCINE. *See* IMMUNIZATION.

SALMONELLA, a large group of rod-shaped germs that are capable of movement. They invade the intestinal tract and they include among others the *typhoid* and *paratyphoid* germs and those that contaminate food by insanitary handling. Foods so poisoned are seized by governmental authorities as being unfit for human consumption. Antibiotics are recommended to combat Salmonella infections. *See also* BACTERIA.

SALPINGITIS, inflammation and infection of the Fallopian tubes, which extend from the ovaries to the horn of the uterus. It is due to *gonorrhea* in 70 percent of cases, and often causes pelvic pain and sterility. Since fever and lower abdominal pain are signs of acute salpingitis, it must be distinguished from appendicitis or tubal pregnancy so that antibiotic treatment is not delayed. *See also* FALLOPIAN TUBES.

SALT, *sodium chloride,* commonly used to season foods. An average of one-half ounce (14.175 grams) of salt is consumed daily, either naturally present in foods or added for taste. Salt may be iodized for consumption in regions where the iodine content of water and foods is deficient.

Normal salt solution, like blood plasma, may be injected as a replacement in cases where the body fluids are lost. Salt is needed by the body to balance the mineral content of the blood plasma, to provide a source for the gastric digestive juice, and as a supply for the bones. Salt retention and elimination are regulated by the *cortex* of the *adrenal glands.*

In extreme heat and after profuse perspiration, the body loses sodium chloride. The resulting symptoms are cramps, weakness and nausea, which are relieved by adding a small amount of salt to the drinking water or taking salt tablets.

An excess of salt in the diet may cause *edema,* increased weight and high blood pressure. For these disorders, doctors order a salt-free diet and also a list of foods which are naturally low in salt.

Chemically, a salt is a combination of an acid with a base; it is a *cation* (electropositive element) combined with an *anion* (electronegative element). Many drugs are administered in the forms of their salts.

A strong salt solution is a good emetic to produce vomiting after swallowing a poison, and a weak salt solution is an old household remedy to strengthen the gums.

SANDFLY FEVER, a viral disease resembling *dengue,* characterized by fever, headache, pains in the eyes, and weakness, followed by complete recovery. It is transmitted by the night bite of the bloodsucking sandfly and occurs most frequently in the Mediterranean area. The onset is sudden, with fever which usually subsides in 2–4 days. Insecticides are recommended to combat the fly, and an insect repellent should be applied after sundown. Neither vaccines nor antibiotics are effective against the fever. *See also* FLIES; KALA-AZAR.

SANITARY NAPKINS. *See* FEMININE HYGIENE.

SAN JOAQUIN FEVER. *See* COCCIDI-OIDOMYCOSIS.

SARCOID, resembling flesh. When the term is applied to skin diseases, it refers to a growth resembling *sarcoma. Sarcoidosis* is a granular growth found in the lung which tends to heal spontaneously. *See also* BOECK'S SARCOID.

SARCOMA, a malignant tumor. It involves bone, cartilage, fibrous and connective tissue, but not the skin, mucous membrane or epithelial tissue. The various forms are named *osteosarcoma, chondrosarcoma, fibrosarcoma,* and *liposarcoma.* The growth invades adjacent tissues and spreads rapidly to distant organs via the bloodstream (metastasis).

Osteosarcoma
(Shown in Spinal Column cross-section)

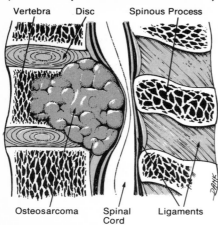

Vertebra   Disc   Spinous Process

Osteosarcoma   Spinal   Ligaments
Cord

Sarcoma—When this malignancy affects bone, it is called osteosarcoma. Occurring on a vertebra, the growth presses against the spinal cord, as shown here. This affects the central nervous system, causing sensory and motor disorders.

The diagnosis is made by a biopsy (microscopic examination of a specimen). *See also* CANCER; TUMOR.

SATYRIASIS, a sexual disorder in men characterized by insatiable sexual desire. The desire may be controlled temporarily by use of bromides, barbiturates, or tranquilizers. A similar condition in women is called *nymphomania. See also* NYMPHOMANIA; SEXUAL ABNORMALITIES.

SCAB, a dried crust over a sore, wound, ulcer or pustule formed by the drying up of the discharge.

SCABIES. *See* LICE AND SCABIES.

SCANNING, a technique by which organs and tissues of the body are rendered visible by various methods for observation and analysis, including use of radioactive isotopes, the Polaroid camera and other special devices. *See also* NUCLEAR MEDICINE.

R<small>ESEARCH REPORT</small> *follows* CONGENITAL HEART DISEASE; HEART ATTACK; NUCLEAR MEDICINE.

SCARLATINA. *See* SCARLET FEVER.

SCARLET FEVER

S<small>CARLET FEVER WAS ONCE</small> one of the dreaded contagious diseases of childhood and is still capable of doing irreparable damage if not properly treated. Thanks to antibiotics, it is now rare.

causes
Scarlet fever is an infection of the throat or tonsils by *Streptococcus* bacteria—actually a strep throat—combined with a rash caused by the susceptibility, especially of children, to the chemical toxins produced by the bacteria.

symptoms
Scarlet fever begins with an acutely sore throat, a rapidly rising fever, swelling of the glands in the neck, nausea and vomiting. From 12 hours to two days after

these symptoms, the characteristic rash appears. It starts at the base of the neck, in the armpits and the groin, and moves down the trunk to the extremities. The rash is made up of tiny red spots that turn white when pressed. Although the victim's cheeks may flush with fever, the rash rarely appears on the face and never around the mouth.

complications
The complications of untreated scarlet fever are the same as those of strep throat: the possibility of rheumatic fever and kidney involvement.

treatment
The antibiotic prescribed for the treatment of strep throat, if promptly admin-

Scarlet Fever (Scarlatina)

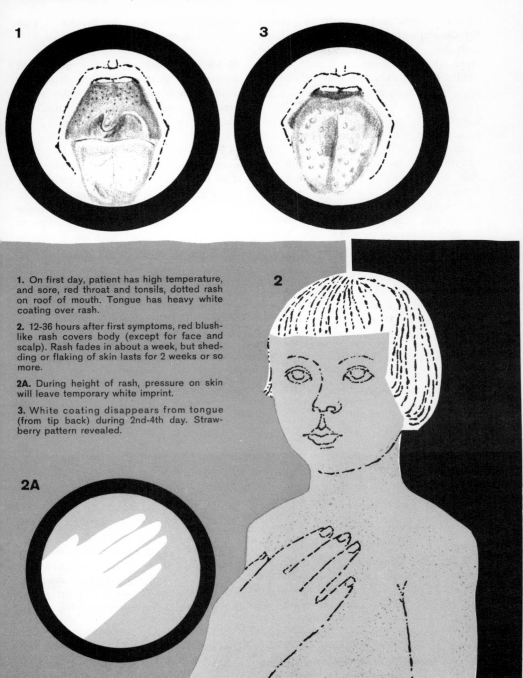

1. On first day, patient has high temperature, and sore, red throat and tonsils, dotted rash on roof of mouth. Tongue has heavy white coating over rash.

2. 12-36 hours after first symptoms, red blush-like rash covers body (except for face and scalp). Rash fades in about a week, but shedding or flaking of skin lasts for 2 weeks or so more.

2A. During height of rash, pressure on skin will leave temporary white imprint.

3. White coating disappears from tongue (from tip back) during 2nd-4th day. Strawberry pattern revealed.

istered, is practically certain to prevent the development of scarlet fever. If the rash does appear during the course of medication, the disease will probably be mild, of short duration and without debilitating consequences.

prevention
Since strep throat is contagious, and since susceptibility to infection with streptococcus bacteria is higher among children of school age than among infants or adults, it is advisable to isolate the victim from other children in the family and provide him with disposable dishes, cutlery, tissues and his own towel. Should an epidemic of scarlet fever occur in school—practically unheard of nowadays—the local school nurses or pediatricians will inform parents of necessary preventive measures. The most effective way to prevent the development

of scarlet fever is to get medical advice at the first complaint of sore throat.

SCARS, permanent marks in healed wounds or diseases resulting from deposits of fibrous connective tissue to replace the original destroyed tissues. *See also* KELOID.

SCHICK TEST, a precaution to determine whether a child is susceptible to *diphtheria*. A small amount of diluted diphtheria toxin is injected into the skin on the front of the forearm. Just a slight swelling at the spot which disappears after a few days indicates the person is immune. A positive reaction is indicated when the area remains red and sore for several days, followed by a brownish spot for several more days. The test is used also for adults during epidemics. *See also* TESTS *and* **medigraph** DIPHTHERIA.

SCHISTOSOMIASIS

O NE OF THE MOST WIDESPREAD parasitic diseases—endemic in Africa, the Far East, South America and the Caribbean, and a threat to more than half a million people—is *schistosomiasis.* The disease has a highly destructive effect on many of the body's organs. It is especially prevalent in warmer parts of the world where people work in and drink contaminated waters.

causes
The parasitic worms known as schistosomes are also called *trematodes* or *flukes.* They are leaf-shaped flatworms and include several different types, of which *Schistosoma mansoni* is one of the most damaging. After the eggs are eliminated in human feces, they hatch in water into free-swimming embryos, seeking out as their *essential* host certain species of freshwater snail. Once inside the snail's body, the parasites multiply and

metamorphose into minute fork-tailed larvae. They then leave the snail host in search of their human victims (this type of schistosomiasis does not involve any other warm-blooded creature) and penetrate the skin head first, shedding their tails as they make their way into the bloodstream. In the process of maturing and mating, they attack the blood vessels of the liver, spleen, bladder and intestines. The newly hatched eggs in the intestinal tract are eliminated in the stool which finds its way into waters where people swim—such as the Caribbean, or where they work—such as irrigation ditches, and the cycle of infection begins anew.

symptoms
One of the first signs of schistosomiasis is the skin irritation that results from penetration by the larvae. In about four weeks—as the parasites move through

Schistosomiasis

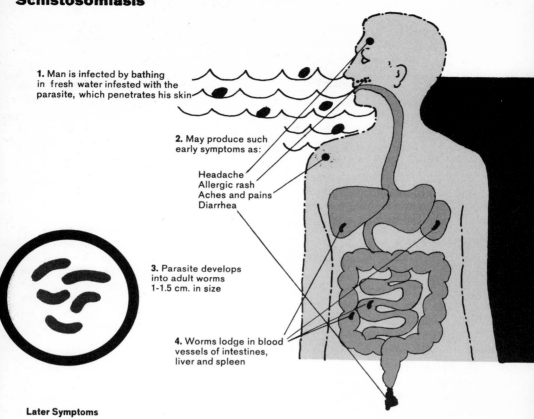

1. Man is infected by bathing in fresh water infested with the parasite, which penetrates his skin

2. May produce such early symptoms as:

Headache
Allergic rash
Aches and pains
Diarrhea

3. Parasite develops into adult worms 1-1.5 cm. in size

4. Worms lodge in blood vessels of intestines, liver and spleen

Later Symptoms

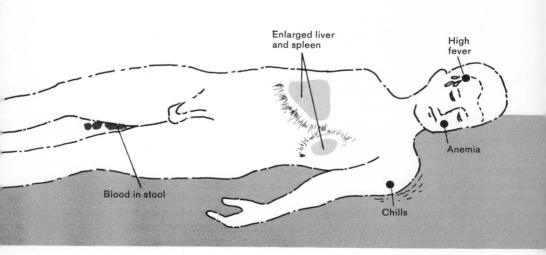

Enlarged liver and spleen

High fever

Anemia

Chills

Blood in stool

various parts of the body in their life cycle—they produce fever, fatigue, dysentery symptoms and abdominal pain.

complications

If the disease goes untreated, or if infestation is chronic, the liver and spleen become enlarged. Chronic blood loss in the stools may lead to anemia, and clogging of the vital organs by eggs and mature worms may be fatal.

treatment

Diagnosis is based on laboratory examination of urine and feces as well as on the results of a rectal biopsy. Medicines can effect a total cure if administered promptly. If the infestation has been permitted to progress to the point where various organs have been damaged, prospects for recovery are poor.

prevention

The elimination of this plague depends largely on effective public health measures which will completely clear contaminated waters of snails and make proper provision for the disposal of human wastes. Waters where the local population wade or work or where tourists are likely to bathe should be regularly tested for contamination and if infested, declared off-limits by local authorities.

SCHIZOPHRENIA, the most common mental disease, afflicting about 25 percent of all mental hospital admissions and about 60 percent of their permanent inmates. The major cause may be heredity, although the disease can skip several generations.

The principal symptoms are: a split personality, escape from reality into a dream world, and emotional indifference. The victims' behavior is determined by their imagined thoughts, not by their real surroundings, and their answers to questions often sound silly and meaningless. Their speech may be garbled and unintelligible and their lack of concern with a serious situation, such as a death in the family, is astonishing.

The onset of schizophrenia is most common in adolescence or early adult life and the course is regressive, with increasing mental deterioration throughout life. There are three principal types: *hebephrenic* (simple mental regression), *catatonic*—with alternating phases of stupor and excitement, and *paranoid*—with hallucinations and delusions of persecution, sometimes leading to violence.

Current methods of therapy offer help for schizophrenics. These include the use of drugs, electro- and insulin shock, and psychotherapy. As a result, from one third to one half of the victims are released from hospitalization after treatment. *See also* ABULIA; AMBIVALENCE; CATALEPSY; CATATONIC; DELUSIONS; HEBEPHRENIA; MENTAL HEALTH.

SCIATICA. *See* SCIATIC NEURITIS.

SCIATIC NERVE, the longest and strongest nerve in the body, measuring ⅘ of an inch in breadth. It is a continuation of the *sacral plexus* inside the pelvis and passes out through a bony opening to the back of the thigh, dividing into two branches to supply the leg and foot. It controls the muscles of the back of the thigh and of the leg and foot and also the corresponding skin areas.

Because of the length of the sciatic nerve, it is exposed to many types of injury. Inflammation or injury to the nerve causes pain that travels from the back or thigh, right down the leg to the foot and toes. Muscles of the leg can be paralyzed by such a disorder. *See also* NERVOUS SYSTEM; SCIATIC NEURITIS.

SCIATIC NEURITIS, often called *sciatica,* inflammation of the sciatic nerve. The gnawing pain is usually felt in the back of the thigh and down the legs, descending from the buttocks and often

Origins and Pathway of the Sciatic Nerve

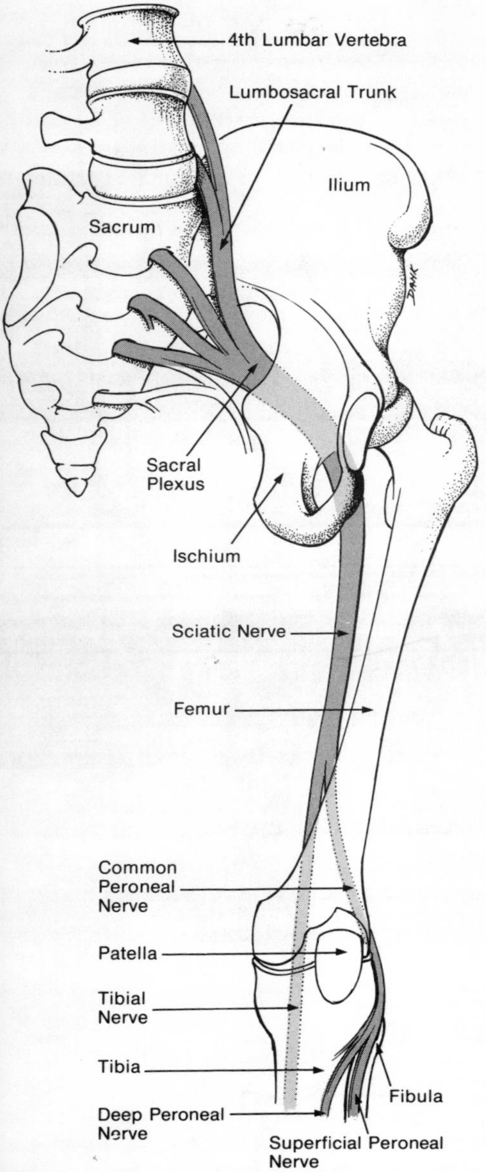

4th Lumbar Vertebra

Lumbosacral Trunk

Ilium

Sacrum

Sacral Plexus

Ischium

Sciatic Nerve

Femur

Common Peroneal Nerve

Patella

Tibial Nerve

Tibia

Fibula

Deep Peroneal Nerve

Superficial Peroneal Nerve

Sciatic Nerve—The body's longest nerve passes down in back of the thighbone (femur). Just above the kneecap (patella) it divides into the common peroneal and tibial nerves that help supply impulses to the lower leg and foot.

Major Causes of Sciatic Neuritis

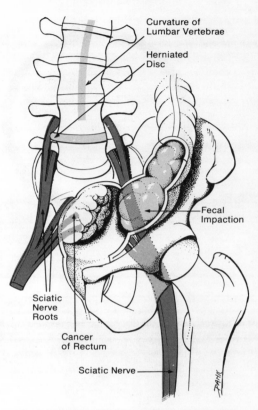

Curvature of Lumbar Vertebrae

Herniated Disc

Fecal Impaction

Sciatic Nerve Roots

Cancer of Rectum

Sciatic Nerve

Sciatic Neuritis—The roots of the sciatic nerve are within the pelvic cavity. Thus a number of disorders within that area can affect the nerve, causing a persistent pain through the buttocks, thigh and leg. Some are illustrated here. Others include arthritis of the lower spine, a fall on the back and sacroiliac disease.

accompanied by numbness in the region of the ankle. When due to spinal root involvement, it is aggravated by change of posture, coughing, sneezing, or defecation.

It has many causes. Constipation or sitting on a cold bench may cause a sciatica of short duration, soon relieved by a laxative or warmth. The cause of chronic sciatica is often difficult to determine. Among the many causes are a

Scleroderma

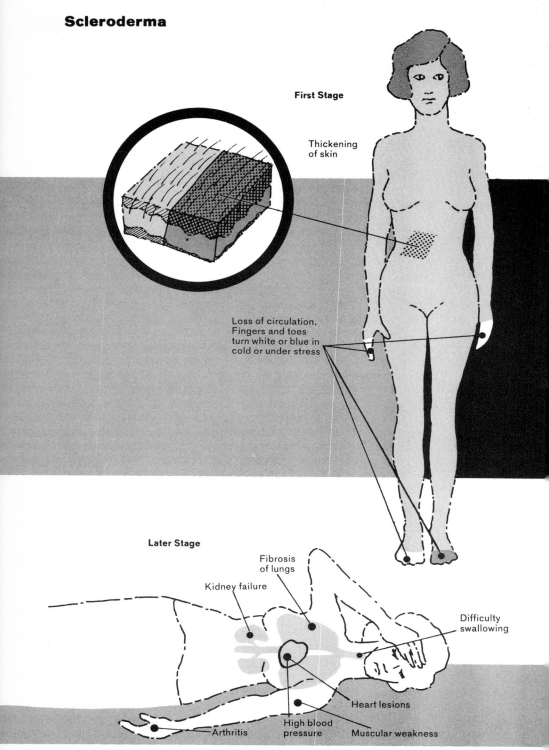

First Stage

Thickening of skin

Loss of circulation.
Fingers and toes
turn white or blue in
cold or under stress

Later Stage

Fibrosis
of lungs

Kidney failure

Difficulty
swallowing

Heart lesions

Arthritis

High blood
pressure

Muscular weakness

slipped or ruptured vertebral disc, a fall on the back, arthritis affecting the sacrum and the lower vertebrae, sacroiliac disease, a tumor of the vagina or rectum pressing on the sciatic nerve inside the pelvis, abnormal curvature of the lower spine, muscular spasms, or absorption of toxins.

Curative treatment requires removal of the specific cause. Relief may be obtained by bed rest, placing the body and lower limbs in a position that causes the least strain, and by application of heat to the painful area. Various drugs provide temporary relief and control of the pain. *See also* BACKACHE; NERVOUS SYSTEM; NEURALGIA; SCIATIC NERVE *and* **medigraphs** NEURITIS; SLIPPED DISC.

SCLERODERMA

SCLERODERMA, ALSO KNOWN AS *progressive systemic sclerosis* and sometimes referred to as "hidebound skin," is a chronic disease in which the skin and subcutaneous tissues become fibrous, rigid and thickened. The condition may be localized and comparatively superficial, or it may involve internal organs. It is more common in women and its onset characteristically occurs during the middle years.

causes
The cause is unknown, although recent studies indicate faulty immunity responses and the possibility of an allergen involvement.

symptoms
Scleroderma usually begins with indication of *Raynaud's disease*. Over a period of several months or even years, affected areas of the skin become shiny and hard, and subcutaneous tissues become so rigid that immobility of the extremities results. If the face is affected, resulting rigidity causes a masklike appearance. Accompanying symptoms of arthritis and ulceration at the joints cause visible deformities.

complications
When the condition is progressively diffused, internal organs may be seriously impaired. Scleroderma of the esophagus may disable swallowing; thickening of lung tissue may result in respiratory malfunction; heart and kidney involvement may eventually be fatal.

treatment
There is no cure for scleroderma at this time, but various measures can be undertaken as soon as symptoms occur so that the victim can be made more comfortable. In some cases, corticosteroid therapy is helpful. Where joints and muscles are affected, physiotherapy can postpone, and perhaps prevent, total immobilization.

SCLEROSIS, a hardening of some part of the body due to a localized overgrowth of tough fibrous tissue. The tissues most often affected are the arteries and the nerves. *See also* ARTERIOLAR NEPHROSCLEROSIS; LATERAL SCLEROSIS *and* **medigraphs** ARTERIOSCLEROSIS; MULTIPLE SCLEROSIS.

SCOLIOSIS. *See* SPINAL CURVATURE.

SCORPION STINGS. *See* ANIMAL BITES AND WOUNDS.

SCOTOMA, a blind or semiblind area in the visual field. *See also* EYE.

SCRATCHING, rubbing and scraping an itching area. Scratching may irritate or tear the skin and often aggravates the itching, but it also provides a pleasant sensation.

SCROFULA, obsolete term for tuberculosis of the *lymph glands* in the neck, forming a cheesy deposit and abscesses and fistulas.

SCROTUM, the pouch behind the penis that holds the two testicles below the junction of the two pelvic bones in front. Outside, it consists of translucent elastic skin lined with a membrane containing muscle fibers. The two testicles are separated by a ridge inside the scrotum and the left hangs lower than the right. The lower temperature of the scrotum as compared with that inside the body is essential for the growth and development of the *spermatozoa* (male sperm cells). Shortly before birth the testicles descend from the inguinal canal to their permanent location in the scrotum.

The most common disorder of the scrotum is *testicular varicocele* (varicosity of the testicular veins). Surgery is required to correct this often painful condition, which can become serious if left untreated. *Orchitis* is a serious disorder of the testicles associated with mumps. *See also* HYDROCELE; TESTICLES *and* **medigraphs** ORCHITIS; VARICOCELE.

SCRUB TYPHUS, *tsutsugamushi disease, Japanese river fever,* a rickettsial infection—found in Japan, Taiwan, the Philippines, New Guinea, and northern Australia—transmitted by the bite of mites. During World War II thousands of cases broke out among the troops stationed in the South Pacific. The symptoms are chills, fever of 104°–105°F. (40°–40.5°C.), headache and insomnia. About the fifth day, a red rash breaks out on the trunk. The temperature drops by the end of the second week, followed by slow convalescence. One attack of the disease confers immunity. A characteristic sign is the formation of a small ulcer (*slough*) with the mite attached to the skin. Various drugs and antibiotics provide effective treatment. Mite repellents also are used but must not be used near the eyes or other sensitive areas. *See also* RICKETTSIAL DISEASES.

SCURVY

SCURVY IS A DEFICIENCY DISEASE, which may be chronic or acute, in which the bones and teeth are affected by internal and external bleeding. Thanks to widespread awareness of nutritional needs and to advances in food technology, this disorder is now rare and when it does occur, is easily corrected.

causes

Scurvy is caused by a deficiency of vitamin C (*ascorbic acid*) in the diet. The deficiency may occur because of ignorance; because of stubborn adherence to some food fad; or because of a gastrointestinal disorder requiring a bland diet. It may also result from severe infection or extensive burns, and it may be a consequence of a temporary inability of the body to metabolize vitamin C properly when taken by mouth.

symptoms

An infant not receiving a daily ration of orange juice after the sixth month, or its equivalent in some form of ascorbic acid, will manifest some of the following symptoms: weight loss, crankiness, bleeding gums, swellings at the long bones and signs of acute pain when attempts are made to move the legs.

Adults suffering from vitamin C deficiency show signs of debility, weight loss, aches and pains. As scurvy develops, the gums bleed, teeth loosen, and internal hemorrhages cause black and blue areas

Scurvy

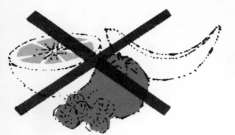

Lack of Vitamin C in diet causes Scurvy

Among best sources of Vitamin C are orange and lemon juice, tomatoes, cabbage, strawberries, cantaloupe

Signs of Scurvy

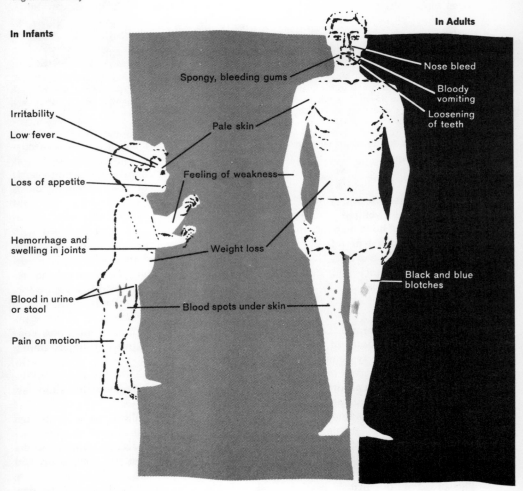

In Infants

In Adults

Spongy, bleeding gums

Nose bleed

Bloody vomiting

Loosening of teeth

Irritability

Low fever

Pale skin

Loss of appetite

Feeling of weakness

Hemorrhage and swelling in joints

Weight loss

Black and blue blotches

Blood in urine or stool

Blood spots under skin

Pain on motion

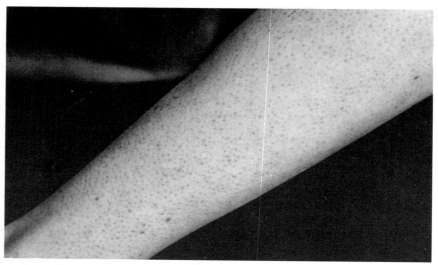

Scurvy—Masses of blood spots under the skin around hair follicles are a sign of scurvy. Bones and teeth are also affected by this disease. Since it is caused by a deficiency of vitamin C, scurvy is easily treated with large doses of the vitamin. It is prevented by inclusion in the diet of fresh citrus fruits and vegetables, raw cabbage and other foods rich in vitamin C.

painful to the touch to appear on various parts of the body.

complications

Untreated infantile scurvy can be fatal because of the eventual involvement of heart, lungs and bone marrow. In chronic adult cases, teeth will fall out and the blood loss occasioned by hemorrhages will lead to anemia and its attendant problems.

treatment

Scurvy in both infants and adults is treated with large doses of vitamin C or ascorbic acid until symptoms disappear. Megadoses may be given by injection for those victims with an absorption problem. Infants may be treated for the deficiency with larger than usual amounts of orange juice.

prevention

In the 18th century, when scurvy was widespread in the British navy because sailors had no access to fresh food during the long sea voyages, it was discovered that lime juice prevented—or as was thought then "cured"—the symptoms. It is now known that a diet containing citrus fruit, fresh green vegetables, raw cabbage, green pepper, strawberies, cantaloupe, or processed food enriched with vitamin C, will prevent scurvy. It should be kept in mind that ascorbic acid can be taken in tablet form when the required foods are not available or are forbidden during a long illness.

Megadoses of vitamin C as a means of preventing respiratory infection continue to be a controversial subject among scientists.

SEASICKNESS. *See* MOTION SICKNESS.

SEBACEOUS CYST, *wen,* a benign tumorlike accumulation of the fatty secretion from a sebaceous gland. It occurs most commonly on the face, scalp and back.

The sebaceous glands are in the dermis (corium), the second layer of skin, and they produce *sebum,* a greasy lubricating substance that helps to keep skin soft and elastic and to prevent penetration by microorganisms. They have separate pores to the outer skin, or they may open into hair follicles. When there is an obstruction of a sebaceous gland's outlet, the sebum it secretes builds up and a retention cyst results. These cysts usually grow until removed.

A cyst that fills with dry sebum or a sebumlike material is a *milium.* These milky white nodules frequently appear on the eyelids and other parts of the

Sebaceous Cyst

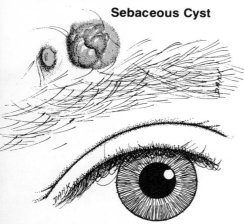

Sebaceous Cyst—The body's sebaceous glands contribute to the skin's elasticity and softness. When an outlet is blocked, the greasy sebum the glands produce builds up and develops into a cyst—most often on the face, scalp and back. Though such cysts are usually benign, they will continue to grow until removed by a physician.

upper face, and sometimes on the scrotum.

Though most cysts are harmless, they occasionally may become malignant or infected, or interfere with function of a gland. Hence, sebaceous cysts should be excised—but only by a physician. *See also* CYST.

SEBACEOUS GLANDS, the oil-producing glands of the skin. *See also* GLANDS; SEBORRHEA; SEBUM; SKIN.

SEBORRHEA, excessive oiliness of the skin due to an oversecretion of *sebum* (skin oil); a dry form is due to dried skin cells. It is most common in adolescence and often associated with acne. The dry form commonly leads to excessive dandruff. Dietary causes include milk, excessive fat, chocolate, sugar and cod liver oil. An oversecretion of *testosterone*—the male sex hormone—has been blamed.

Persons with an oily skin should wash the face frequently with abundant soapy lather. Application of face creams should be avoided, as they increase the oiliness and clog the pores to form blackheads. In dry seborrhea and especially for dandruff scales, a tar soap is useful as a shampoo for its effectiveness in removing scales. Drugs also have been used to reduce the secretion of sebum in seborrhea. *See also* DANDRUFF; OILY SKIN; SKIN *and* **medigraph** SEBORRHEIC DERMATITIS.

SEBORRHEIC DERMATITIS

SEBORRHEIC DERMATITIS is a chronic scaly inflammation of the skin directly connected with an excessive discharge of sebum from the sebaceous glands. The excessive discharge is called *seborrhea* and results in an abnormally oily skin. The inflammation occurs only in adults, since the discharge of sebum is regulated by the activity of sex hormones. The condition may be mild,

chronic, or acute. In some cases, it accompanies acne; in others, it may precede psoriasis.

causes
The underlying cause is unknown. There are indications that it is an inherited disorder of the immune responses, especially since victims of this type of dermatitis are more vulnerable to various bacterial

Seborrheic Dermatitis

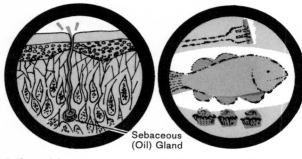

Sebaceous (Oil) Gland

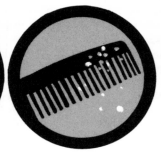

1. Caused by too much production of oil by glands of skin

2. Chocolate, seafood, fatty and fried foods may stimulate overproduction of oil

3. Milder forms range from dandruff to acne — but they are not necessarily preliminary to development of seborrheic dermatitis

Where Disease May Strike...

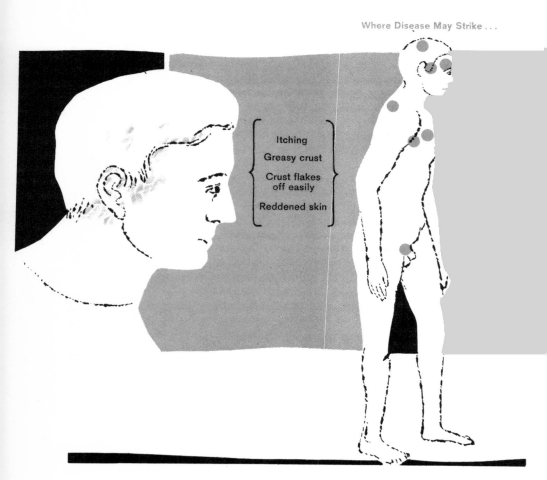

Itching

Greasy crust

Crust flakes off easily

Reddened skin

skin infections. It may be triggered or aggravated by a particular food or by an emotional crisis. Obese people are at a higher risk than the average.

symptoms

A mild or superficial attack may be limited to the hairline or eyebrows, or it may cover the outside of the ears, the chest and the area of the back between the shoulder blades. The skin becomes inflamed and scaly; itching may be mild or severe or it may not be present at all. In its acute manifestations, the lesions will appear on the face and the neck, and in overweight people they commonly occur in the body folds.

treatment

Like most kinds of dermatitis, this one is difficult to treat because of the different responses to medication. Most cases improve with the use of hydrocortisone lotions. Keeping the skin scrupulously clean and dry, and exposing the affected areas to air may keep the distressing symptoms at a minimum.

prevention

In some instances, people with this skin disorder have been able to ward off attacks by trial and error avoidance of particular foods. Medicated soaps should be used only on a doctor's advice.

SEBUM, skin oil secreted by the *sebaceous glands,* a thick semifluid substance composed of fat, horny tissue and skin debris. Its normal function is to lubricate the scalp and skin of the face and prevent dryness. An excessive secretion of sebum may clog the pores and cause blackheads, acne and dandruff. *See also* DANDRUFF; SKIN *and* **medigraphs** ACNE; SEBORRHEIC DERMATITIS.

SEDATIVES, drugs that quiet the nerves. They comprise mostly the *tranquilizers, bromides, barbiturates,* and *chloral hy-*drate. *See also* TRANQUILIZERS *and* **medigraph** BARBITURATE ABUSE.

SEDIMENTATION RATE, the time required for the red blood cells in a specimen of withdrawn citrated (treated with *sodium citrate* to prevent coagulation) blood to settle at the bottom of a test tube, serving as an index of its concentration. The rate is somewhat more rapid in females and is increased during menstruation, in pregnancy, and in a number of diseases. *See also* TESTS.

SEIZURES, sudden onset of abnormal symptoms, such as fits in *epilepsy,* shortness of breath in *asthma,* or heart pain in *angina pectoris.*

SELENIUM, *selenium sulfide,* an antiseborrheic drug for external use against dandruff. It is applied topically to the scalp for five minutes, after which the hair is thoroughly washed. *See also* DANDRUFF.

SEMEN, the fluid produced by the male reproductive organs which carries the *spermatozoa* (male sex cells) that impregnate the woman. It is a thick whitish liquid that carries the spermatozoa secreted by the testicles suspended in the secretions of the seminal vesicles, the *bulbourethral (Cowper's) glands,* and the prostate to provide a medium in which the spermatozoa can live and move. When ejaculated into the vagina, each cubic centimeter of semen contains 60–70 million spermatozoa, one of which may be destined to combine with the female egg and initiate pregnancy. The prostatic secretion promotes the motility of the spermatozoa. *See also* EJACULATORY SYSTEM; PROSTATE; REPRODUCTIVE SYSTEM; SEMINAL DUCTS; SEMINAL VESICLES; TESTICLES *and* **medigraph** STERILITY.

SEMINAL DUCT, *vas deferens,* the excretory tube of the testicle which carries the semen from the tail of the *epididymis* through the *inguinal canal* in the groin to the *ejaculatory duct* at the base of the prostate, which opens into the *urethra* (tube of the penis). Contractions of the muscles in the vas deferens, ejaculatory duct, seminal vesicles and the prostate force the semen into the urethra, from which it is squirted into the vagina by further contractions. *See also* EJACULATORY SYSTEM; REPRODUCTIVE SYSTEM.

SEMINAL VESICLES, two membranous pouches divided into lobes lying between the fundus (base) of the bladder and the rectum which serve as reservoirs for semen and add their own fluid to the *spermatozoa* coming from the testicles. Each vesicle consists of a single tube, coiled upon itself, varying in length from 4–6 inches when uncoiled. The seminal vesicles are connected with the *vasa deferentia* and the *ejaculatory ducts*. During ejaculation, the musculature of the seminal vesicles contracts to help force the semen into the *urethra* (tube of the penis). *See also* EJACULATORY SYSTEM; REPRODUCTIVE SYSTEM.

SENESCENCE, the condition of aging, the mental and physical changes that take place in the mind and body with advancing years. *See also* AGING.

SENILITY, abnormal physical and mental deterioration and impairment associated with old age. *See also* AGING.

SENSITIVITY TRAINING, in psychology, education of a person's capacity to respond to stimulation as by sight, sound, touch, taste or thoughts. The blind can be taught to become highly sensitive to stimulation by the other senses.

SENSITIZATION, the process of rendering a person allergic to a certain protein contained in a food, drug, pollen or other substance by exposing the person repeatedly to a small amount of that substance. *See also* ALLERGY.

SEPTAL DEFECT, a gap in the partition between two spaces, such as the two chambers of the nose or the two atria of the heart. *See also* BIRTH DEFECT *and* **medigraphs** CONGENITAL HEART DISEASE; DEVIATED SEPTUM.

SEPTICEMIA, blood poisoning or bacteria in the blood. *See also* BACTEREMIA.

SEPTIC SORE THROAT, *acute tonsillitis,* an acute infection of the throat caused by the *Streptococcus hemolyticus,* a dot-shaped germ arranged in chains that breaks down blood. The illness begins suddenly with a chill, fever up to 105°F., severe swelling and soreness of the throat, stiff neck, hoarseness and painful swallowing. Complications are ulceration of the throat and formation of abscesses in the neck glands, and later, infection of the heart valves and kidneys, rheumatic fever or middle ear infection. Contaminated milk from infected cows is the main source of the infection. Antibiotics combat it. Rest in bed, hot wet packs on the neck, and aspirin to reduce high temperature are advised. Diagnosis is aided by results of a throat culture. *See also* QUINSY; THROAT; TONSILS *and* **medigraph** TONSILLITIS.

SEPTUM, a natural partition separating two anatomical cavities—such as the chambers of the heart or the nasal cavities. *See also* HEART; NOSE *and* **medigraphs** CONGENITAL HEART DISEASE; DEVIATED SEPTUM.

SERUM, the yellowish liquid which exudes from coagulated blood when the clot shrinks. It is a complex fluid containing water, albumin, globulins, metabolic substances, salts, lipids, hormones, enzymes, and in some cases antibodies. The serum from specifically immunized horses and

Blood Pathway in Interatrial Septal Defect

Normal Heart   **Interatrial Defect**

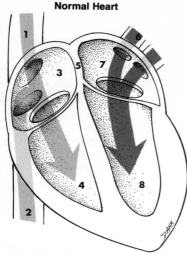
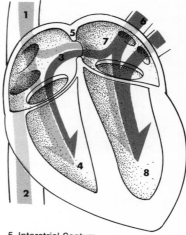

1 Venous Blood from Head
2 Venous Blood from Body
3 Right Atrium
4 Right Ventricle

5 Interatrial Septum
6 Arterial Blood from Lungs
7 Left Atrium
8 Left Ventricle

Septal Defect—An opening between the heart's atria (3, 7) normally closes after birth. Thus blood from the right side is pumped into the lungs for oxygen, returns to the left atrium (7) and ventricle (8), and is pumped into body circulation.

When the opening fails to close, there is abnormal blood flow between the two upper chambers. This leads to heart and lung damage and eventually to poor oxygenation of the blood. When possible, early surgical repair brings best results.

other animals is used as the basis of many *antitoxins*. See also ANTITOXIN; BLOOD; PLASMA; SERUM SICKNESS.

SERUM SICKNESS, a severe *allergic reaction* following injection of a serum, characterized by hives, swelling, joint pains, fever and prostration. *See also* ALLERGY; SERUM *and* **medigraph** TETA-NUS.

SEVEN-YEAR ITCH, popular name for *scabies,* a parasitic infection of the skin caused by a mite. *See also* **medigraph** LICE AND SCABIES.

SEX EDUCATION, instruction about the sexual facts of life involving men and women, including the physiology of sex. It should be introduced to young children so that they will not be misled by mis-

informed peers. Lack of sexual knowledge may expose children to the hazard of venereal disease through casual sexual encounters with people of the same or opposite sex.

The parents' attitude toward sex is reflected in their children. If they recognize it as natural and beautiful, their children will respect them and be guided accordingly in their attitudes toward boys and girls and later toward the women or men they marry. If the parent associates sexual intercourse with disgust and loathing, the children may also develop an abhorrence or fear of sex.

Sex education should be handled in the same way as any other educational subject—honestly, objectively, and without any prejudice. Sometimes, books serve better than lectures. From them the boy and girl can learn the true facts about

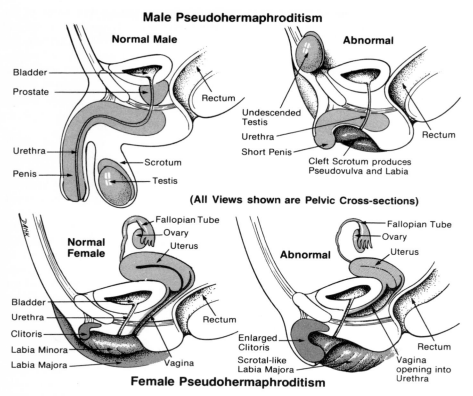

Male Pseudohermaphroditism

Normal Male

Bladder
Prostate
Rectum
Urethra
Scrotum
Penis
Testis

Abnormal

Undescended Testis
Urethra
Short Penis
Rectum
Cleft Scrotum produces Pseudovulva and Labia

(All Views shown are Pelvic Cross-sections)

Normal Female

Fallopian Tube
Ovary
Uterus
Bladder
Urethra
Rectum
Clitoris
Labia Minora
Labia Majora
Vagina

Abnormal

Fallopian Tube
Ovary
Uterus
Enlarged Clitoris
Scrotal-like Labia Majora
Rectum
Vagina opening into Urethra

Female Pseudohermaphroditism

Sexual Abnormalities—True hermaphroditism, in which a person has both male and female sex gland tissue, is extremely rare in humans. More common is pseudohermaphroditism, in which an individual has all or part of the external characteristics of one sex, but internally the sex glands of the other sex. Thus a male pseudohormaphrodite has undescended testicles and male cells, while external genitalia may resemble that of a female or consist of an incompletely developed penis. A female with the condition has female cells and ovaries, but outwardly a clitoris so enlarged it resembles a penis. There are many variations combining all or some of these factors.

the anatomy and physiology of their bodies and the purpose and performance of sexual functions. The diagrams and pictures in legitimate sex books are highly educational. Deprived of this knowledge, a child is apt to read pornographic literature or see licentious sex films which give him (or her) false ideas concerning sexual relations and marriage.

Many schools have courses on sex education which are taught by competent instructors. Such courses provide a basis for more compatible human relations. *See also* ADOLESCENCE; BIRTH CONTROL; FEMININE HYGIENE; MALE PUBERTY; VENE-

REAL DISEASE *and* **medigraphs** GONORRHEA; SYPHILIS.

SEXTUPLETS. *See* MULTIPLE BIRTH.

SEXUAL ABNORMALITIES. The principal anatomical sexual abnormality is *pseudohermaphroditism,* in which the gonads are of one sex but characteristics of the opposite sex are also present. Thus the male pseudohermaphrodite has undescended testicles and a crude vagina; the female, ovaries and a rudimentary penis. Surgery can help masculinize or feminize some of these people.

Much more common are *impotence* (inability to produce erection or ejaculation), *frigidity* (lack of sexual desire in the woman), *premature ejaculation* (completion of the male orgasm before the female attains orgasm) *homosexuality* (sexual intercourse with a person of the same sex), *lesbianism* (abnormal attraction of one woman for another), *incest* (intercourse with a blood relative), the *Oedipus complex* (a man's sexual love for his mother), the *Electra complex* (sexual love of a woman for her father), *exhibitionism* (sexual pleasure from showing the naked body), *narcissism* (self-love), *sadism* (cruelty to the loved person), *masochism* (pleasure from being tortured), *sodomy* (intercourse by the rectum), *fellatio* (sucking the penis), *cunnilingus* (sucking the vulva and vagina with the lips), *pedophilia* (sexual fondness for children), *satyriasis* (excessive lust in the man), *nymphomania* (excessive lust in the woman), and *transvestism* (a craving to wear the clothes and be accepted as a member of the opposite sex). *See also* ADRENAL GLAND DISORDERS; ANDROGYNY; BISEXUAL; EXHIBITIONISM; FRIGIDITY; HERMAPHRODITE; HOMOSEXUALITY; IMPOTENCE; KLINEFELTER'S SYNDROME; MASOCHISM; MASTURBATION; NYMPHOMANIA; PEDERASTY; PREMATURE EJACULATION; SADISM; SATYRIASIS; TRANSVESTITE *and* **medigraph** SIMMONDS' DISEASE.

SEXUAL INTERCOURSE, *coitus,* the mutual performance of the sexual act by a man and a woman. After a period of mutual fondling and caressing—called *love play*—the man inserts his erect penis deep into the vagina, moving it so as to achieve the maximum sensation of intimate contact. The woman responds by rolling her hips and secreting a lubricating mucus around the vaginal opening. When the climax (*orgasm*) is reached, the male seminal vesicles, prostate and ejaculatory duct contract so as to force the semen into the urethra (tube of the penis), thence into the vagina. At the end of a mutual orgasm, both partners feel completely relaxed and may fall asleep.

If intercourse is performed during the fertile period of the menstrual cycle, pregnancy may result. *See also* REPRODUCTIVE SYSTEM.

SEXUAL LIFE, the duration of sexual interest. It begins at puberty in both sexes, reaching its peak in the early 20's, and continues past the menopause in many women and into old age in many men. Some babies have been born to women past the menopause and have been fathered by men in their 80's and 90's. Formerly, older women enjoyed sexual intercourse especially because they were relieved of the fear of pregnancy and this also held true of elderly men, who did not need to worry about "getting an older woman pregnant." Today, modern means of conception control have freed younger people from the fear of unwanted pregnancy. This freedom, however, has also resulted in increased sexual license. *See also* ADOLESCENCE; AGING; BIRTH CONTROL; MIDDLE AGE CHANGE AND PROBLEMS; REPRODUCTIVE SYSTEM *and* **medigraph** MENOPAUSE.

SEXUAL PRECOCITY, the occurrence of masculinization or femininization before the age of puberty. In both sexes it is usually due to overactivity of the pituitary gland and sexual hormones. Young people who are taught to dance, sing and act in public frequently develop sexual precocity, the cause of which is psychological. *See also* PRECOCITY.

SHAKING PALSY. *See* PARKINSON'S DISEASE.

SHELTERED CARE HOME. *See* NURSING HOME.

SHIGELLOSIS. *See* DYSENTERY.

SHINGLES

SHINGLES IS AN ACUTE INFECTION of a particular sensory nerve, accompanied by pain and an outbreak of blisters along the affected neural path. The technical term for the disorder is *herpes zoster* ("girdle of blisters"). A related disorder is known as *herpes simplex,* more commonly called cold sores or fever blisters.

causes

Shingles is caused by the same virus that causes chickenpox. The disease appears to occur only to those adults who had chickenpox as children, but certainly not to all of them. The mechanism of latency and reactivation of the virus is not yet understood.

symptoms

Onset of the infection is signaled by fever and severe pain in the affected nerve. The nerve most commonly involved is one of the trunk nerves; a semicircle of blisters similar to half a belt extends around half the chest or abdomen. Herpes zoster may also attack one of the cranial nerves, causing the symptoms to appear on the face and forehead and, in some cases, within the eye itself.

complications

Any indication of eye involvement should receive immediate medical attention since the formation of blisters on the cornea may lead to blindness and the need for a corneal transplant. A doctor's supervision is also required when the victim is over 60 because of systemic complications.

treatment

Although there is no specific treatment for shingles, where severity of pain is a problem, it can be alleviated. Analgesics may be necessary for weeks or even months after the blisters have dried up and disappeared, since the neuralgia may persist. It is also advisable to keep the blisters covered with a sterile powder especially after they break open and provide possible entry to bacteria.

prevention

Current investigations may result in the development of a vaccine that will immunize children against the chickenpox virus and in turn protect adults against shingles.

RESEARCH REPORT

MONKEY VIRUS MAY SHED LIGHT ON CHICKENPOX AND SHINGLES

A close relationship has recently been established by scientists sponsored by the NATIONAL INSTITUTE OF ALLERGY AND INFECTIOUS DISEASES between a virus that causes *chickenpox* in monkeys and a virus that is responsible for both chickenpox and *shingles*—or *herpes zoster*—in humans. Since both disease-bearing agents belong to the same virus family, researchers believe that the animal virus can be used in experiments which may clarify some of the mysteries connected with the human virus. Chief among these is the fact that *varicella-zoster* (V-Z) produces shingles *only* in those human adults who have previously had chickenpox as children and in whom the virus continues to lie dormant.

How and why this latency and reactivation occur may now be explained by studies of the *Delta herpes virus* (DHV) which has been responsible for several epidemics of chickenpox among the monkeys at the DELTA REGIONAL PRIMATE CENTER in Covington, Louisiana. It was at the Center that DHV was first isolated and shown to have a serological relationship to V-Z.

Immunological studies are now using DHV as the basis for experimental vaccines that may protect people against smallpox and the more serious herpes zoster.   NIH216

Shingles (Herpes Zoster)

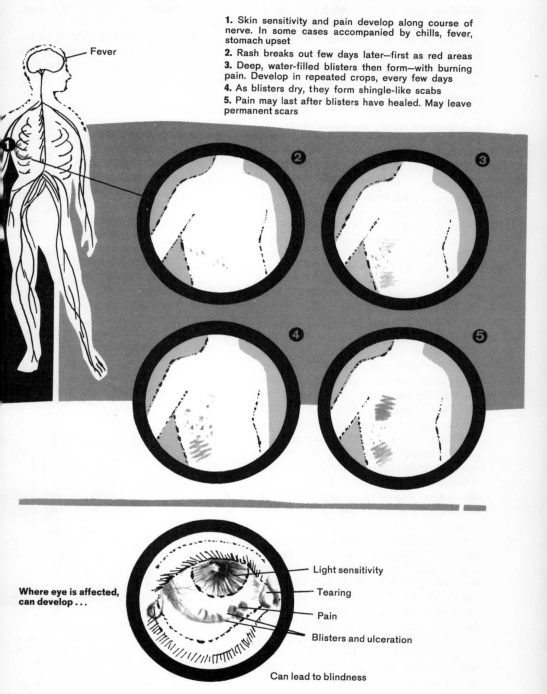

1. Skin sensitivity and pain develop along course of nerve. In some cases accompanied by chills, fever, stomach upset

2. Rash breaks out few days later—first as red areas

3. Deep, water-filled blisters then form—with burning pain. Develop in repeated crops, every few days

4. As blisters dry, they form shingle-like scabs

5. Pain may last after blisters have healed. May leave permanent scars

Fever

Where eye is affected, can develop . . .

Light sensitivity

Tearing

Pain

Blisters and ulceration

Can lead to blindness

SHOCK, a state of collapse manifested by sudden failure of the peripheral circulation in the small blood vessels and capillaries and a sharp fall in the blood pressure. It is most often caused by an injury or accident, surgical operation, hemorrhage, extensive burns, a severe illness, too much ether anesthetic and overdoses of other depressing drugs, insulin overdosage in diabetes, or great emotional stress. The principal sign is a fall of blood pressure accompanied by exhaustion, pallor, thirst, cold clammy skin and a weak rapid pulse. Unless the victim is given emergency and follow-up treatment, death may result. *Surgical shock* during operations is the result of a combination of trauma, ether or other anesthetic, and the preexistent illness. A *secondary shock* due to damage of the tissues may follow the initial shock from a wound, burn, operation or injury, and may appear an hour or more later.

Life may be saved in cases of shock by immediate first aid treatment with a follow-up of professional emergency measures. First, the head should be lowered and the feet elevated, so that the flow of blood in the brain and heart will be maintained. The nearest physician or hospital aid should be summoned as an emergency call. If breathing has stopped, artificial respiration should be performed by a first aid operator. In shock following burns, the victim, if conscious, should be given salt and soda in water (one quart of cool water, one teaspoonful of salt, and one-half teaspoonful of baking soda) to replace the salty liquids lost from the tissues. When the doctor arrives, he may decide to give a blood or plasma transfusion. For low blood pressure and weak heart action, the doctor may give a hypodermic injection of a stimulant.

If shock occurs during surgery, the anesthetist is ready to order immediate cessation of the operation, lower the head of the table (*Trendelenburg's position*), and inject saline solution intravenously.

For insulin shock due to overdosage, sugar is the immediate remedy.

Electric shock treatment (ECT) or insulin shock therapy is sometimes employed for mental depression. *See also* ELECTRICAL INJURIES; ELECTRIC SHOCK TREATMENT; FIRST AID; HEAD INJURIES; INSULIN SHOCK THERAPY; LOW BLOOD PRESSURE; RESUSCITATION *and* **medigraphs** DIABETES; MENINGITIS; MYOCARDIAL INFARCTION.

SHOULDER, the rounded part of the body above the upper arm connected with the chest and neck that includes and covers the ball-and-socket shoulder joint. It is formed by the hemispherical head of the *humerus* (upper arm bone) joined to the shallow cavity of the *scapula* (shoulder blade), a structure that allows a considerable range of movements. The two bones are held in position by ligaments, strong muscles and tendons.

Front View of Shoulder

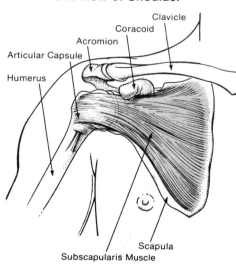

Shoulder—This versatile ball-and-socket joint is formed by the meeting of the upper arm bone (humerus) and the shoulder blade (scapula). The acromion and coracoid extensions of the scapula form the cavity into which the head of the humerus fits. An articular capsule reinforced by tendons and ligaments encloses the joint.

Back View of Shoulder

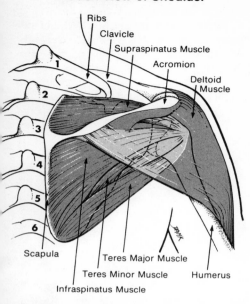

Shoulder—The deltoid muscle produces forward, backward and outward movements of the arm. External and internal rotation depend on the supraspinatus, infraspinatus, teres minor and subscapularis muscles. Constructed to allow varied movement, the shoulder lacks the stability of the hip and is the joint most often dislocated.

The shoulder joint is easily injured and may become stiff and painful from a number of causes. It is subject to dislocation, requiring manipulative reduction by a surgeon and a special type of bandaging for retention. Recurrent dislocation is common in athletes and acrobats. The most common disorder is *frozen shoulder* —due to inflammation of the *subscapular* and *subdeltoid bursae,* causing severe pain and immobility in the shoulder and arm. Another disorder is *acute brachial radiculitis,* manifested by sudden onset of acute pain in the shoulder radiating to the arm or neck and atrophy of the shoulder girdle. *See also* ARM; ARTHRITIS; JOINT; SHOULDER-ARM-HAND PAIN *and* **medigraphs** BURSITIS; FRACTURES AND DISLOCATIONS; OSTEOARTHRITIS; RHEUMATOID ARTHRITIS.

SHOULDER-ARM-HAND PAIN, *frozen shoulder, bursitis,* is due to injury or infection of the *subdeltoid* and *subscapular bursae.* This disorder causes severe pain and partial immobility in the shoulder, arm and hand. Gentle exercise and movement are essential. Carrying the arm in a sling results in freezing the shoulder joint and aggravating the bursitis. Application of heat is helpful but the most effective treatment is with certain steroids and related drugs. *Shoulder-hand syndrome* is manifested by severe constant pain in the shoulder and arm, limited joint motion, diffuse swelling of the lower part of the arm, fibrosis and wasting of the muscles, and loss of calcium from the bones of the arm, forearm and hand. The cause is unknown. *See also* SHOULDER.

SICCA SYNDROME, *Sjögren's disease,* dry inflammation of the cornea, conjunctiva, larynx and nose, with reddish spots on the face and enlargement of both *parotid* (salivary) *glands.* It is most common in menopausal women and is accompanied by rheumatoid arthritis and deficient secretion of saliva. The cause is unknown.

SICKLE CELL ANEMIA

S ICKLE CELL ANEMIA is an inherited blood disease in which a defect in the manufacture of hemoglobin causes the blood cells to be sickle-shaped rather than round, and to be destroyed in the bloodstream with consequences that are frequently fatal. It is estimated that approximately ten percent of all American blacks carry the sickle cell trait without themselves suffering from the disease.

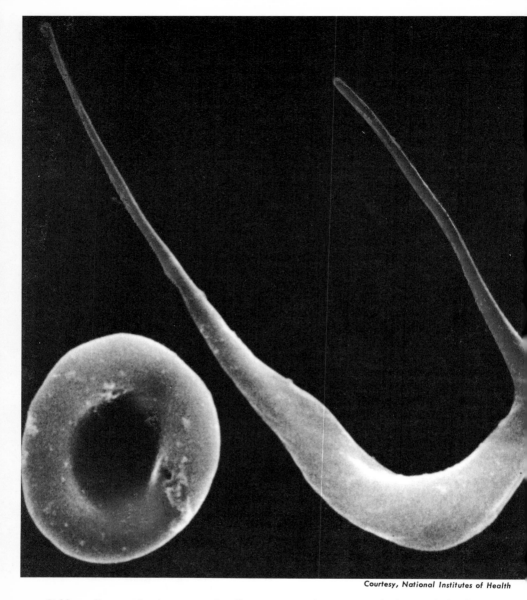

Courtesy, National Institutes of Health

Sickle cell anemia is a genetic disease transmitted from parents to offspring. This disease affects blacks almost exclusively. In this disorder, red blood cells assume an abnormal "sickle" shape instead of the normal "doughnut" shape *(see photograph above)*. The abnormal cells tend to congregate in the hands and feet, where they induce excruciating pain. Victims of sickle cell anemia most commonly die in childhood from complications such as multiple thromboses and infarcts of internal organs. Gallstones frequently occur and ulcers of the legs are common. Abdominal pain and distress is another common symptom. Medical science has still not found a cure for sickle cell anemia, but intensive study now under way may someday find the solution. Many people carry the *trait* for sickle cell anemia without having the disease itself. It is necessary to inherit the trait from *both* parents to exhibit the symptoms of this dread disease. If two "carriers" marry, there is a one-in-four chance of having a child with the disorder.

It is important for prospective spouses (particularly blacks) to know if they are carriers of the sickle cell trait. This can now be determined by blood tests. Right, a medical researcher conducts such a test (called a *red cell osmotic fragility study*). Below, while waiting for blood test results, these conscientious people watch an educational film about the sickle cell research program. A doctor sits at left to answer any questions. Since the sickle cell trait is known to confer resistance to malaria, scientists believe this aberration first arose in Africa as a bodily defense against that infectious disease. Unfortunately, a person inheriting the trait from both parents develops sickle cell anemia.

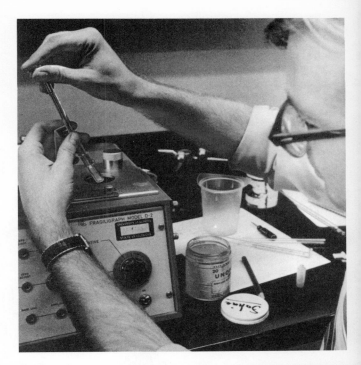

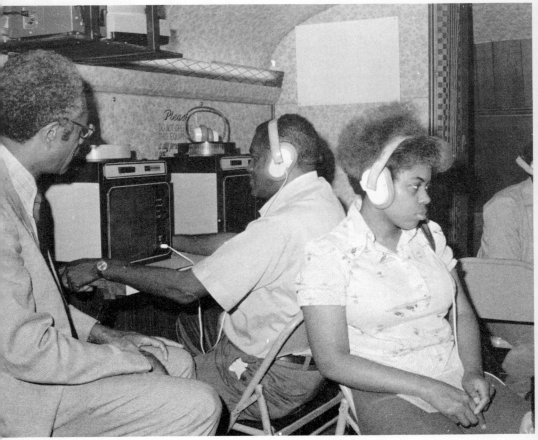

Sickle Cell Anemia

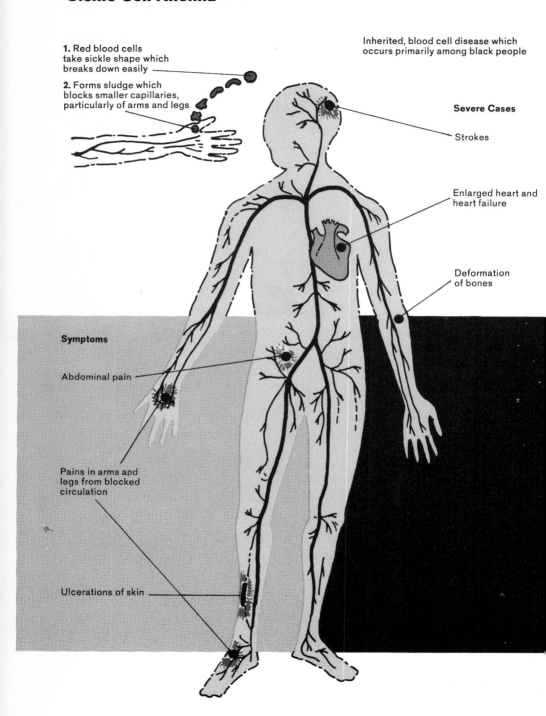

1. Red blood cells take sickle shape which breaks down easily

2. Forms sludge which blocks smaller capillaries, particularly of arms and legs

Inherited, blood cell disease which occurs primarily among black people

Severe Cases

Strokes

Enlarged heart and heart failure

Deformation of bones

Symptoms

Abdominal pain

Pains in arms and legs from blocked circulation

Ulcerations of skin

The hemoglobin aberration evolved in Africa and in other parts of the world—such as the lowlands of Sardinia over a long evolutionary period—where malaria was endemic. It is known that the sickle cell trait provides protection against infection with malignant malaria. The fact that this threat of malaria is nonexistent in the United States is expected to result in the eventual disappearance of the sickle cell trait.

causes

The disease itself is genetically determined: the offspring of two parents who carry the trait have a 25 percent chance of being born with the disease. The anemia results from the presence of an abnormal hemoglobin in the blood cells which turns to sludge or a gel when it is deoxygenated.

symptoms

People with the sickle cell trait rather than the full-blown disease may not suffer from severe symptoms except under circumstances where the oxygen level is low—as in high altitudes, or under anesthesia during surgery. Where the disease exists, it is apparent by the time a child is two years old. Chronic anemia is coupled with severe pain, and the blockage of circulation because of clotting eventually involves the heart, lungs and kidneys.

complications

Victims of sickle cell anemia are extremely vulnerable to blood poisoning caused by bacterial invasion to which they have little or no resistance. Stroke and heart failure are among the most common causes of death. The disorder has an extremely high mortality rate: half its victims are dead before the age of 20; half do not live beyond the first year. Progressive renal damage is a common complication in persons who survive the disease beyond fifty years.

treatment

There is no specific way of treating sickle cell anemia. Treatment is given to relieve disabling attacks of pain and fever, and partial exchange transfusions are effective in preventing crises. People with the sickle cell trait should take the precautions necessary for preventing a crisis if they expect to travel to high altitude areas or if they anticipate surgery, no matter how minor.

prevention

Genetic counseling is available to all potential parents who wish to find out whether one or both carry the sickle cell trait. If both are carriers, there is a one-in-four chance (in each pregnancy) that the offspring will have the disease. New techniques for prenatal blood testing now make it possible to determine whether the fetus has the anemia, in which case an elective abortion can terminate the pregnancy.

RESEARCH REPORT

SURGICAL PATIENTS WITH SICKLE CELL ANEMIA NEED SPECIAL ANESTHETIC MANAGEMENT

Patients with *sickle cell anemia* who require surgery for other reasons should be watched closely for adverse postoperative effects. Anesthesiologists from HAHNEMAN MEDICAL COLLEGE AND HOSPITAL in Philadelphia point out that because such patients often suffer from chronic anemia, subnormal lung function, and impaired liver and kidney function, proper anesthetic management should be assessed both before and after surgery.

The immediate postoperative period is a critical one since the incisional pain, the effects of potent muscle relaxants and especially the reduction in arterial oxygen tension that normally follow surgery are special dangers for the sickle cell patient. In such a case, depending on the site of the operation, the arterial oxygen tension may not return to preoperative levels for days. NIH1025

SIDEROSIS, chronic inflammation of the lungs due to prolonged inhalation of iron salts, common in iron miners and arc welders. *See also* INHALING OF DANGEROUS SUBSTANCES; LUNGS; PNEUMOCONIOSIS.

SIDS. *See* SUDDEN INFANT DEATH SYNDROME.

SILICONE, an organic compound in which all or part of the carbon has been replaced by *silicon,* a nonmetallic element of the carbon group that forms many complex compounds that are an essential part of the earth's surface. In a soft solid form, silicone is used to build up tissue in plastic surgery.

SILICOSIS

ONE OF THE LUNG DISEASES categorized as *pneumoconioses* ("dust diseases"), silicosis is an incurable occupational disorder commonly associated with such jobs as sandblasting, quarrying and mining. A rapidly developing form of silicosis is endemic among workers in plants that manufacture and pack abrasive soap powders. According to the occupation of the victim, silicosis has had many names in the past including miner's mold, potter's asthma, stonecutter's cough and grinder's rot.

causes
The disease is caused by prolonged inhalation of the finely divided dust particles of *silicon dioxide,* commonly called *silica.* The dust of hard glassy minerals —found in a variety of forms and especially in quartz and sand—enters the lungs and accumulates in the tissues. The chronic irritation produces fibrous growth and scarring, thus reducing the lungs' elasticity and respiratory competence, leading to complications.

symptoms
Silicosis is an insidious disease because in many cases it develops very slowly and with few detectable symptoms. It may take ten years of exposure to the dust to cause a rock cutter or a sandblaster to begin to suffer from shortness of breath and a constant cough. In the early stages of the disease the cough may be dry, but soon enough it begins to produce mucus, perhaps tinged with blood. Loss of appetite, chest pain and a general feeling of weakness are other symptoms.

complications
The damaged lung tissue becomes highly vulnerable to such complications as emphysema, chronic bronchitis and pneumonia. The risk of pulmonary heart disease is always present and may eventually be fatal.

treatment
There is no treatment for silicosis. When the disease is in its earliest phase, removal of the victim from exposure to further damage can halt the progress of the lung scarring. Rehabilitation and change of occupation are strongly advised at this point.

prevention
All workers exposed to the dangers of silicosis should have routine chest x-rays and other tests administered by specialists so that the disease can be detected at the soonest possible moment. Prevention can be accomplished only by the combined efforts of trade unions and government agencies working toward the stringent application of laws requiring ventilation, protective clothing, job rotation and other health safeguards in those industries where some exposure is inevitable.

Silicosis

Lung disease caused by inhalation of rock (silica) particles

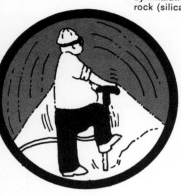

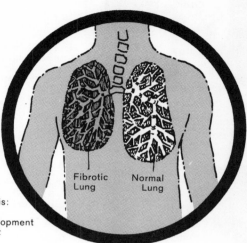

Rock particles irritate lung, causing fibrosis: shrinking of lung and development of nodules in it

Fibrotic Lung

Normal Lung

Symptoms

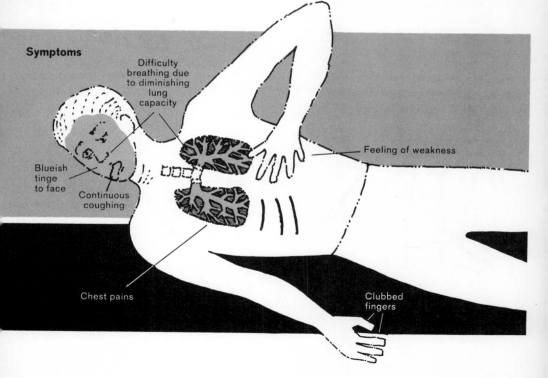

Difficulty breathing due to diminishing lung capacity

Feeling of weakness

Blueish tinge to face

Continuous coughing

Chest pains

Clubbed fingers

Hypogonadism and Simmonds' Disease

(Underactive Pituitary Gland Disorders)

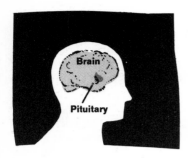

Front part of pituitary gland is attacked by tumor, impairment of blood supply or inflammation. Result may be underproduction of sex—and other—hormones.

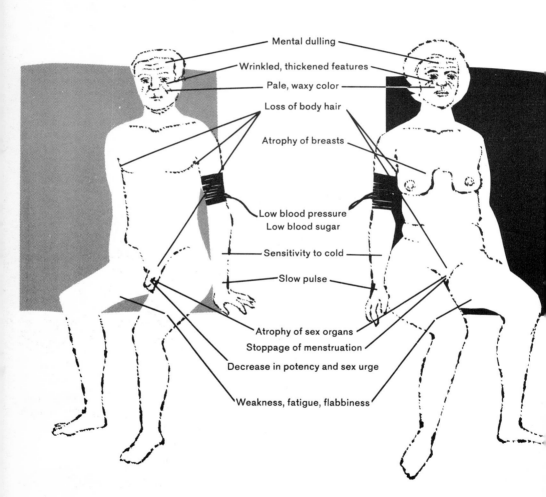

- Mental dulling
- Wrinkled, thickened features
- Pale, waxy color
- Loss of body hair
- Atrophy of breasts
- Low blood pressure
- Low blood sugar
- Sensitivity to cold
- Slow pulse
- Atrophy of sex organs
- Stoppage of menstruation
- Decrease in potency and sex urge
- Weakness, fatigue, flabbiness

SIMMONDS' DISEASE

THE PITUITARY GLAND is a small bulb, about one-third of an inch long, located at the base of the brain. It is attached to the *hypothalamus*—which is considered the control center of the body —by a short stalk and a network of nerves and blood vessels. The anterior and posterior lobes of the pituitary secrete different hormones that regulate the activities of the other endocrine glands. In addition to producing the growth hormone, the pituitary manufactures the secretions that activate the thyroid, the adrenals and the gonads. Underactivity of this master gland (*hypopituitarism*) results in a variety of disorders including *diabetes insipidus, dwarfism, hypogonadism* and *Simmonds' disease.*

causes

The cause of an insufficiency of one of of several of the pituitary secretions may be congenital, or the consequences of accident, injury, infection, or tumor. Disturbance of hormone production may also result from severe hemorrhage following a difficult childbirth, or it may be a manifestation of some unknown disorder of the hypothalamus.

symptoms

One of the disorders caused by underfunctioning of the anterior lobe of the pituitary gland is *pituitary dwarfism,* in which growth and sexual development are retarded but intelligence is normal. *Hypogonadism* is a condition in which undersecretion of one of the pituitary hormones results in underactivity of the gonads, the glands that are crucial in normal sexual maturation and functioning. When the onset of the disturbance occurs in adulthood because of accident, injury, tumor, or systemic infection, it results in libido loss and discontinuation of menstruation in women, and in shrink-ing of the genitals and impotence in men. *Simmonds' disease,* first described in 1914 by the German doctor whose name it bears, is another hypopituitary disorder that may occur after surgery, infection, or an extended labor preceding delivery. Simmonds' disease is characterized by sudden weight loss, general debility, a slow pulse, pallor and low blood pressure. This can progress to premature senility and apathy.

treatment

Considerable progress has been made in recent decades in the treatment of some of the diseases associated with pituitary hypofunction. Since the 1950's, dwarfism has been treated with injections of human growth hormone which is made available to medical centers throughout the United States by the National Pituitary Agency. Where tumor is the cause of malfunction, surgery or radiation therapy or both can have a positive effect. Other cases may require closely supervised injections over a long period of various hormones to compensate for natural deficiencies.

SINGULTUS. *See* HICCUPS.

SINUSES, hollows inside bones and other anatomical structures. The term is usually applied to the sinuses connected with the nose by narrow passages and lined with mucous membrane. These are: the *frontal sinuses* above the eyebrows, the *maxillary sinuses* in the upper jaw bones, and the *ethmoid sinus* located deep behind the nose.

The sinuses have three useful functions: by reducing the weight of their bones, they maintain the balance of weight between the heavier skull and the lighter neck; by secretion of mucus and the wavy motion of their lining hairs, they block dust and germs from entering the throat and breathing passages; and they give resonance to the voice and heighten and broaden the vocal tones for speakers and singers. Through the nasal passages, the sinuses are vulnerable to the *pollens* that cause hay fever and to the *viruses* of colds and influenza that cause complicating sinusitis. *See also* ANTRUM; NOSE *and* **medigraphs** HAY FEVER; MENINGITIS; SINUSITIS.

SINUSITIS

S INUSITIS IS AN INFLAMMATION of the mucous membranes that line the *sinuses* (the air spaces of the bones of the skull that open into the nose). Enlarged adenoids, nasal deformities such as a deviated septum, polyps and occupational exposure to extremes of temperature place people at a higher risk to this type of inflammation.

causes
Chronic or mild sinusitis may be the result of exposure to polluted air or of an allergy to certain dusts. Acute sinusitis may be a consequence of an upper respiratory infection during which vigorous nose-blowing spreads the germs into the sinuses. It may accompany diseases such as influenza and measles, or it may flare up because of an infected tooth. In some instances, sinusitis is an expression of emotional stress; in others, swimming and diving without noseplugs may be the immediate cause.

symptoms
When the frontal sinuses are affected, the common symptom is a headache with most of the discomfort concentrated at the forehead and above the eyes. The swollen membranes may discharge mucus through the nose and the pressure resulting from the swelling may lead to a feeling of dizziness.

complications
If the sinuses become blocked and cannot drain properly, bacterial infection may spread to the eyes, ears and throat. In severe cases, it may spread to the brain in the form of *meningitis,* or to the bones in the form of *osteomyelitis.* Since the use of antibiotics, these complications are extremely rare.

treatment
A mild case of sinusitis usually clears up with the use of medicated nose drops or spray mists that shrink the swollen membranes and encourage drainage. Neither of these treatments should be used regularly over a long period without a doctor's supervision, since they may have an adverse cumulative effect. Aspirin and a heating pad usually alleviate the discomfort of headaches. Antibiotics may be prescribed to prevent secondary infection.

In an acute attack, bed rest may be advisable for a few days. Chronic sinusitis that interferes with normal functioning may require periodic irrigation and drainage of the sinuses, the avoidance of air pollutants and the elimination of smoking. Surgery in which the sinus openings are enlarged to facilitate drainage and ventilation is recommended only in extreme cases, since it does not necessarily provide a permanent cure.

prevention
When sinusitis is obviously the result of such factors as polyps or a structural deformation of the nose, corrective surgery is advisable. Where the inflammation is connected with an allergy, desensitization should be considered. Recurrent attacks of sinusitis can sometimes be prevented by the routine use of a humidifier and/or air conditioner.

Sinusitis

A. The Sinuses—and Where Pain from Them Strikes

1. Frontal Sinus — Directly outward to forehead.

2. Ethmoid Sinus—Back of the eyes and nose.

3. Sphenoid Sinus — Back of the head and neck.

4. Maxillary Sinus — Beneath eyes and up to forehead.

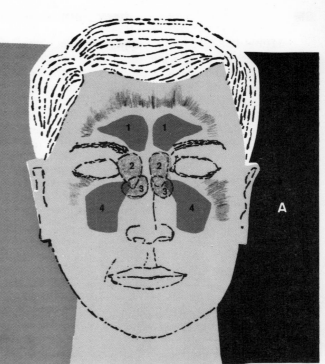

A

B. Cross-section View of Acute Sinusitis

1. Infection creates pus in sinus.

2. Thick yellow or green discharge seeps down into nose and throat.

3. Infection blocks normal air passage through sinus, congests nasal lining, creates feeling of pressure, tenderness, pain in surrounding area.

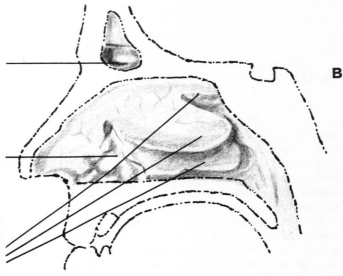

B

SIPPY DIET, a special dietary regimen for patients with *peptic ulcer* who are emaciated and unable to eat bulky foods. It consists of nothing but milk for the first few days, plus crackers, cereals and eggs on the third or fourth day. The amounts are increased gradually and later puréed vegetables are added. On the 28th day, if there has been satisfactory tolerance, the patient is placed on a regular diet. During the period of dietary restriction, vitamin and mineral supplements may be added to supply the recommended daily allowance. *See also* DIET, SMOOTH; NUTRITION; PEPTIC ULCER.

SITZ BATH, a form of *hydrotherapy* in which the person sits in a tub with the hips immersed in cool, warm or hot water, sometimes recommended for relief of hemorrhoids or painful menstruation.

SJOGREN'S DISEASE. *See* SICCA SYNDROME.

SKELETAL SYSTEM, the 206 bones and the connecting joints of the human body which serve as a bony framework to protect internal organs and for attachment of muscles and ligaments to provide motion for the body. It consists of the 28 bones of the skull (8 cranial, 14 facial and 6 ossicles of the ear); the hyoid bone in the neck; 26 vertebrae; 24 ribs; the sternum (breastbone); the shoulder girdle (2 clavicles and 2 scapulae); the 2 fused bones of the pelvic girdle; and 30 bones in each extremity. Not included are the tiny sesamoid bones located in the tendons of pressure points such as the toes and fingers.

The bony skeleton acts as a support and protective framework for the vital organs of the body. For example, the skull protects the brain; the spinal column shields the spinal cord and maintains the erect posture; the ribs shelter the heart, lungs and liver; and the pelvic bones help protect the kidneys and internal sexual organs. The long bones are designed for leverage as in the upper and lower limbs; the small bones for flexibility, as in the fingers.

The paired bones include the 12 ribs on either side, 8 wrist bones, 5 hand bones, 14 finger bones, 7 ankle bones, 5 foot bones, 14 toe bones, 3 auditory ossicles, and the parietal, temporal, palatine, lacrimal, nasal, upper jaw, cheek, lower nasal concha (shell-shaped), collarbone, shoulder blade, hip, arm bone, outer and inner forearm, thigh, kneecap, calf, and shin bone. The single bones include the 26 vertebrae—7 in the neck (cervical), 12 in the thorax, and 5 in the loins or lumbar region, the sacrum (five fused vertebrae), the coccyx (four fused vertebrae); the frontal bone; occipital; sphenoid wedge; ethmoid (a sieve-shaped bone); lower jaw; *vomer* (nasal septum); hyoid (lingual) bone; and the breastbone. In additional there are a variable number of sesamoid bones—from 8–18—which are small rounded masses embedded in certain tendons and usually related to joints.

Certain features of some of the bones deserve special mention. The *cranium* lodges the brain and the spinal cord emerges from the *occipital bone* through a large hole called the *foramen magnum.* The *temporal bone* contains the middle and internal ear structures for hearing and equilibrium, and the mastoid process. Infection of this process requires antibiotic therapy and sometimes surgery. The *sphenoid bone* has a hollow called the *sella turcica* because it resembles a Turkish chair; it lodges the two-lobed dominating pituitary gland of internal secretion. The front lobe of the pituitary gland regulates the growth of bone and controls the length of the long bones. If it is overactive, the individual will become a giant; if underactive, a dwarf. The *frontal bone* has a large socket on either side of the eyeball, at the back of which is an opening for the

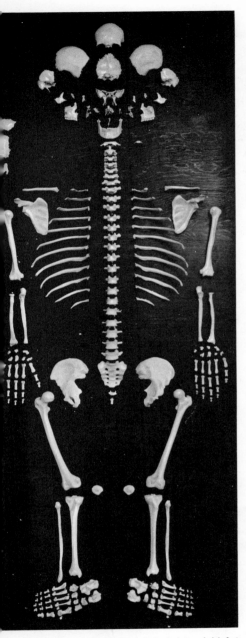

Skeletal System—A disjointed skeleton laid flat reveals the interesting variety of bones in the body. Note the assortment forming the head. These include the large cranial and medium facial bones and the six tiny ossicles of the ears. The long bones of the arms and legs allow leverage, while the small bones of the wrists, hands and feet provide flexibility. The curving ribs protect lungs, heart and liver; the arch of the long column of vertebrae shields the spinal cord.

optic nerve. Sinuses in the frontal, ethmoid and upper jaw bones are frequently infected as a result of colds or influenza and may require drainage or antibiotic therapy. The *hyoid bone* (horseshoe-shaped situated at the back of the tongue) is broken during hanging and chokes the victim to death. The *vertebrae* contain a large hole in the center for the spinal cord and a hole on either side as an outlet for the spinal nerve. The *collarbone* is the most frequently fractured in the body. The two lowest ribs on either side are not attached in front and are called *floating ribs.* The vertebrae, separated by cartilaginous discs, provide the most common cause of backache due to displacement from slipped discs. The *sacrum* was so named on the basis of an ancient superstition that it lodged the soul. The *coccyx* is a vestigial tail carried over from our ancestral apes. The tuberosities of the *ischium* (lower back part of the hip bone) are covered with muscles to support the weight of the body while sitting. The neck of the *thigh bone* is frequently broken in elderly persons but can now be repaired by an operation to pin the fragments together. The ligaments of the *ankle bones* are commonly involved in sprains.

The bones are held together by *ligaments,* which often cause trouble when torn by athletic activities such as football and skiing. The knee joint is the area most commonly involved.

Muscles and *joints* provide the means of moving the bones for performance of various physical activities. Coordinated contraction of groups of muscles pull the bones in the desired directions. There are several types of joints: the ball-and-socket joint such as the hip and shoulder; the hinge joint such as the knee; the pivot joint such as that for rotation of the skull on the spine; and the gliding or sliding joints such as the wrist and ankle. The joints are lubricated by *synovial fluid* resembling the white of egg and they are

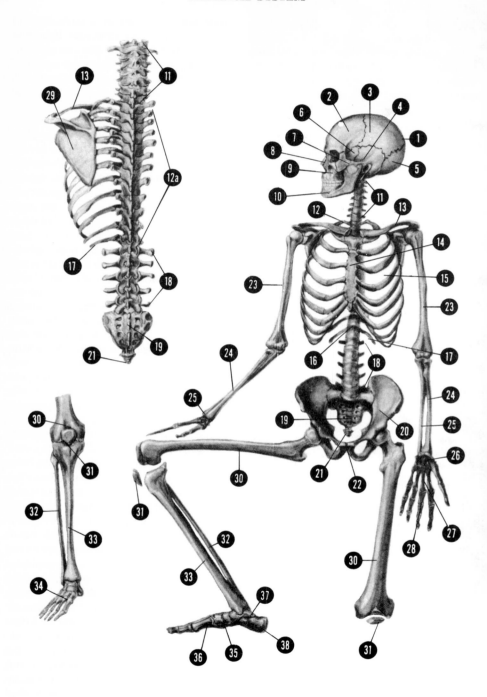

protected from friction by *bursae,* which are small sacs containing fluid. Certain joints are of especial interest. The first vertebra in the neck, called the *atlas* because it carries the weight of the head, rotates around the *axis,* so named because it provides the pivot for this movement. The shoulder joint is frequently dislocated and is also one of the most common sites of bursitis. The hip joint is often involved in arthritis and tuberculosis.

Bone is the hardest and strongest structure in the human body and is normally tough and elastic, not brittle. It is hollow

1	Cranium
2	Frontal
3	Parietal
4	Temporal
5	Occipital
6	Sphenoid
7	Zygomatic
8	Nasal
9	Maxilla
10	Mandible
11	Cervical vertebrae
12	First rib
12a	Thoracic vertebrae
13	Clavicle (collarbone)
14	Sternum
15	Thoracic cage
16	Twelfth thoracic vertebra
17	Twelfth rib
18	Lumbar vertebrae
19	Sacrum
20	Ilium
21	Coccyx
22	Symphysis pubis
23	Humerus
24	Radius
25	Ulna
26	Carpal bones of wrist
27	Metacarpal bones of hand
28	Phalanges
29	Scapula (shoulder blade)
30	Femur
31	Patella
32	Fibula
33	Tibia
34	Foot bones
35	Tarsal
36	Metatarsal
37	Astragalus
38	Calcaneus (heelbone)

inside and composed of a large amount of spongy bone, so it is also light and easily maneuvered by the muscles attached to it. Bone is composed of two kinds of tissue, called *compact* and *cancellous.* The compact tissue is dense in texture like ivory; the cancellous is a network like lattice. The bone is nourished through a system of *Haversian canals,* whose branches lodge blood vessels which carry blood and nutritive elements needed for growth and repair. Especially in childhood and pregnancy, a balanced diet should supply adequate amounts of calcium- and phosphorus-containing foods such as milk and cheese. Generally a pint of milk daily is recommended for persons of all ages. Supplements of vitamins D and C are given to protect the bones as is a calcium supplement when more of that mineral is needed. The strength of bone has been compared with that of steel, granite and white oak. Experimentally, the tensile strength of the dog's thigh bone was found to be at least 25,000 pounds per square inch as compared with 20,000 pounds for cast iron and 10,000 pounds for white oak.

The bones develop from *cartilage* (gristle) by a physiological process called *ossification.* The first step inside the body of the cartilage is enlargement of the cartilage cells and arrangement in rows, followed by deposits of chalky (calcium) material which provide the strength of the bone. Near the surface underneath the periosteum, a vascular membrane called the *perichondrium* forms and supplies the *osteoblasts* (bone formers) while the *osteoclasts* (bone destroyers) excavate passages through the bone layer for deposition of the new bone. When fragments of a fractured bone are replaced and held together by means of a splint or a cast, bone regeneration forms a *callus* (natural splint) to heal the injury by the same process as in its original development. The osteoblasts manufacture a gelatinous substance called *collagen,* which forms the basis of cartilage, in which salts of calcium and phosphorus are deposited to impart the stony quality of bone. When there is a gap separating the fragments, a graft can be obtained from a bone bank.

A layer of *periosteum* (so-called because it surrounds bone) composed of connective and elastic tissues and carrying blood vessels, envelops the bone and adheres closely to it, supplying the necessary nourishment. In young bones, the periosteum is thick and vascular and serves as the *nidus* (nest) for growth of new bone.

The *marrow* fills up the cylindrical hollows of the bones and in different locations is of the yellow or red variety. The red blood cells are formed by the red marrow as are also many of the white blood cells. When the red marrow is underactive, a condition of *pernicious anemia* may result. If it is overactive in conjunction with the spleen, a malignant disorder called *splenomyelogenous leukemia* is a usual result.

The normal deposit of calcium and phosphorus in the bones, to give them firmness and strength, requires the presence of vitamin D. Without this vitamin the bones are soft and bend under pressure. Years ago, before the routine administration of cod liver oil or other sources of vitamin D to babies and children, *rickets* was common and many children were bowlegged because their legs bent under the weight of their bodies. Nowadays this deformity has largely disappeared except in underdeveloped areas. In fact, excessive vitamin D is sometimes fed with detrimental results. The recommended daily allowance is 400 U.S.P. units. Direct exposure to sunlight has the same effect as vitamin D in the form of fish liver oils or irradiated ergosterol.

Another soft bone disease is called *osteomalacia.* It is due to a deficiency of calcium and phosphorus associated with lack of vitamin D. In this condition the calcium bone content may be reduced to about 50 percent of normal and the phosphorus to about 60 percent. Osteomalacia responds rapidly to large doses of a calcium supplement and vitamin D.

There are many other diseases of the bones including among others *tuberculosis,* particularly of the hip; *osteomyelitis* (infection of the inside bone with pus-forming germs); *osteoporosis* (with thinning of the compact bone substance); *acromegaly* (with increased size of the bones of the hands, feet and face); *Paget's disease* (a deforming bone malady with a greatly enlarged skull and leg bones bowing under its weight); *leontiasis ossea* (with a leonine appearance of the face due to overgrowth of the facial bones); *achondroplasia* (an abnormal bone development in a typical congenital dwarf); *hypertrophic osteoarthropathy* (with new bone development, clubbed fingers, and symptoms of arthritis); *osteoma* (a benign bone tumor located particularly in the skull); *exostosis* (the most common benign tumor of bone); *myeloma* (a tumor of bone marrow); *osteosarcoma* (a malignant bone tumor affecting chiefly children and young adults with early metastasis to the lungs and usually fatal in children under 12); and *metastatic cancer* spread from distant organs of the body. *See also* BODY; CARPAL BONES; CARTILAGE; COLLAGEN; COMPOUND FRACTURE; CRANIUM; DISC; DISLOCATION; FINGER; HIP; JAW; JOINT; LEG; LIGAMENTS; MANDIBLE; MARROW; ORTHOPEDIC SURGERY; OSSIFICATION; OSTEITIS; OSTEOMALACIA; OSTEOPOROSIS; PAGET'S DISEASE; PARATHYROID GLANDS; PELVIS; SKULL; SPINE; VERTEBRA; WRIST *and* **medigraphs** CELIAC DISEASE; CUSHING'S SYNDROME; FRACTURES AND DISLOCATIONS; HYPERPARATHYROIDISM; OSTEOARTHRITIS; OSTEOMYELITIS; RICKETS. RESEARCH REPORT *follows* FRACTURES AND DISLOCATIONS; VITAMINS.

SYNTHETIC HORMONE EFFECTIVE IN HEREDITARY BONE DISEASE

The hereditary crippling bone disease in children, *osteogenesis imperfecta*, may now be arrested and effectively treated with a new drug under investigation at DOWNSTATE MEDICAL CENTER in Brooklyn. The drug is a *synthetic* version of *calcitonin*, a thyroid gland hormone which, by retarding the flow of calcium from bone to blood, has already proved its effectiveness in the treatment of Paget's disease and osteoporosis, two conditions also characterized by high bone resorption rates.

The basic mechanism underlying osteogenesis imperfecta seems to be the fact that calcium resorption by the blood occurs at a faster rate than calcium accretion in the bones. Therefore, the calcium in the diet leaves the bones before proper hardening and growth can take place. This abnormality results in softness and porosity of the skeleton, leading to multiple fractures as well as severe deformities such as curvature of the spine and legs of uneven length. Softening of the bones of the inner ear frequently leads to deafness as one of the characteristics of the disease.

In the Brooklyn studies, five children ranging in age from about four to 13 years who were admitted to DOWNSTATE UNIVERSITY HOSPITAL received injections of synthetic calcitonin three times a week for six weeks. During this period, the radioactive calcium studies that were made indicated that the hormone therapy had effectively increased the patients' calcium balance and reduced the bone turnover in their skeletons.

The encouraging results, which showed no adverse reactions, toxic effects, or allergic responses, have led the reseachers to conclude that long-term calcitonin therapy may suppress the flawed metabolic processes underlying osteogenesis imperfecta, and that such therapy can be initiated at an earlier stage of the child's development to forestall the possibility of fractures and deformities.

The five children who are undergoing the hormone therapy seem to break fewer bones and show a temporary growth spurt as well as increase in bone density.   NIH214

SKENE'S GLANDS. *See* VULVA.

SKIN, the surface layers of thin tissue which cover the body; protect the underlying tissues from injury, drying and the invasion of foreign germs; and help to regulate the body temperature. It is the largest single organ of the body, weighs about six pounds, and if spread flat would cover an area of about 16–20 square feet.

The skin consists of flat *epithelial cells* cemented together to form a solid membrane, elastic fibers, numerous small blood vessels called *capillaries,* small nerves and nerve endings, sweat and oil glands, and hair follicles from which the hair roots grow to full length. It contains four main layers (from outside inwardly):

1. The *epidermis* (*cuticle*) the outermost layer, which is thick and horny, contains no blood vessels or nerves, is nourished by *lymph* (a clear liquid exuding from the deeper blood vessels), and containing in its deepest layer *melanin* (dark pigment).
2. The lucid clear transparent layer is next.
3. Then comes the granular layer of flattened cells.
4. The *dermis* (*corium*), the deepest layer, is tough, flexible, and consists of felted connective tissue, with a varying amount of elastic fibers and numerous blood vessels, lymphatics, and nerve terminals with special sensory organs for the senses of touch, temperature, and pressure. The skin cells of the corium grow and multiply continuously, pushing the worn-out cells toward the outer layer and replacing them.

In old age, the skin becomes drier and wrinkled when blood circulation decreases. Vitamin A is important for the nutrition of the skin. A deficiency of vitamin B_6 may cause excessive oiliness.

Appendages of the skin are the nails, hair, sweat glands and sebaceous (oil) glands. There are numerous skin diseases, treatment of which constitutes the branch of medicine known as *dermatology. See also* ALBINISM; ALLERGY; BARBER'S ITCH; BODY ODOR; COMEDONES; DERMABRASION; DERMATOGLYPHICS; DERMATOLOGIST; DRY SKIN; ECTHYMA; ECZEMA; ERYSIPELAS; EXANTHEM; EXCRETION; FISH-SKIN DISEASE; FOLLICULITIS; HAIR; ITCHING; KELOID; KERATOSIS; LUPUS VULGARIS; MEL-ANOSIS; NAILS; OILY SKIN; PERSPIRATION; PORES; RINGWORM; ROSACEA; SEBACEOUS CYST; SEBORRHEA; SEBUM; SKIN CARE; SPOROTRICHOSIS; SUNBURN; TATTOO; VITILIGO *and* **medigraphs** ACNE; CARBUNCLES, FURUNCLES AND FOLLICULITIS; CHICKENPOX; COLD SORES; CONTACT DERMATITIS; FUNGUS INFECTIONS OF THE SKIN; HANSEN'S DISEASE; HIVES; IMPETIGO; LICE AND SCABIES; LUPUS ERYTHEMATOSUS; PILONIDAL CYST; PITYRIASIS ROSEA; PSORIASIS; ROCKY MOUNTAIN SPOTTED FEVER; SCLERODERMA; SEBORRHEIC DERMATITIS; SHINGLES; SKIN CANCER; VITAMIN A DEFICIENCY; WARTS.

SKIN CANCER

S KIN CANCERS ARE AMONG the most common and the most curable of all types of malignancy. Although approximately 300,000 new cases are reported each year in the United States, skin cancer mortality is the lowest of all categories of cancer deaths, amounting to about one percent of the total for both men and women.

Skin Cancer—Growths or moles on the skin that ulcerate or change in size or texture should be investigated for possible malignancy. Surgery plus x-ray therapy, freezing with liquid nitrogen and administration of a special drug are among the treatments for skin cancer. It is the most common and most curable of malignancies.

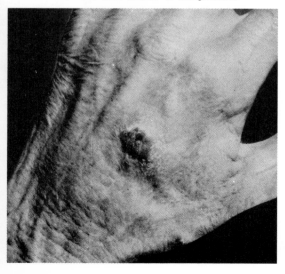

causes

It is currently assumed that a genetic factor as yet unidentified predisposes some people to skin cancer. The typical victim is a fair-complexioned adult who has been overexposed to the sun. Thus farmers, seamen and others whose work keeps them out of doors are at high risk. Other causes include contact with chemicals such as arsenic and coal tar products, and exposure to x-rays. The dangerous levels of radiation and occupational carcinogens are sometimes regulated by federal laws. A self-inflicted cause of skin cancer is the pursuit of a suntan involving overexposure to the sun and consequent coarsening and aging of skin texture.

symptoms

The onset of skin cancer is signaled by the development of a pale lump which becomes inflamed, then ulcerates and is covered by a crust, or by the sudden appearance of sharply delineated red patches. The areas most commonly af-

Skin Cancer

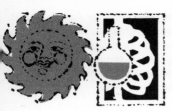

Contributing Factors
X-ray radiation, contact with
industrial chemicals, chronic
irritation; too much sunlight

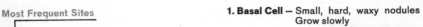

Two Types of Skin Cancer

1. Basal Cell — Small, hard, waxy nodules
Grow slowly

Most Frequent Sites

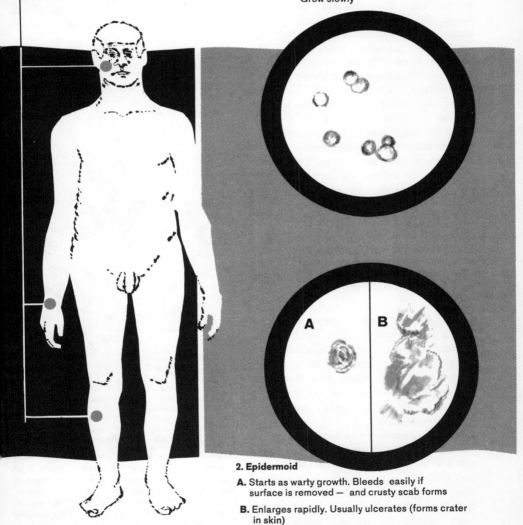

2. Epidermoid

A. Starts as warty growth. Bleeds easily if
surface is removed — and crusty scab forms

B. Enlarges rapidly. Usually ulcerates (forms crater
in skin)

fected are the exposed parts of the body: face, backs of hands, forearms and neck.

Changes in the size or texture of moles, scars, birthmarks, or other accustomed blemishes on the skin surface may also indicate the beginning of a cancer. Such malignancies are usually not painful.

treatment

Ninety-five percent of all skin cancer patients are completely cured of the disease through early diagnosis and proper treatment. Of the two main types of skin cancer cells—*squamous* and *basal*—the latter rarely spreads to other parts of the body. However, basal skin cancer can penetrate to the bone if it is not arrested by therapy. Squamous cell cancer is rarer but riskier, since it does tend to spread to other tissues. Current treatment for both types of malignancies consists of surgery and x-ray therapy. Malignant tissue may be destroyed by other methods, including the application of caustic chemicals, freezing with liquid nitrogen, or cauterizing with an electric "knife." The use of the drug *5-fluorouracil* has been effective in the treatment of some skin cancers. In some cases, combination therapy over an extended period may be necessary for complete cure.

SKIN CARE, *cosmetology,* embodies simple home hygiene, the avoidance of harmful cosmetics, and the application of scientific methods to beautify the skin by trained beauty specialists. For most people, nightly washing of the face with soap and warm water and drying with a heavy towel suffices.

Excessive exposure to sunlight and the use of too many cosmetics have a damaging effect on the skin. Reliable face powders, rouge and lipstick are permissible for their cosmetic effect, provided that they are washed off at night. Reputable beauty parlors are staffed with trained operators who can provide tem-

porary improvement in appearance. Maintenance of general health is very important in skin care. *See also* BATHING; BODY ODOR; COSMETICS; DEODORANTS AND ANTIPERSPIRANTS; DEPILATORY; DRY SKIN; OILY SKIN; SKIN.

SKIN TUBERCULOSIS. *See* LUPUS VULGARIS.

SKULL, the bony framework of the head, including the *cranium* (which holds the brain and pituitary gland) and the

The Skull
Cranial Bones

Facial Bones

1 Frontal	7 Lacrimal
2 Parietal	8 Nasal
3 Occipital	9 Inferior Nasal Concha
4 Temporal	10 Maxilla
5 Sphenoid	11 Zygomatic
6 Ethmoid	12 Mandible

Skull—The wavy lines on the cranium indicate sutures—the blending of the various bones. Each temporal bone (4) contains the essential organ of hearing, canals that control balance, and the mastoid process. The frontal bone (1) and the maxilla (10) contain sinuses. A large hole in the occipital bone (3) allows the bulb of the lower brain to pass into the spinal cord.

bones of the face and jaws. It consists of 8 cranial bones, 14 facial bones and 6 ossicles of the ears.

The eight cranial bones are the two *parietal*—on the sides of the skull, the two *temporal*—in the region of the ears, the single *frontal*—at the forehead and front of the skull, the *occipital*—at the back of the skull, the bat-shaped *sphenoid*, which forms a wedge, and the cubical *ethmoid* between the eye orbits.

Each temporal bone lodges inside its structure the *cochlea* (the essential organ of hearing), the three *semicircular canals* which control balance and equilibrium, and the *mastoid process* which is involved in *mastoiditis* complicating middle-ear infections. The frontal bone has two frontal air sinuses located behind and above the eyebrows. The occipital bone has a large hole below—the *foramen magnum*—through which the bulb of the lower brain passes into the spinal cord. The skull is also perforated by other holes for passage of the cranial nerves.

The 14 facial bones consists of the 2 *nasal bones* which form the bridge of the nose; the 2 upper jaw bones (*maxilla*), each of which carries eight teeth and is hollowed by a large sinus; the 2 cheek bones (*zygomatic*); the lower jaw bone (*mandible*), which carries 16 teeth; the hard palate bones (*palatine*); the spongy scroll-shaped *inferior nasal concha* (shell inside each nasal cavity); the plow-shaped *vomer,* which forms part of the nasal partition; and 2 tiny *lacrimal* (tear) bones.

The roof (vault) of the skull is formed by the frontal and parietal bones and the base of the occipital, temporal, sphenoid and ethmoid bones. The skull is subject to fractures and various diseases which may also affect the brain. *See also* BRAIN; CONCUSSION; CRANIUM; FONTANEL; HEAD INJURIES; HYDROCEPHALUS; JAW; MANDIBLE; SKELETAL SYSTEM *and* **medigraphs** FRACTURES AND DISLOCATIONS; RICKETS.

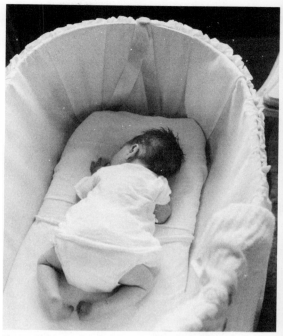

Sleep—Babies this young sleep most of the time. The need gradually decreases through later infancy and the childhood years, usually averaging 7–8 hours per night in adult life.

SLEEP, a period of rest—averaging eight hours—with partial suspension of consciousness and physical and mental activity. Physiological activity is reduced and the body is enabled to repair itself by eliminating wastes and replenishing depleted tissues with needed constituents. The pulse rate slows down, blood pressure falls, breathing is slower and deeper, the temperature drops to its lowest level for the day, the basal metabolism is reduced, and the *cerebrum* (higher brain) is inactive except for dreams.

The amount of sleep needed varies mostly according to age, but everyone should have enough to awaken rested and refreshed. The normal adult requires seven or eight hours of sleep; the aged, six hours; children 2–3 years old, 12–13 hours; and infants, almost all of the time. For persons who tire easily, an afternoon nap of about an hour is helpful. Coffee or tea drunk late at night often causes sleeplessness. The habit of taking sleeping pills is bad, as they depress vital functions and produce dependence upon them. *See also* DREAMS; HYPNOTICS; INSOMNIA; NARCOLEPSY; NIGHTMARE; REST; SLEEPWALKING; SNORING *and* **medigraph** ENCEPHALITIS.

SLEEPING SICKNESS. *See* ENCEPHALITIS.

SLEEPLESSNESS. *See* INSOMNIA.

SLEEPWALKING, *Somnambulism,* a condition in which the victim walks, talks and has full possession of his senses but no recollection after awakening. Sleepwalking usually arises from a psychological complex buried in the subconscious mind. Somnambulism generally ceases when a doubt or fear is relieved; sometimes this requires psychiatric treatment. *See also* SLEEP.

SLIPPED DISC

RUPTURING OF ONE OF THE PADS OF cartilage that act as shock absorbers between the spinal vertebrae is informally designated "slipped disc." The formal term for this condition is *prolapse of an intervertebral disc*. It occurs most commonly in the lower back because of the strain of lifting; less often in the neck because of a whiplash injury.

causes
Inside the pads of intervertebral cartilage and fiber is a firm, spongy and elastic tissue known as the *nucleus pulposus*. Under ordinary circumstances, the discs (pads) accommodate themselves to the movement of the spine. However, during an excessive strain, the cartilage may weaken, allowing the nucleus to bulge and protrude at the back of the vertebral body. The bulging tissue impinges on one or another of the nerve roots in the spinal canal, causing severe pain.

symptoms
A slipped disc is most likely to occur in the lower back, creating acute discomfort by pressing on the sciatic nerve thus involving the buttocks, thighs, calves and feet. The resultant sciatica makes walking almost impossible. Even when the person is sitting or lying still, the pain may be activated or intensified by coughing or sneezing. The slightest movement may unpredictably result in excruciating twinges of pain.

When the slipped disc occurs in the neck, the pain is experienced at the back of the neck and spreads through the arms to the fingers. Head movements thus become extremely limited.

treatment
If the lumbar region is affected, prolonged bed rest on a hard mattress over a bed board may lead to self-correction of the condition. Heat applications and pain killers are usually part of treatment, and in some instances traction may be applied to the legs to relieve the pressure on the nerve. If the slipped disc is located between the cervical vertebrae, heat, bed rest and traction are also used. The neck may be immobilized by a rigid collar to reduce the incidence of pain. Cases that do not respond to these measures may require surgical correction. In an operation called a *laminectomy,* a portion of the arch of the vertebra is cut away and the herniated portion of the disc that is impinging on the nerve is removed.

prevention
The best precaution against a slipped disc is to learn the proper way to lift and carry bulky or heavy objects and to avoid

Slipped Disc

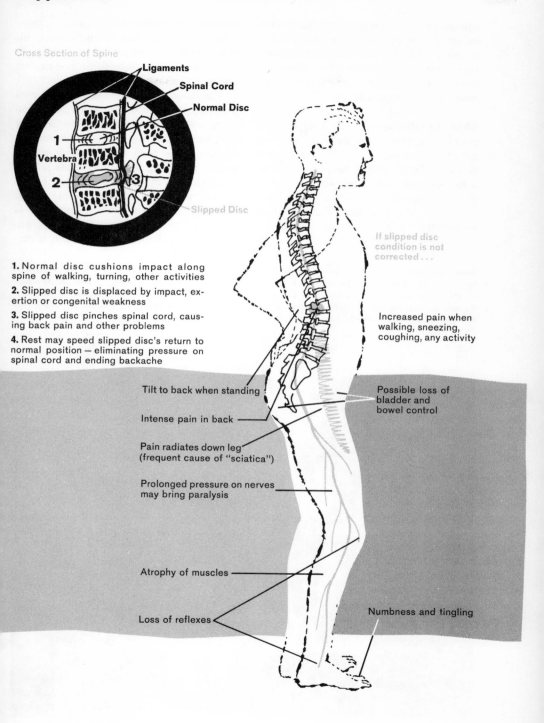

Cross Section of Spine

Ligaments

Spinal Cord

Normal Disc

1

Vertebra

2

3

Slipped Disc

1. Normal disc cushions impact along spine of walking, turning, other activities

2. Slipped disc is displaced by impact, exertion or congenital weakness

3. Slipped disc pinches spinal cord, causing back pain and other problems

4. Rest may speed slipped disc's return to normal position — eliminating pressure on spinal cord and ending backache

If slipped disc condition is not corrected . . .

Increased pain when walking, sneezing, coughing, any activity

Tilt to back when standing

Intense pain in back

Pain radiates down leg (frequent cause of "sciatica")

Prolonged pressure on nerves may bring paralysis

Possible loss of bladder and bowel control

Atrophy of muscles

Loss of reflexes

Numbness and tingling

unnecessary straining of the back. The temptation to lift a hefty grandchild or a weighty valise should be resisted in one's later years, and if there is a tendency to lower back discomfort, a supportive back brace might be considered.

SMALLPOX (*variola*), an acute, highly contagious, often fatal disease that once ravaged mankind in epidemics. Its first signs are chills, high fever, severe headache and backache, followed by a rash which eventually covers the entire body and turns into pus-filled blisters. These in turn dry up to form scabs which very often leave pockmarks. The disease may also be accompanied by vomiting, convulsions and diarrhea. Complications include other skin infections such as boils and abscesses, ear infections, pneumonia and heart failure.

Thanks to a persistent vaccination program by the World Health Organization (whose efforts were aided by the fact that the disease is not transmitted by animals), smallpox has been eradicated from the world, except for Ethiopia, where it is in a comparatively mild form and is expected to be eliminated before long. Hence, vaccination against smallpox is no longer a requirement for school entrance in the United States, nor is a cer-

Smallpox—Before this scene took place in 1796, the world was helpless in the face of epidemics of often-fatal smallpox. A rural British physician, Edward Jenner, inserted a fluid into scratches on the arm of an eight-year-old boy. It was from a cowpox pus-filled blister on the hand of a dairymaid, and it was the first successful smallpox vaccination. Despite opposition when he published his findings, the vaccination became accepted practice during Jenner's lifetime.

© 1960, Parke, Davis & Company

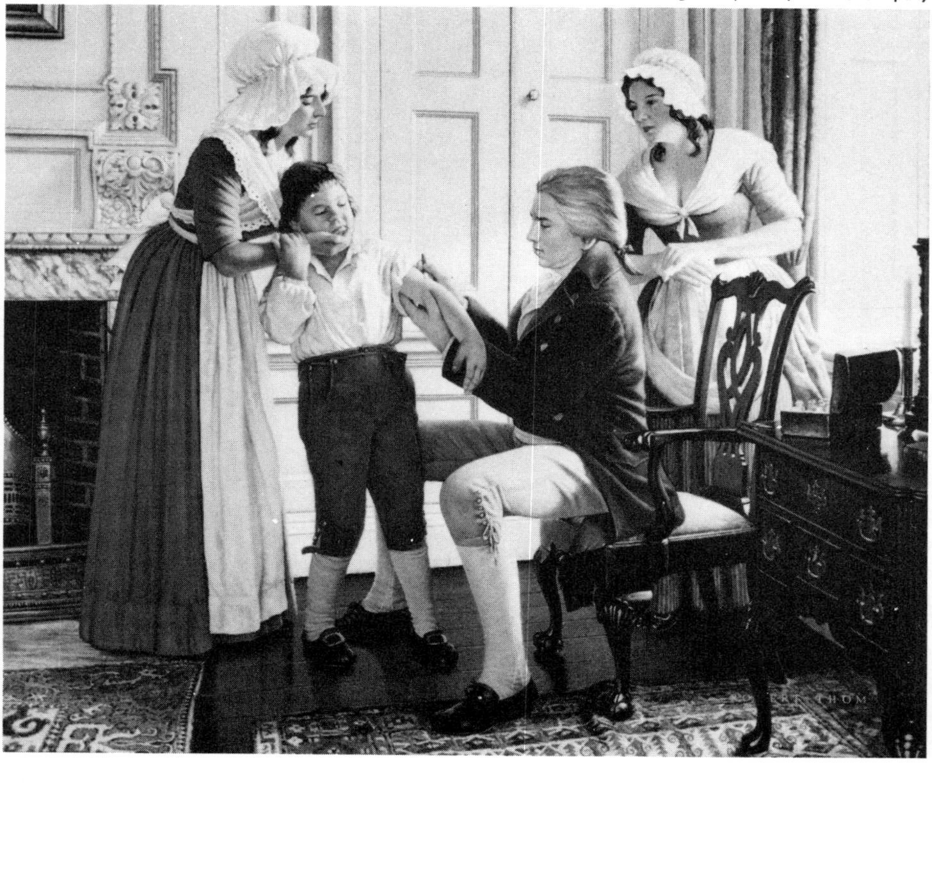

tificate of vaccination required on reentering the U.S. from abroad. *See also* INFECTIOUS DISEASES.

SMEARS, specimens of blood, pus, urine, and so on, spread on a glass slide for microscopical examination. *See also* PAP SMEAR TEST; TESTS.

SMEGMA, the thick cheesy ill-smelling secretion which accumulates under the foreskin of the penis in uncircumcised males and around the sensitive clitoris in females. It may cause irritation if excessive and not washed off.

SMELL, one of the five senses of sight, hearing, smell, taste and touch. It involves the perception of aromas and odors by sensory organs in the mucous membrane of the nose. The sensation is carried from the nose via the *olfactory nerves* to the olfactory *bulb* in the *rhinencephalon* of the brain, where its nature is identified. The sense of smell is heavily involved with taste. Fine discriminations in taste are actually achieved through the sense of smell.

Loss of the sense of smell is called *anosmia,* increased sensitiveness to odors *hyperosmia,* and a distorted sense of smell *parosmia.* An instrument that tests the sensitiveness of the nose to odors is known as an *olfactometer.* Some mentally ill people complain of *olfactory hallucinations*—they "smell' substances which are not present.

In dogs, cats and other animals, the olfactory lobes and the sense of smell are very highly developed. Because of this faculty, dogs are employed in tracking down fugitives and identifying certain concealed narcotic drugs. *See also* ANOSMIA; NOSE; OLFACTORY SENSE; TASTE.

SMOG, a fog made heavier and darker by city smoke, as from automobile gas exhaust. It is a hazardous example of air pollution and aggravates asthma and

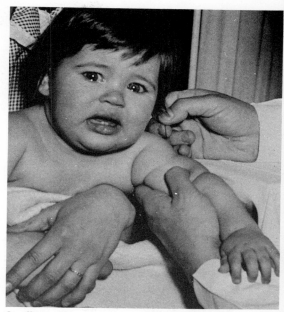

Smallpox—This was once a common occurrence as infants were given immunity against smallpox. A persistent vaccination program has eliminated the disease from most of the world.

bronchitis. *See also* AIR POLLUTION; TEMPERATURE INVERSION.

R^{ESEARCH}E P O R T *follows* AIR POLLUTION.

SMOKING AND LUNG CANCER. Cigarette smoking is largely responsible for the rapidly increasing occurrence of cancer of the lung and larynx. Cigarette advertising on television is prohibited in the United States and all packages there must carry a warning that it may be injurious to health. The carcinogenic tars in cigarettes are mostly to blame. It has also been established that nonsmokers who work in smoke-filled rooms are vulnerable to lung cancer as well. The smoking habit can be cured by will power and also by substituting a disagreeable lozenge for the cigarette whenever there is a desire to smoke. The fight against smoking will save many lives. *See also* CANCER; CANCER PREVENTION; CARCINOGENS; TOBACCO *and* **medigraph** LUNG CANCER.

SNAKE BITES

DEATH FROM SNAKEBITE in Europe is a rare occurrence since only the *adder* (viper) is poisonous. In India on the other hand, about 30,000 people die each year of the bites of *cobras, kraits, seasnakes* and *vipers.* No more than about 15 fatalities from snakebite occur annually in the United States where there are four kinds of poisonous snakes: *rattlesnakes, copperheads, moccasins* and *coral snakes.* The first three are known as "pit vipers" because of the concavity between the eye and the nostril on each side of the head. The coral snake is a type of cobra that has teeth behind its fangs. Most of the poisonous snake bites reported in this country are caused by rattlesnakes.

causes
The bite of a pit viper is *hemotoxic,* that is, the venom paralyzes the *circulatory system* by destroying the red blood cells and immobilizing the clotting mechanism. The venom of the coral snake is *neurotoxic* and directly affects the *nervous system.*

symptoms
The venom of a pit viper is deposited beneath the skin when it inflicts one or more puncture wounds with its fangs. The bite is acutely painful and is followed *rapidly* by swelling of the affected area which begins to turn reddish-blue because of the destruction of red blood cells. Within a period of 1–2 hours, the victim becomes weak, nauseous and short of breath. The vision dims and the pulse becomes rapid.

The bite of a coral snake causes less local pain but does greater damage. Pain and swelling at the site of the wound may be mild, but the effects on the nervous system become evident in slurred speech, blurred vision and drowsiness. Heavy sweating, salivation, respiratory distress, nausea and vomiting precede the onset of paralysis.

complications
If treatment is not administered within a few hours, the victim of either type of bite may go into convulsions, becoming comatose as the venom is increasingly absorbed and respiration fails. In all cases of snakebite, symptoms are aggravated by acute fear and anxiety since these emotions have a marked effect on hormone secretions which in turn affect cardiovascular responses.

treatment
Emergency measures consist of keeping the victim as still, calm and reassured as possible while the area of the bite is immobilized and if possible positioned below the level of the heart. The nearest doctor or hospital should be telephoned immediately so that antivenin will be available for treatment on arrival. Specialists feel that only a medically trained person should administer antivenin because of the victim's possible sensitivity to the horse serum which it contains. Such sensitivity may result in death from anaphylactic shock unless Adrenalin and antihistamines are available.

The damaged tissue at the site of the wound may be surgically removed to prevent gangrene. The incised area may require eventual reconstruction and skin grafting. Antibiotics are always given as part of treatment even when the bite is not poisonous, on the assumption that all snakes have disease-causing bacteria in their mouths. Tetanus shots are also administered if the victim has not had any for five years.

prevention
All campers, hikers and workers who travel on foot through snake-infested wooded or swampy areas should wear

Snake Bites (Poisonous Snakes)

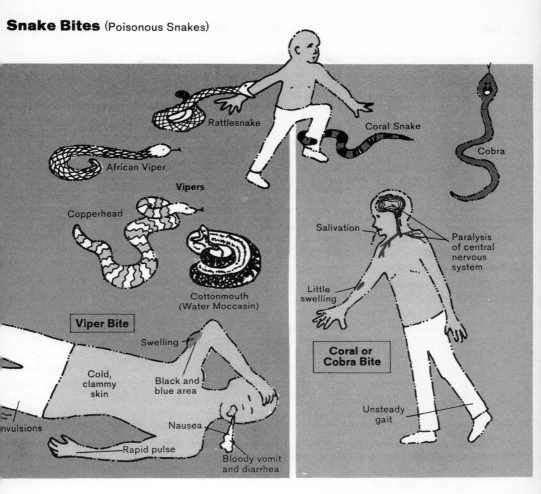

Rattlesnake

Coral Snake

Cobra

African Viper

Vipers

Copperhead

Cottonmouth
(Water Moccasin)

Salivation

Paralysis
of central
nervous
system

Little
swelling

**Coral or
Cobra Bite**

Unsteady
gait

Viper Bite

Swelling

Cold,
clammy
skin

Black and
blue area

Convulsions

Nausea

Rapid pulse

Bloody vomit
and diarrhea

1 Put tourniquet
above site of bite
to prevent spread
of infection

2 Make incision
crosswise thru
bite with
sterilized knife

3 Use suction cup or
mouth to suck all
blood or venom in
wound

Quick Action Can Prevent Snake Bites from Becoming Fatal

4 Kill snake to
bring to doctor
for identification

5 No exertion or
stimulants for
snakebite victim

6 Rush victim to
doctor to administer
antivenom serum

1331

boots, long pants and protective gloves. They should also be proficient in first-aid treatment if the areas are at a considerable distance from transportation to a doctor or hospital.

SNEEZING, a reflex action similar to a cough, manifested by a sudden uncontrollable violent expulsion of air through the nose and mouth. It may be caused by air pollution, inhaling an irritant, a cold, hay fever or influenza. Standing barefoot on a cold floor or staring at a bright light may also start sneezing. When sneezing, a person must be careful to cover his nose and mouth with a handkerchief or tissue because the expelled mucus and droplets often carry viruses and bacteria that may infect nearby persons.

A sneeze can often be suppressed by pressing the fingers between the end of the nose and the upper lip. Persistent sneezing may be relieved by application of an ephedrine solution. *See also* COLD, COMMON *and* **medigraph** HAY FEVER.

SNORING, habitual breathing through the mouth during sleep so as to cause a rough audible sound, due to vibration of the soft palate. It may be due to adenoids, a deflected nasal septum, partial obstruction of the nose or throat, the habit of sleeping with the mouth open or on the back instead of the side, or an unconscious falling backward of the tongue or soft palate. The snoring habit is hard to break and annoys others who must sleep in the same room. The best way to stop snoring is to correct any functional causes. If this does not work, the person should try to sleep on the side and keep the mouth closed. *See also* ADENOIDS *and* **medigraph** DEVIATED SEPTUM.

SNOW BLINDNESS, temporary loss of vision resulting from the glare of bright sunlight upon surrounding snow. It is due to fatigue of the retina and is relieved by rest in a dark room. Snow blindness af-

fects people walking or driving in high altitudes and may cause accidents if the afflicted person is driving a car. *See also* EYE.

SODIUM BICARBONATE, an antacid used in the relief of hyperacidity of the stomach and gastric ulcer; also, baking soda used in cooking. Since its action is brief, it may be followed by an acid rebound and upset the acid-base balance of the system. Sodium bicarbonate has largely been replaced in treatment by other antacids. *See also* BICARBONATE OF SODA.

SODOMY, a sexual act performed by inserting the penis into the rectum of the partner. Legally, the term *sodomy* includes any abnormal sexual act. *See also* SEXUAL ABNORMALITIES.

SOLAR PLEXUS, a network of nerves in the abdomen behind the stomach, which is sensitive to blows, a reason that boxers seek to punch it to gain a knockout. It belongs to the *sympathetic nervous system. See also* NERVOUS SYSTEM.

SOMNAMBULISM. *See* SLEEPWALKING.

SOPORIFIC, producing sleep, applicable to boredom or to hypnotic drugs such as *opiates, barbiturates, bromides* and *tranquilizers.*

SORE THROAT, *pharyngitis,* a symptom of many illnesses including colds, influenza, tonsillitis, quinsy, diphtheria, measles, scarlet fever, rheumatic fever and syphilis; also due to heavy smoking and cold damp weather. Temporary relief may be obtained by swallowing honey or sucking a soothing lozenge. *See also* PHARYNX.

SPACE MEDICINE, medical care and study of astronauts, who live in sealed cabins under conditions different from those on earth. They are subject to weightlessness, cold, lack of natural oxygen, restriction of movement and many other unnatural conditions. The cabin is pressurized and, in addition, the astronaut is provided with a specially fitted space suit. An artificial atmosphere containing oxygen is created inside the spaceship and the exhaled carbon dioxide is neutralized chemically. Food and liquids are supplied in plastic containers which can be squeezed to eject their contents directly into the mouth. Urine is voided into a container built in the space suit. The Soviet astronauts use various artificial means to manufacture water inside the capsule and salt is added. Tablets are added as vitamin and mineral supplements to the diet and necessary drugs are supplied. Shielding substances are used to protect the astronauts from heat, sunburn and ionizing radiation, especially to the eyes.

The space physician on earth continuously studies the physiological changes of the astronauts in flight, who radio to earth such measurements as blood pressure, pulse rate, rate of breathing and electrocardiograms. In space flights orbiting the earth, there are no significant changes.

Since astronauts are carefully selected for their adaptability to a different environment, it is not surprising that they usually do not suffer from psychological disturbances. The ordinary person is more likely to become maladjusted when his way of life is suddenly changed. On their return to earth, the astronauts are screened for a short period and examined by physicians for their health and the possibility that they might have contracted new types of viruses and bacteria in outer space.

Progress in space medicine has led to advances in general medicine and the development of instrumental procedures such as *microinstrumentation* and *biotelemetry*. The possibilities of studying plant and animal life on other planets, radioactivity, and lethal viruses and bacteria are of great interest to both astronomers and physicians.

SPANISH FLY. *See* CANTHARIDES.

SPASM, a cramp or sudden involuntary muscular contraction, either single or multiple. The most common spasm is of the calf and leg muscles occurring at night. A *tonic spasm* is a sustained contraction, while a *clonic spasm* contracts and relaxes alternately. A general spasm over the whole body is called a convulsion or fit—such as occurs in *epilepsy*. Spasms may be caused by muscular fatigue, a psychological reaction, or irritation of the nerves that supply the spasmodic muscles. Spasms commonly affect infants and young children and last only a few seconds. Sudden chilling of the body while swimming may cause severe disabling cramps or spasms.

Some of the more serious spasms are: of the coronary arteries in the heart, causing *angina pectoris;* of the bronchial tubes in the lungs, causing *asthma;* of the gullet, causing difficulty in swallowing; of the midriff, causing hiccup; of the pyloric end of the stomach, causing severe pain; of the gallbladder ducts, causing *colic;* of the bladder, causing difficult and painful urination; and of the large arteries of the brain, causing a minor stroke. A deficiency of the parathyroid gland in the neck causes painful prolonged muscular spasms, called *tetany*. *Habit spasms* (tics) may develop in children as a form of imitation. *Winking spasm* (*blepharospasm*) is a spasmodic twitching and blinking of the eyelids; *nodding spasm,* associated with wryneck. *Writer's cramp* is an occupational spasm of the hand of psychological origin. The twitching and grimacing of *chorea* are not true spasms. See also CLONUS; CONVULSION; CRAMPS; HABIT SPASM; HICCUPS; MUSCLE DISEASES AND DISORDERS;

NERVOUS SYSTEM *and* **medigraphs** BRON-
CHIAL ASTHMA; EPILEPSY; STROKE.

SPASTICITY, tightness and tension of a
muscle or group of muscles, impairing
their natural function and increasing
their deep reflexes. Spasticity is typical
of *Parkinson's disease, amyotrophic lateral sclerosis,* the paralyzed side after
apoplexy, and in association with certain
other diseases of the nervous system.
See also AMYOTROPHIC DISEASES; APO-
PLEXY; GAIT; NERVOUS SYSTEM; PARAL-
YSIS *and* **medigraphs** CEREBRAL PALSY;
MERCURY POISONING; PARKINSON'S DIS-
EASE; STROKE.

SPEECH, the utterance of spoken words
representing ideas or feelings. Speech is
produced by vibrations of the vocal cords
associated with corresponding movements
of the mouth, throat, tongue, teeth and
soft palate. The center of speech is located in the cortex—the gray matter of
the left rear convolution of the frontal
lobe of the brain, adjoining the motor
centers for the body (on the right side in
lefthanded persons). When this center
is destroyed—as may occur in a stroke
affecting the right side—speech is lost
and the condition is called *motor aphasia.*

Most children learn to speak by listening to their parents talk and associating
words with actions. They adopt the
words, accents, inflections, and manner-
isms of those around them. In most cases,
the child can speak well enough to com-
municate feelings, wishes and thoughts
by the end of the first year. The facility
of speech is an index of the child's mental
development.

Hoarseness in speaking may be due to
laryngitis, inhaling tobacco smoke, or too
much talking or singing; it may also be
temporarily due to a cold or influenza.
In most cases of laryngitis, inhalation of
warm steam from a vaporizer is helpful.

A *lisp* is a manner of speaking in which
the sibilant letters s and z are pronounced
like th. This is sometimes caused by an
abnormal shortness of the membrane
connecting the base of the tongue to the
floor of the mouth and can be corrected
by surgery. If the lisp is a careless habit,
it can be corrected by practice. *Stammering* and *stuttering* are habits of interrupted and hesitant speech with inability
to enunciate the syllables without repeated effort. This condition is of psychological origin and may require training
and the help of a speech therapist.

Aphonia or complete loss of the voice
may indicate a serious disease of the
larynx or hysteria. Speech defects caused
by *harelip* or *cleft palate* are corrected
by surgical closure of the gap. *See also*
APHASIA; APHONIA; BIRTH DEFECT; BRAIN;
CLEFT PALATE; DEAF MUTISM; DUMBNESS;
LARYNGITIS; LARYNX; STUTTERING; VOCAL
CORDS AND VOICE *and* **medigraphs** ALCO-
HOLISM; AMPHETAMINE ABUSE; BOTULISM;
CEREBRAL PALSY; MESCALINE ABUSE; MUL-
TIPLE SCLEROSIS; PARKINSON'S DISEASE;
POLIOMYELITIS; STROKE.

R_{EPORT}ESEARCH *follows* MENTAL RETARDATION.

RESEARCH
EPORT

SUCCESSFUL NEW SPEECH
THERAPY USES COMPUTER-BASED
SYSTEM

Computer-based feedback instruments are now being used for correcting the faulty speech articulation
of patients who have not been helped
by traditional therapy. Through the
combined efforts of speech patholo-
gists, physiologists, dentists, and electrical engineers at the UNIVERSITY OF
ALABAMA, the OUTPATIENT CLINICAL
RESEARCH CENTER has devised a new
diagnostic and treatment system known
as *PAGIS.*

In this system, electrodes or "beads"
embedded in a thin plate are placed
against the roof of the patient's
mouth to detect tongue contacts. A
video-based system determines lip
and jaw movements by scanning the
"beads" attached to the face and one
tooth.

As the patient speaks, a display
panel lights up when he touches dif-

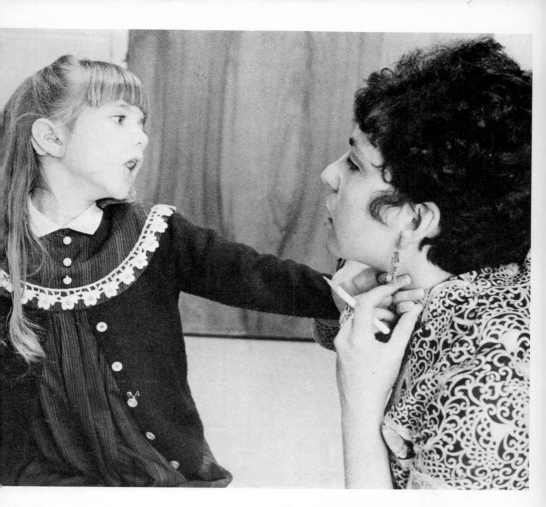

Children with serious speech and hearing difficulties can now be helped to overcome their problems through the services and facilities of special speech-hearing therapy centers. Many such centers are to be found throughout the United States. At all these centers, comprehensive "work and play" exercises are employed to diagnose and correct a wide range of speech and hearing defects. Since the trained specialists administer all therapeutic programs under the guise of games, children undergoing remedial treatment find the experiences fun. Enjoyment is important in helping these children overcome their impediments. Playing games with toys, mirrors, and earphones becomes a painless way of learning to hear and speak better. Initially, children brought to the centers are tested for auditory (hearing) discrimination and receptivity. Some

hearing difficulties in children may be due simply to a lack of normal reaction to auditory stimuli (sound). Various exercises serve to enhance these reactions and to develop improved coordination between visual and auditory reactions (that is, between seeing and hearing). Proper hearing is an essential step in overcoming speech defects. Therapy games are specially designed to stimulate speech and language production. Through group experiences and activities, the boys and girls are encouraged to participate in "spontaneous speech practice." The therapy programs also include systematic exercises to improve the muscular control of the speech-producing organs. Above, a therapist conducts a test with this young girl, who feels with sensitive fingertips the therapist's vocal chord vibrations as an aid in producing her own speech sounds.

Young children cannot be expected to understand the importance of correct speech. Therefore, it is essential to devise remedial programs which the children can enjoy. Children will respond much more readily to therapy presented in a game format than to a more formal therapeutic approach they might construe as dull or tiresome.

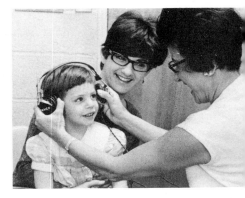

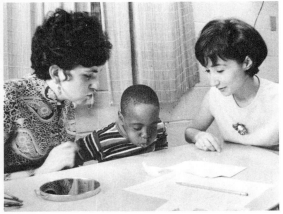

Two students in speech correction and audiology *(left)* conduct a test for muscular coordination. The boy is asked to blow the piece of paper as far as he can. Above, the therapist adjusts a pair of earphones on the child preparatory to a test for receptivity to sound. Below, the clinicians supervise a "spontaneous speech practice" session for a group of children with defective speech. Improvements in speech can be dramatic when remedial training is made enjoyable.

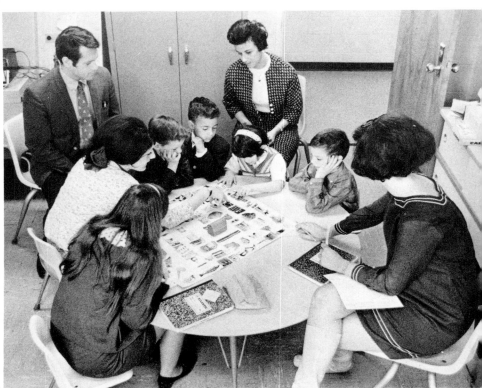

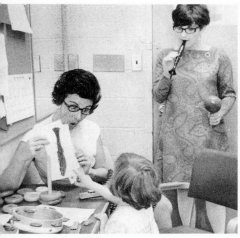
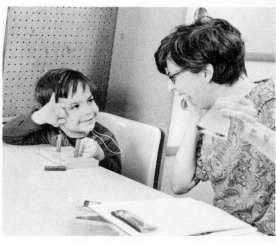

Many speech disorders are due either to actual hearing difficulties or to an impairment or disturbance of auditory perception. Professional speech therapists have devised various ingenious tests which simultaneously measure hearing acuity and allow the children to have fun. Above left, therapists administer a test to determine hearing response. The child is taught to identify musical sounds and to associate them with specific musical instruments, such as the recorder, castanets, and tambourines shown here. Above right, with the help of the student therapist, a young boy learns to place a peg in a hole whenever he hears a sound. The experiment tests the child's awareness of the presence and absence of sound. Below, a group activity session aimed at teaching children to play and work together cooperatively. The therapists are leading a game of "this is my right hand." This could be called "painless learning."

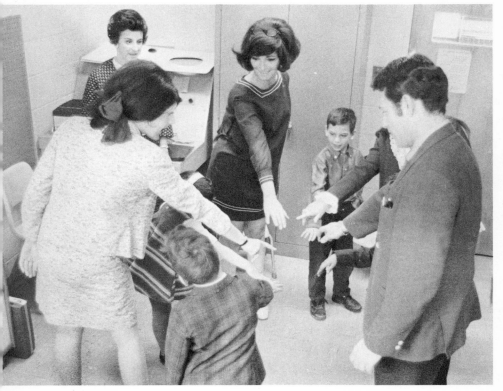

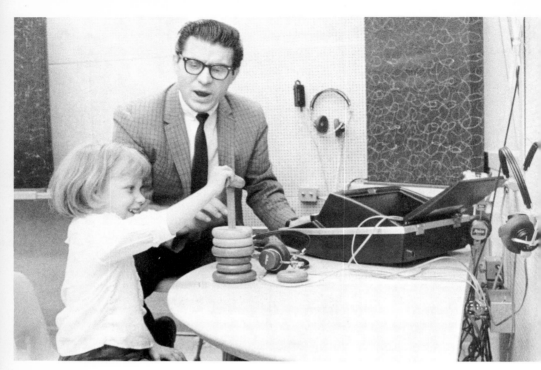

Putting "donuts" on a stick is part of one hearing tests (above). Note the earphones and sophisticated measuring instruments. Be- low, a boy practices looking, listening, and then saying a word. The therapists reinforce every response he makes.

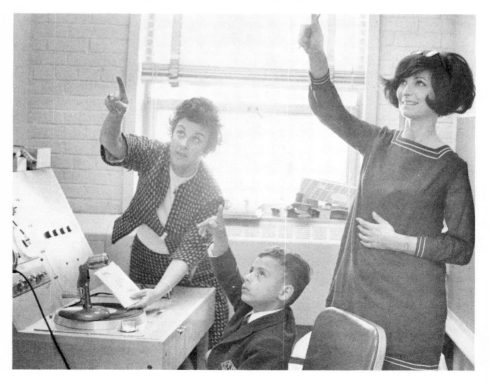

○ ferent parts of the roof of his mouth, allowing him to see and feel what
○ happens in his mouth during faulty articulation. Adjacent to this panel is
○ a computer-produced pattern of activities in the mouth during proper artic-
○ ulation. The patient then attempts to change his own visualized pattern so
○ that it conforms to the correct one. During these attempts, he can see,
○ hear, and feel the results, and as the new movements become part of a
○ habitual sensory pattern, the correct procedures replace the faulty ones.
○   In one case, a patient who had un-
○ dergone three years of traditional
○ speech therapy for the correction of a faulty "s" sound—with no success
○ —began to produce the correct sound after only one hour of PAGIS treat-
○ ment.   NIH815

SPERM, one of the secretions of the testicles. Also defined as the *spermatozöon* —male sex cell—which penetrates the female egg to produce pregnancy. It has a well-defined head, a midsection, and a swimming action which enables it to reach the female sex cell when ejected into the vagina during intercourse. *See also* RE-PRODUCTIVE SYSTEM.

SPERMATIC CORDS, two cords by which the testicles are suspended in the scrotum from the abdominal inguinal ring in the groin. The left cord is longer than the right, therefore the left testicle hangs lower. The spermatic cord is composed of arteries, veins, lymphatics, nerves, and the excretory duct of the testicle, connected by *areolar* tissue (filled with small openings or spaces) and covered by layers of membrane from the testicle. A thin muscle, the *cremaster,* passes alongside the spermatic cord and to a small extent moves the testicle toward or away from the body depending on the external temperature.

The spermatic cords—particularly the left—are subject to *varicocele* (varicosity of the veins). *See also* REPRODUCTIVE SYSTEM; SPERM; TESTICLES *and* **medigraph** VARICOCELE.

SPERMATOGENESIS, the manufacture of millions of spermatozoa (sperm cells) by the testicles, carrying the inherited characteristics in their chromosomes and capable of swimming to the female egg and starting pregnancy after ejaculation into the vagina. *See also* REPRODUCTIVE SYSTEM; SPERM; TESTICLES.

SPHINCTER, a ringlike muscular band which closes an opening or passage when contracted. Typical sphincters close the anus, bladder, vagina, the opening of the gullet into the stomach, the *pyloric* opening of the stomach into the duodenum (first part of the small intestine), and the openings of the *biliary* and *pancreatic* passages, respectively. There are many other sphincters.

SPHYGMOMANOMETER, an instrument for measuring the blood pressure. It is equipped with a tube containing a column of mercury calibrated to indicate the pressure when the level is indicated by the sound of the pulse passing through the constricted artery in the arm; it also contains an inflatable cuff and a rubber bulb. It is part of the standard equipment in a doctor's office. *See also* BLOOD PRESSURE; MEDICAL INSTRUMENTATION *and* **medigraph** HIGH BLOOD PRESSURE.

SPIDER BITES. Although all spiders have poison glands for killing their prey, only a few are a danger to man. In the United States, the *black widow* and the *brown recluse spiders* are capable of inflicting a serious bite.

BLACK WIDOW SPIDER, a common arachnid in North and South America. The highly venomous female is about half an inch long and derives its name from the fact that it sometimes eats its mate after copulation. The abdomen is about the size of a marble and has a red or yellowish hourglass-shaped marking on the underside. The spider spins her web in various protected sites, including dark corners of basements, outhouses, and beneath privy seats. When disturbed, the black widow bites, most often on the genitals, the buttocks or thighs.

The bite is felt as a sharp prick, soon followed by swelling and redness, after which the nerve poison spreads rapidly throughout the body. The victim soon suffers from dizziness and weakness, the legs tremble, and often the victim has stomach cramps with rigid abdominal muscles. Other symptoms include difficulty in urination, slow and feeble pulse, and labored breathing and speech. In severe cases delirium, stupor and convulsions may follow. Usually the acute symptoms subside within 48 hours. The death rate is estimated at about five percent.

Although the black widow is not an insect, it is readily killed by effective insecticides. Because it reacts so viciously, it should never be disturbed. A specific

Spider Bites—The female black widow spider most often bites on the genitals, buttocks or thighs. The venomous bite of the brown recluse spider causes great pain, high fever and chills.

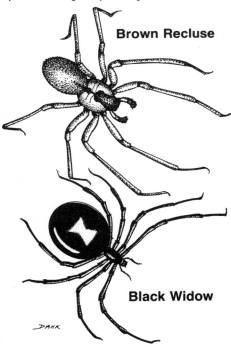

Brown Recluse

Black Widow

antivenin is prepared from the serum of immunized horses and should be injected into the shoulder muscle—never intravenously. Under the supervision of a physician, the victim should avoid all exertion and alcoholic beverages. Analgesics are given to relieve the pain, and injection of a relaxant, accompanied by hot baths or hot packs, brings relief from severe muscle spasms.

BROWN RECLUSE SPIDER, a dangerous arachnid found in the southern and midwestern United States. Although this spider usually lives under stones or in the bark of trees, it may occasionally secrete itself in cellars or closets where humans will be most likely to encounter it.

The bite of the brown recluse spider is exceedingly venomous, and affects both the nervous system and the bloodstream. Symptoms appear 6–8 hours after the bite, with inflammations and tenderness at the site. After 12–24 hours, high fever, chills, and sometimes nausea and vomiting develop. At about 36 hours, a measles-like rash may erupt over the entire body. After two days, the skin around the site of the bite turns white (because of impaired blood supply), and *necrosis* (death of the cells) sets in. The pain becomes so excruciating that even narcotics may be unable to give relief.

Fortunately, bites by the brown recluse spider are rare. They usually occur when the spider becomes trapped in sheets or blankets. Therefore, campers, especially, should examine their sheets and blankets carefully before using them. Sheets and blankets which have been in a closet for a long time should also be carefully examined before use.

Treatment is with powerful analgesics and sedatives to relieve the pain, and with corticosteroids, antihistamines, and antibiotics to counteract the venom. Drugs have been used to minimize necrosis and gangrene. In many cases, surgical excision of the necrotic area is the preferred treatment, and this usually relieves the pain. Plastic surgery may then be necessary to restore the appearance of the area.

The spider can be controlled by spraying likely hiding places with potent insecticides. *See also* ANIMAL BITES AND WOUNDS; FIRST AID.

SPINA BIFIDA, *split spine,* a congenital birth defect in which the spine in the *lumbosacral* region fails to close and the membranes covering the spinal cord—containing cerebrospinal fluid and sometimes nervous tissue—protrude as a *hernia.* Each year, approximately 6000 babies are born with spina bifida and the specific form of the defect varies. The functions of the lower spinal nerves may be disturbed, sometimes resulting in paralysis of the legs and loss of control over the bladder and bowels. If the nerve supply of the skin is inadequate, ulcers may develop. Sometimes spina bifida is accompanied by *hydrocephalus* (water on the brain). Surgical repair of the split spine should be undertaken as early as possible with good results in more than half of the cases. *See also* BIRTH DEFECT; GENETIC COUNSELING; HYDROCEPHALUS.

Spina Bifida

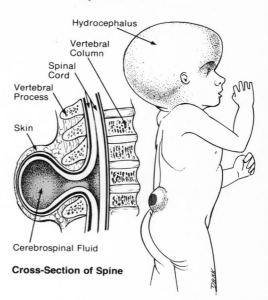

Cross-Section of Spine

Spina Bifida—This disabling condition results when certain vertebrae fail to develop fully during pregnancy. This causes a gap in the vertebral column through which the spinal cord protrudes, as shown. Varying degrees of both loss of bladder and bowel control and paralysis below the opening occur. Hydrocephaly (water on the brain) is sometimes also present with the disorder.

SPINAL CORD, an elongated, nearly cylindrical extension of the central nervous system from the brain and *medulla oblongata,* about 18 inches long and as thick as the little finger, passing through the hollow of the spinal column and giving off 31 pairs of spinal nerves. Since the vertebral column is much longer than the spinal cord, many of the spinal nerves which serve the lower parts of the body emerge from the cord at higher levels and continue downward through the rest of the spinal column.

Like the brain, the spinal cord is covered by three *meningeal membranes.* The cord is composed of H-shaped gray matter in the center, extending forward as the *anterior nerve roots* and backward as the *posterior nerve roots,* and solid

white tracts of nerve fibers descending from the brain or ascending to it. The anterior nerve roots are motor in function and control the various muscles; the posterior nerve roots are sensory and carry messages to the brain. The spinal cord controls *reflex actions,* which never reach the brain. Some of the reflexes include the self-protective action of jumping away from a hot object or other source of pain, control of the bladder and rectum, erection of the penis during sexual excitement, the peristaltic (wormlike) movements of the intestines during digestion, the control of breathing and the heartbeat, and the knee jerk diagnostic sign.

The principal diseases to which the spinal cord is exposed are *anterior polio-*

Spinal Curvatures

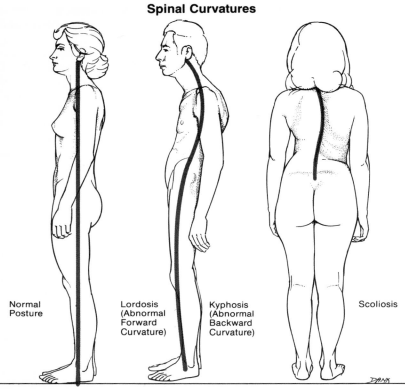

Normal
Posture

Lordosis
(Abnormal
Forward
Curvature)

Kyphosis
(Abnormal
Backward
Curvature)

Scoliosis

Spinal Curvature—A drawing compares a torso with a normal spine (*left*) to those with malformations of the spinal structure. Excessive curving of the spine backward in the chest area is kyphosis, which can be congenital or caused by disease. Abnormal increase of the forward curve of the lower spine is lordosis. The center figure shows both in a condition called double curvature. Lordosis and kyphosis also occur separately in individuals. Scoliosis (*right*) is a displacement sideways of a section of spine, usually the upper, and can be caused or aggravated by poor posture.

myelitis (infantile paralysis), in which the anterior motor nerve roots are destroyed; *transverse myelitis,* extending across the spinal cord; *multiple sclerosis,* with patches of scar tissue in the brain and spinal cord; *amyotrophic lateral sclerosis,* with hardening of the lateral white columns and spastic paralysis of the legs; and *syringomyelia,* in which the senses of heat and pain are lost in certain areas but the senses of touch and pressure are retained.

Acute spinal meningitis is an infection of the membranes surrounding the spinal cord, for which various antibiotics are effective. The spinal cord may be injured also by fractures of the vertebrae, concussion, and the pressure of tumors causing temporary paralysis. *See also* BACKACHE; BRAIN; GLIOMA; KNEE JERK; MEDULLA; MENINGES; NERVOUS SYSTEM; PARALYSIS; SPINAL INJURIES; TABES DORSALIS *and* **medigraphs** MENINGITIS; MULTIPLE SCLEROSIS; POLIOMYELITIS.

SPINAL CURVATURE. The spinal column, composed of 33 vertebrae—connected blocks—is shaped somewhat like the letter S if seen from the side. The portions in the neck and loin region are curved convex forward; in the thoracic and lowest region, concave forward. The spine has springiness and elasticity which protect the brain and other organs from constant shocks and jolts.

There are four principal deviations from the normal spinal curvature: scoliosis, kyphosis, lordosis, and round shoulders.

Scoliosis is a lateral curvature of the spine, named according to the location and direction of the convexity, most often in the thoracic region. Usually there are two curves, the original and a compensatory curve—for example, an original right thoracic with a compensatory left curve in the loin region. In most instances scoliosis is due to bad posture and can be corrected by training and exercises.

Kyphosis is an angular curvature of the spine pointing backward, usually situated in the thoracic region and involving a number of vertebrae. It is found in hunchbacks and is caused by tuberculosis, arthritis or injury and is aggravated by improper posture.

Lordosis is an increased forward curvature of the lower spine in which the person is inclined to sway backward. It may be associated with pregnancy, enlargement of the abdomen in obesity or cirrhosis of the liver, and disease of the hip joint. However, it is a normal ana-

tomical characteristic of some ethnic groups, notably African blacks and their descendants.

The *round-shouldered curvature,* due to faulty posture, manifests itself as drooping of the shoulders and increased concavity of the thoracic spine. It is common in weak, poorly developed young women and can be corrected by tennis and other forms of athletics. Spinal curvature may weaken the ligaments and lead to displacement of vital organs— such as a floating kidney for example. *See also* BACKACHE; KYPHOSIS; LORDOSIS; POSTURE.

SPINAL INJURIES include broken neck, broken spine, fractures of other vertebrae and dislocations sometimes caused by wrestling, twisting dances and unskillful manipulation. As the spinal cord may be involved and ligaments may be torn, such injuries can be serious.

Any break of the vertebrae in the spine —resulting from causes such as falls, automobile accidents, a sudden violent jerk or assault, excessive effort to lift or move a heavy load, or war injury—is a spinal fracture. The most severe are broken neck and broken spine. Such fractures may cause paralysis in one or more parts of the body. In some cases the spinal cord is injured with serious consequences. Spinal fracture is suspected when the victim is unable to stand or walk. The diagnosis is established by x-ray examination.

In first aid, the person suspected of suffering from a spinal fracture should be moved as little as possible to avoid further injury and displacement of the fragments. The victim should be left lying down and covered with a blanket until the ambulance or a doctor arrives, when the victim is usually removed on a board. If the neck is broken, the head must be kept motionless. When there is shock, the head should be lowered. In the operating room the surgeon attempts to replace the broken bone fragments and

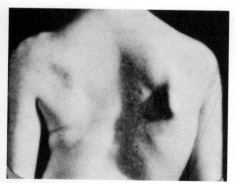

Spinal Curvature—This type of sideways curvature is called scoliosis. Sometimes it begins in infancy, but it is more common in adolescence. Prolonged poor posture or a bone-affecting disease such as rickets can be the cause.

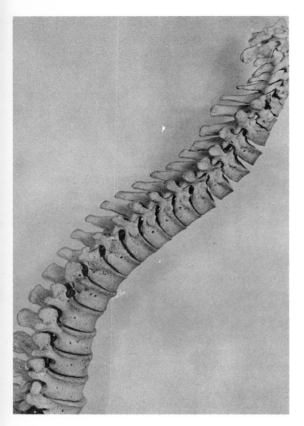

Spine—This is how the spinal column adjusts when a person bends forward with the head erect. The two topmost vertebrae are specially adapted to support the head and its movements. These 24 vertebrae are separated by discs, not shown in the model. The pads of fibrocartilage absorb shocks and promote flexibility of the spine.

bind them in place until healing occurs. *See also* BACKACHE; NECK, BROKEN; PARALYSIS; RUPTURED DISC; SPINAL CORD *and* **medigraphs** FRACTURES AND DISLOCATIONS; SLIPPED DISC; WHIPLASH INJURY OF THE NECK.

SPINAL TAP, *lumbar puncture,* withdrawal of a specimen of *cerebrospinal fluid* from the loin region of the spine for diagnostic examination. A sterile hollow special needle is inserted between the third and fourth lumbar vertebrae until

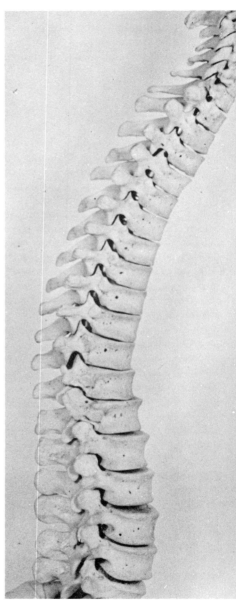

Spine—A closeup of a model of an erect spine emphasizes its extraordinary structure. The top seven bones are the cervical vertebrae of the neck. Next are the twelve thoracic vertebrae of the chest region. The next five are the large lumbar vertebrae that form the lower back and bear the weight of the trunk. Not visible are the sacrum and coccyx at the base of the spine.

the clear fluid pours out into the test tube. If the fluid spurts out, there may be pressure in the brain. Pus in the spinal fluid indicates *meningitis;* blood may indicate an injury or simply that the needle accidentally struck a vein while it was being inserted. A positive Wassermann reaction establishes the diagnosis of syphilis of the nervous system—such as *general paresis* or *tabes dorsalis.* The nature of the infection may be indicated by the cell count or a culture of the spinal fluid. *See also* PARESIS *and* **medigraphs** MENINGITIS; SYPHILIS.

SPINE, the vertical column of 26 *vertebrae*—attached blocks—that maintains the body in its erect position. There are 7 vertebrae in the neck region, 12 in the *thorax,* 5 in the *loin,* the *sacrum* (lower back), and the *coccyx* at the lower end of the spine. (In a baby, there are 5 bones in the sacrum and 4 in the coccyx, but these are fused together by the time a person reaches adulthood.)

The spine is shaped like the letter S with two curvatures. In the neck and loin region, the spine is curved convex forward; in the thorax and lowest end, concave forward. It is springy and elastic, thus protecting the brain and other organs from shocks and jolts. The vertebrae are separated from each other by cartilaginous *intervertebral discs,* which further absorb shocks and facilitate turning and twisting motions without friction.

The spine is composed of such heavy bones and protected by such powerful muscles that it is strong enough to carry the weight of the skull and body. Anthropologists believe that the erect human spine is an evolutionary development from the horizontal posture of ancestral hominoids. *See also* BACKACHE; COCCYX; DISC; LUMBAR; RUPTURED DISC; SACRUM; SKELETAL SYSTEM; SPINA BIFIDA; SPINAL CORD; SPINAL CURVATURE; SPINAL INJURIES; SPINAL TAP; VERTEBRA *and* **medigraphs** FRACTURES AND DISLOCATIONS;

The Spleen

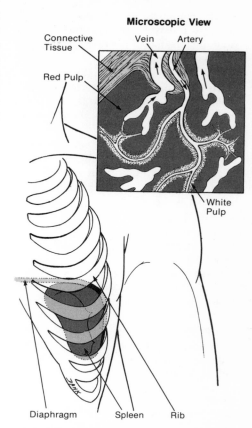

Microscopic View

Connective Tissue

Red Pulp

Vein   Artery

White Pulp

Diaphragm   Spleen   Rib

Spleen—This dark purple organ is at the lower left of the rib cage, behind the stomach. It manufactures white blood cells that help fight infection, stores blood and helps cleanse the blood of foreign materials. The inset shows an enlarged section of the spleen's pulpy tissue. The arteries are surrounded by white pulp, while the veins pass through red pulp. If the spleen is removed, the liver and bone marrow assume its functions.

OSTEOARTHRITIS; SLIPPED DISC; WHIPLASH INJURY OF THE NECK.

SPLEEN, a large organ situated behind the left lower ribs and extending behind the stomach and midriff. It is oblong and flattened, soft, dark purplish, full of blood and lymphatic vessels, weights about seven ounces, and measures five inches in length, three inches in breadth, and 1½ inches in thickness. The spleen is not an indispensable organ, as people survive after its removal. Its functions are not fully understood. Physicians know that the spleen manufactures *lymphocytes* (small white blood cells), stores broken-down red blood cells to replenish hemoglobin when needed, and is concerned with the metabolism of the *purine bodies* (that yield uric acid).

At times the spleen contracts, discharging a quantity of blood into the general circulation. For this reason the spleen is helpful in maintaining the proper volume of blood in the circulation. The spleen is insensitive to pain and can be transplanted outside the abdomen. It is believed to play an important part in the defensive mechanism against infection. *See also* BANTI'S SYNDROME; BLOOD; BLOOD CONDITIONS; LYMPHATIC SYSTEM; PURPURA; SPLENIC DISEASE; THROMBOCYTOPENIA; WHITE BLOOD CELLS, DISEASES OF *and* **medigraphs** CHAGAS' DISEASE; HISTOPLASMOSIS; HODGKIN'S DISEASE; LEUKEMIA; MALARIA; MONONUCLEOSIS, INFECTIOUS; PERNICIOUS ANEMIA; SCHISTOSOMIASIS; TOXOPLASMOSIS.

SPLENIC DISEASE, principally complications of other primary diseases. *Splenomegaly* (enlargement of the spleen) appears in malaria, Banti's disease, undulant fever, Hodgkin's disease, lymphatic leukemia, pernicious anemia, and certain infectious diseases.

The doctor can feel the enlarged spleen by pressing his fingers up behind the left lower ribs. Extreme enlargement of the spleen is usually associated with severe anemia. Splenomegaly is associated with *purpura hemorrhagica* and *thrombocytopenia*—in which blood platelets are lacking and the clotting time of the blood is delayed; removal of the spleen may be curative in some cases. Steroid therapy and blood platelet transfusions have also proved helpful. *See also* SPLEEN.

SPLINTERS, thin sharp slivers of wood, metal or other material which have been cut or torn off lengthwise and may penetrate the skin accidentally. A splinter should be removed gently with a tweezer. Then an effective antiseptic should be applied to prevent infection. Last, apply an adhesive bandage for protection. *See also* FIRST AID *and* **medigraph** TETANUS.

SPLINTS, pieces of flat wood, metal, plastic, wire or other material for immobilizing the ends of a fractured bone—restricting movements. They may be applied to hold the two fragments together and may be held in place with a suitable bandage. *See also* FIRST AID *and* **medigraph** FRACTURES AND DISLOCATIONS.

SPONDYLITIS, ankylosing, a chronic progressive disease of the sacroiliac joints and their spiny projections and *ankylosis* (welding together) of the bones of the spine. The disease resembles *rheumatoid arthritis*. The main symptoms are low back pain and stiffness and the diagnosis is established by the x-ray signs. Certain analgesics are effective in relief of the symptoms. *See also* ANKYLOSIS; BACKACHE *and* **medigraph** RHEUMATOID ARTHRITIS.

SPONDYLOLISTHESIS, slipped *vertebra,* forward displacement of one vertebra over another, usually of the fifth lumbar over the sacrum or of the fourth lumbar vertebra over the fifth. It is caused by a lateral defect of the vertebral arch or erosion of the articular surfaces due to degenerative joint disease. Because of lack of support, the condition causes backache radiating down the thigh and leg. The pain disappears at rest but returns on exertion. *See also* **medigraph** SLIPPED DISC.

SPOROTRICHOSIS, an infection of the skin and mucous membranes by a fungus (*Sporotrichum schenckii*) that grows on plants and brush, also occurring in horses,

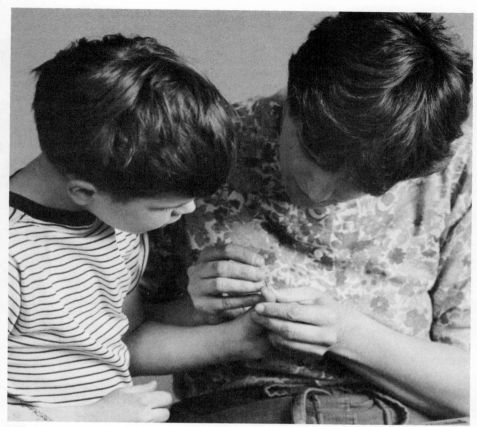

Splinters—A mother carefully works a splinter out of her son's thumb. If the tip of the imbedded sliver is below the surface, it can be gently teased out with a sterile needle, then grasped and pulled out with tweezers. The affected area should be washed before removal and covered with an antiseptic and a small bandage afterwards to avoid infection.

dogs and cats. Farmers, gardeners and miners are most often infected.

A hard rubbery growth appears at the site of the infection about 20 days to three months after contact with the fungus. It hardens, becomes inflamed and gradually breaks through the skin, discharging a small amount of thin pus. The surrounding area becomes discolored and finally turns black. In the *disseminated form,* small lumps under the skin spread over the body. The disease is rarely fatal and usually responds to drug treatment. *See also* SKIN *and* **medigraph** FUNGUS INFECTIONS OF THE SKIN.

SPOTS BEFORE THE EYES, most often an optical illusion. If you close your eyes and then suddenly open them and look up at the sky or a white ceiling, you will see a number of small spots moving before your eyes. They are blood corpuscles moving in the capillaries at the back of the eyes. Persistent spots before the eyes, if confirmed by an ophthalmoscopic examination, may indicate small hemorrhages in the retina due to high blood pressure or kidney disease. Certain drugs have proved helpful in the absorption of such retinal hemorrhages. *See also* EYE *and* **medigraph** CATARACTS.

Sprains and Strains

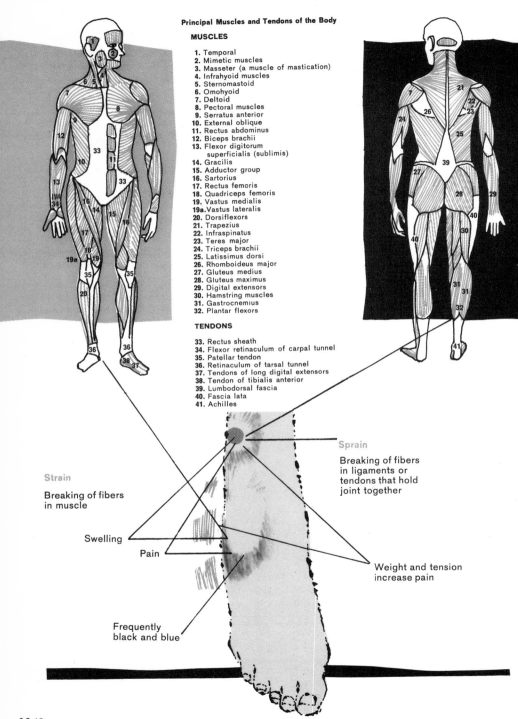

Principal Muscles and Tendons of the Body

MUSCLES

1. Temporal
2. Mimetic muscles
3. Masseter (a muscle of mastication)
4. Infrahyoid muscles
5. Sternomastoid
6. Omohyoid
7. Deltoid
8. Pectoral muscles
9. Serratus anterior
10. External oblique
11. Rectus abdominus
12. Biceps brachii
13. Flexor digitorum
    superficialis (sublimis)
14. Gracilis
15. Adductor group
16. Sartorius
17. Rectus femoris
18. Quadriceps femoris
19. Vastus medialis
19a. Vastus lateralis
20. Dorsiflexors
21. Trapezius
22. Infraspinatus
23. Teres major
24. Triceps brachii
25. Latissimus dorsi
26. Rhomboideus major
27. Gluteus medius
28. Gluteus maximus
29. Digital extensors
30. Hamstring muscles
31. Gastrocnemius
32. Plantar flexors

TENDONS

33. Rectus sheath
34. Flexor retinaculum of carpal tunnel
35. Patellar tendon
36. Retinaculum of tarsal tunnel
37. Tendons of long digital extensors
38. Tendon of tibialis anterior
39. Lumbodorsal fascia
40. Fascia lata
41. Achilles

Strain

Breaking of fibers
in muscle

Sprain

Breaking of fibers
in ligaments or
tendons that hold
joint together

Swelling

Pain

Weight and tension
increase pain

Frequently
black and blue

SPRAINS AND STRAINS

A SPRAIN IS AN INJURY to the soft tissues surrounding a joint. The ligaments that hold the joint in position may be stretched or torn, and the associated tendons and blood vessels will suffer mild or severe damage.

A strain is an injury to a muscle in which the fibers may be stretched or torn. It is a less serious injury than a sprain.

causes

SPRAIN, the result of a wrenching and twisting of a joint—as commonly occurs in a "twisted" ankle, or as occurs in an athletic mishap to a shoulder. Before the widespread use of safety seats and safety belts in automobiles, sprained necks were a frequent result of rear-end collisions causing whiplash injuries.

STRAIN. The area most affected by strained muscles is the lower back because of the frequency with which people lift heavy objects incorrectly or carry them without regard to how the weight is distributed. Strained leg, shoulder and wrist muscles are a risk of various athletic activities; "turned" ankles occur when footing is missed on stairs, or when high heels (or soles) cause loss of balance.

Both sprains and strains commonly result from such home accidents as falling off a ladder, falling down the cellar stairs, or slipping on a newly polished floor.

symptoms

In a severe *sprain,* the pain is so acute that the affected area cannot be moved. Swelling occurs together with discoloration of skin because of the internal bleeding of torn vessels. Since these symptoms may be difficult to distinguish from those produced by a fracture, an x-ray may be necessary before treatment is undertaken.

The chief symptom of a muscle *strain* is pain, rarely accompanied by swelling and discoloration.

treatment

If an ankle or knee joint is *sprained,* the victim should not be permitted to walk, and the injured area should be elevated during the day and raised by several pillows at night. The site of the bruise should be covered with a clean handkerchief or cloth, and an ice pack applied for several minutes at a time every hour for two days. A wrung-out cold wet towel may be used instead of the ice. The sprained area should not be immersed in ice water. If the pain and swelling persist or increase after 24 hours of this treatment, a doctor should be consulted about the advisability of splinting and bandaging or the need for an x-ray.

Most ordinary *strains* are relieved by resting the affected part and the use of heat applications together with pain-relievers. Any back strain that causes severe pain should be diagnosed by a doctor.

prevention

Most sprains and strains can be prevented by exercising a normal amount of care and good sense about athletics, gymnastics, on-the-job risks and safety measures at home and elsewhere.

SPRUE, *tropical sprue,* a chronic nutritional deficiency of the small intestine marked by poor absorption of foods, particularly fats but also sugar and vitamins. It prevails mostly in the tropics but scattered cases also occur in the United States, Europe, and other temperate-climate areas. The illness begins insidiously with loss of appetite and flatulence followed by diarrhea, sore tongue, weakness and emaciation. The stools are bulky, frothy and foul-smelling, and the abdomen is distended and protruded. Brown discoloration of the skin often appears over the bare trunk and limbs. Blood pressure is reduced considerably. Some form of *anemia* is usually present, often resembling pernicious anemia with large red blood corpuscles and a reduction of the white blood cells and the platelets, which may cause purpura and hemorrhages in the skin and mucous membranes.

The standard treatment is a diet low in fat, high in protein and vitamins, and rich in bananas. Associated vitamin deficiencies should be treated with therapeutic doses of the lacking vitamins. Skim milk, calcium and iron supplements, vitamin B_{12}, and corticosteroid therapy have proved helpful. Injections of folic acid and liver extract bring about substantial relief in some cases. As a last resort, blood transfusions may prove life saving in critical cases. Broad-spectrum antibiotics have been used with reported success. *Non-tropical sprue (celiac disease)* is a distinct disorder. *See also* DEFICIENCY DISEASES; FOLIC ACID; MALABSORPTION SYNDROME *and* **medigraph** CELIAC DISEASE.

SPUTUM, a discharge expectorated from the lungs, bronchi, larynx or throat and removed chiefly by spitting. It may consist of saliva, mucus, pus and germs, sometimes with blood. Rusty sputum is common in the early stage of pneumonia, and a bloody discharge raises the suspicion of tuberculosis in the lungs. Microscopic and bacteriologic examinations of the sputum are standard diagnostic procedures.

SQUINT, *strabismus,* common in cross-eyed children, is the practice of looking obliquely at the visual object because the two eyes do not focus equally. In the most common form of strabismus, one eye looks toward the object while the other turns away from it. There are various other types of squint, which require diagnosis by an eye specialist (ophthalmologist).

In most cases strabismus may be cor-rected by training and special eyeglasses. Sometimes—when the muscles attached to the eyeball are of unequal length or strength—a short tight muscle must be cut or stretched. *See also* AMBLYOPIA; EYE.

STAMMERING. *See* STUTTERING.

STANFORD-BINET TEST, an adaptation of the French *Binet-Simon* intelligence (I.Q.) test to North American children and subjects. The test is conducted by asking a series of questions adapted to and standardized at the mental capacity of normal children at various ages. The questions are so worded as to test judgment, not memory. According to the answers given, the mental age of the subject is suggested in the form of a quotient. *See also* BINET-SIMON TEST; INTELLIGENCE; MENTAL RETARDATION.

STAPES OPERATION, a delicate operation on the *stapes*—the innermost of the three *auditory ossicles,* which is shaped like a stirrup. These three ossicles form a continuous chain for the transmission of sound to the hearing organ in the internal ear. The stapes and the other two ossicles may be involved in middle ear infections. *See also* EAR; OTOSCLEROSIS.

STAPHYLOCOCCUS, a dot-shaped germ arranged in clumps like a bunch of grapes. The most virulent variety is *Staphylococcus aureus* (orange colored) —a frequent cause of boils, styes, abscesses, bone marrow infection and sometimes pneumonia. It is the standard germ used in testing the potency of antiseptics. *Staphylococcus albus* is white and *Staphylococcus citreus* lemon yellow. *See also* ANTIBIOTICS; BACTERIA; INFECTION; INFECTIOUS DISEASES.

STARVATION, lack of sufficient food to sustain life. Famine is caused by overpopulation, war, floods, droughts, crop failures, inflation and food hoarding. Millions of people are destined to die of starvation unless the causes of famine are corrected. *See also* MALNUTRTION.

STEATORRHEA, fatty diarrhea, common in *sprue* and *celiac disease.* Bananas and a low fat diet are recommended for sprue, and a gluten-free diet for celiac disease sufferers. *See also* DIARRHEA; SPRUE *and* **medigraph** CELIAC DISEASE.

STEIN-LEVENTHAL SYNDROME, a symptom-complex characterized by enlarged ovaries, absence of menstruation, abnormal uterine bleeding, ovarian cysts, and sometimes retarded breast development, obesity and masculine hairiness. *See also* POLYCYSTIC OVARIES.

STENOSIS, constriction or narrowing of a channel—as in *mitral stenosis,* where the narrowed valve between the left atrium and the left ventricle obstructs the blood flow and reduces the capacity of the heart. *See also* HEART; MITRAL STENOSIS; PULMONARY STENOSIS *and* **medigraphs** ARTERIOSCLEROSIS; CONGENITAL HEART DISEASE; HEART FAILURE; STROKE. RESEARCH REPORT *follows* APOPLEXY.

STERILITY

STERILITY IS THE INABILITY of a male and female to produce children. This state of affairs is also called *infertility.* It is rarely absolute. In many cases thought to be hopeless by the couple themselves, it has turned out that the male's inability to fertilize the ovum or the female's inability to conceive was a condition that could be treated with positive results.

causes
In a small number of cases, sterility in the male may result from impotence or inability to perform the act of copulation. However, most instances are attributable to other circumstances. A failure in the production of a sufficient number of healthy *spermatozoa* may be due to undescended testicles; testicular atrophy resulting from radiation treatment or disease; excessive testicular heat because of tight clothing; chronic drug abuse or alcoholism; glandular disorders; obstruction of the seminal tract; abnormalities of the urethra or prostate; or untreated venereal disease.

A woman who is unable to conceive because her generative organs are structurally or functionally inadequate is said to be *absolutely* sterile. Far more cases are those whose sterility is relative, so that under the proper conditions, conception and pregnancy can occur. Among the many conditions that may prevent conception are deficient ovaries; chronic vaginal or cervical infection; tumors and cysts; glandular disorders that interfere with normal ovulation and menstruation; and psychological factors which in turn affect the endocrine system.

symptoms
Although the symptom is the disorder itself, the underlying causes have to be sorted out and diagnosed by examinations and tests. Obvious problems such as impotence or abnormality of ovulation need to be explored before other anomalies are investigated.

treatment
Treatment of male infertility depends on detailed diagnosis. Where disease, chronic fatigue, nutritional deficiencies, alcoholism, or other obvious causes are involved, proper rehabilitative therapy is undertaken. In a surprising number of cases, male infertility can be traced to the wearing of underclothing that is too tight,

Sterility

Can have many causes . . .

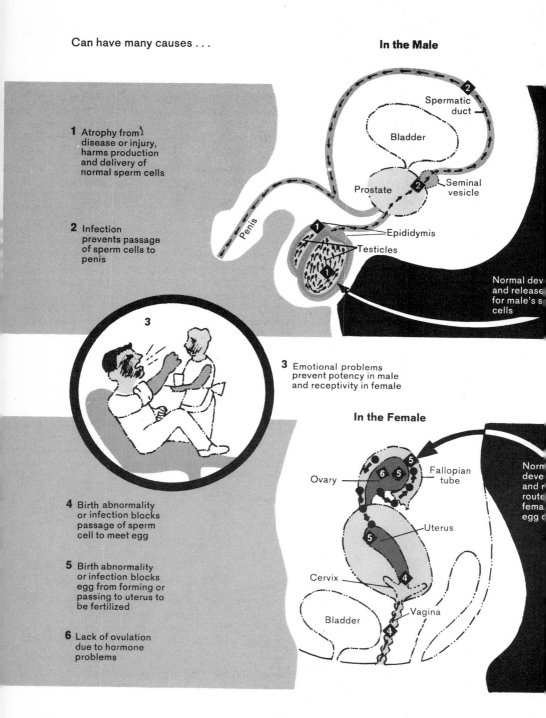

In the Male

Spermatic duct

Bladder

Prostate

Seminal vesicle

Penis

Epididymis

Testicles

Normal dev
and release
for male's s
cells

1 Atrophy from
disease or injury,
harms production
and delivery of
normal sperm cells

2 Infection
prevents passage
of sperm cells to
penis

3

3 Emotional problems
prevent potency in male
and receptivity in female

In the Female

Ovary

Fallopian tube

Uterus

Cervix

Vagina

Bladder

Norm
deve
and r
route
fema
egg c

4 Birth abnormality
or infection blocks
passage of sperm
cell to meet egg

5 Birth abnormality
or infection blocks
egg from forming or
passing to uterus to
be fertilized

6 Lack of ovulation
due to hormone
problems

preventing the testes from hanging freely and overheating the sperm. Where glandular aberrations need correction, thyroid and cortisone treatment may be effective. In some instances, surgical correction of obstruction may be essential.

In female sterility, removal of cysts or tumors may be necessary; surgical correction of a structural defect may be effective. Erratic ovulation as indicated by carefully kept temperature records may be corrected by estrogen and progesterone therapy.

Where sterility results from premature ejaculation, or because of a coital or emotional problem that resists treatment, and adoption is found unacceptable as a solution, artificial insemination using the man's semen—if it is viable—may be the only way for the couple to achieve parenthood.

STERILIZATION, the complete destruction of germs and viruses on surgical instruments, dressings and office equipment, such as hypodermic needles and syringes,

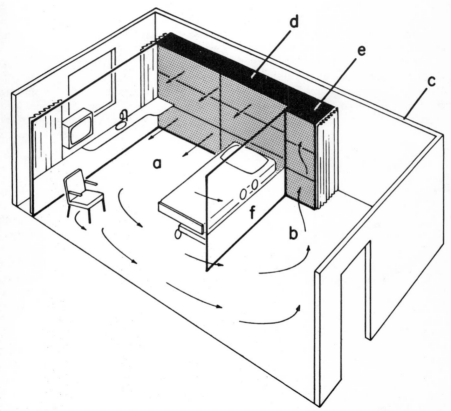

Courtesy, National Institutes of Health

Sterilization—Rooms where the air is kept 99.97 percent sterile provide extra protection for hospital patients who are infection-prone because of their disease or treatment. The clean air is drawn through filters (d) and circulates across the patient module (a). Exhaled air and airborne microorganisms flow to the anteroom (b) and are removed through another filter (e). Glove ports in a heavy vinyl curtain wall (f) allow the staff to tend patients without entering the germ-free area. Anyone who must enter it wears special disposable gown, gloves, boots, mask and cap.

to prevent infection. The approved methods are by heat in the form of wet steam under pressure at 120° C. for 15 minutes, dry heat at 360–380° C. for 3 hours, or immersion in liquid disinfectants.

Before surgery, the skin is usually sterilized by application of an antiseptic.

The term *sterilization* is also applied to operations which render the man or woman incapable of reproduction.

The procedures for making a woman incapable of bearing children include the operation of complete *hysterectomy* (removal of both the uterus and the ovaries), removal of the Fallopian tubes, or x-ray treatments. The simplest procedure is *laparoscopy,* in which the Fallopian tubes are located with a visualizing instrument and cauterized with a forceps inserted through small incisions in the abdominal wall without opening the adomen. The woman can still enjoy sexual intercourse after voluntary sterilization.

Tubal Ligation

Under Observation through a special Scope, the Fallopian Tube is grasped and an Elastic Band slid over a doubled-up Segment

Sterilization—The physician locates the Fallopian tubes with a laparoscope inserted through a small cut at the navel. Through another incision, a foreceps closes off each tube. This sterilization procedure is called laparoscopy.

The standard procedure for voluntary sterilization of a man is *vasectomy*—partial removal and tying of the *vas deferens* (the excretory ducts of the testicles). The operation does not make the man effeminate and he can still enjoy sexual intercourse.

It has been reported that about a million people are voluntarily sterilized in a year, about 80 percent of them men. *See also* ANTISEPTICS; FALLOPIAN TUBES; HYSTERECTOMY; VASECTOMY *and* **medigraph** STERILITY.

STEROIDS, a group of compounds resembling *cholesterol,* widely distributed in the body. Bile acids and sex hormones are steroids.
RESEARCH REPORT *follows* ASTHMA.

STERTOR, noisy breathing or snoring, such as the rasping rattling sound produced when the larynx (voice box) and the air passages are partially obstructed by mucus. *See also* SNORING.

STETHOSCOPE, the instrument used by physicians to hear the sounds produced by breathing, the heartbeat, the passage of blood through the valves, and movements in other parts of the body. It consists of a cup-shaped piece of metal or hard rubber, which is placed against the chest, connected with rubber tubing which conducts the sound to both ears of the examiner. *See also* AUSCULTATION; MEDICAL INSTRUMENTATION.

STIGMA, any mental or physical characteristic or peculiarity which is typical of a particular condition. The *stigmas of degeneracy* are abnormalities of the body which are found in degenerate persons. The *hysterical stigmas* encompass a wide variety of symptoms which are characteristic of hysteria.

STILLBIRTH, the birth of a dead child. Untreated syphilis causes eight times as

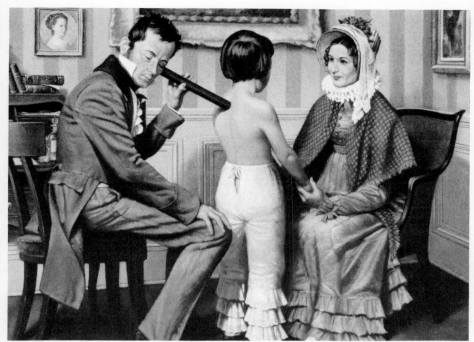

Stethoscope—In 1816, the French physician Theophile Laennec devised the first stethoscope—a hollow wooden cylinder—for listening to sounds in the chest. He learned to accurately diagnose heart and lung conditions by comparing opinions formed during stethoscopic examinations with later findings at autopsies. This led to understanding pulmonary diseases.

many stillbirths as occur in all other pregnancies. Syphilitic stillbirths can be prevented by a routine blood test during the early stage of pregnancy and treatment with an antibiotic when the report is positive. *See also* BIRTH DEFECT; GENETIC COUNSELING.

STIMULANTS, drugs that increase functional activity especially of the brain. Their excessive or injudicious use may be harmful. Coffee and tea are stimulating because of their caffeine content. Prescriptions for stimulant drugs are regulated by the Drug Enforcement Administration of the Department of Justice. Alcohol is not a stimulant. *See also* CAFFEINE; METHAMPHETAMINE *and* **medigraph** AMPHETAMINE ABUSE.

STINGS, the wounds from a bee, wasp, mosquito, spider or various insects. Such bites may transmit serious diseases such as malaria, yellow fever and sleeping sickness. *See also* ANIMAL BITES AND WOUNDS; BEE STINGS; INSECT BITES; MOSQUITO BITES; SPIDER BITES; WASP STINGS.

STOMACH, the large dilated J-shaped receptacle for swallowed food passing to it from the mouth through the gullet. It is situated below the midriff, lying mostly to the left but partly to the right, and extends from the midline to the region beneath the left lower ribs. The stomach has two openings: the *cardiac* where it connects with the gullet, and the *pyloric* where it extends to the first part of the small intestine and is closed by the pyloric valve and sphincter. There are two curvatures: the *lesser* and the *greater* (which is four to five times as long). There are four coats in the wall of the

The Stomach

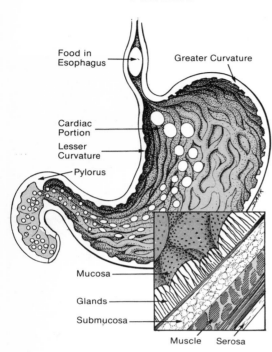

Food in Esophagus

Greater Curvature

Cardiac Portion

Lesser Curvature

Pylorus

Mucosa

Glands

Submucosa

Muscle   Serosa

Enlarged View of Stomach Wall

Stomach—Food enters the stomach at the cardiac opening. Later partially digested food is ejected through the pylorus into the intestine. The inset shows the layers in the stomach wall, the outermost being the serosa. The glands of the mucosa, the inner lining, produce hydrochloric acid and pepsin—which form gastric juice.

stomach: the *serous* (outside covering), the *muscular* coat, the *submucous* coat; and the *mucous* coat that forms the inner lining. The mucous coat contains the stomach glands which secrete the diges-

tive enzyme *pepsin* and hydrochloric acid. The solid food remains in the stomach for several hours, and during that time the muscles contract about every 20 seconds to grind and mix the food with the gastric juice and also to eject the liquid portions through the pylorus into the *duodenum* (first part of the small intestine) as *chyme*. After the stomach has been empty for some time, it contracts and produces uncomfortable sensations called "hunger pangs."

The stomach is subject to various disorders including hyperacidity (excessive acidity), anacidity (lack of hydrochloric acid secretion), gas bloating, dilatation, spasm of the cardiac or pyloric valve, acute or chronic gastritis, gastric ulcer, cancer, adenoma (benign tumor), fistula and gastroptosis (dropped stomach).

Cancer of the stomach is a leading cause of death. It occurs most often in men past 45 and at first causes only minor digestive symptoms such as loss of appetite; later it causes loss of weight. The only hope lies in early diagnosis and radical surgery. *See also* ACHYLIA; ALIMENTARY CANAL; CARDIOSPASM; DIGESTION; DIGESTIVE SYSTEM; ESOPHAGUS; GASTRECTOMY; GASTRIC; GASTROENTERITIS; GASTROPTOSIS; GASTROSTOMY; HYDROCHLORIC ACID; INDIGESTION; PEPSIN; PEPTIC ULCER; PYLORUS; SOLAR PLEXUS *and* **medigraphs** GASTRITIS; HIATUS HERNIA; STOMACH CANCER; ULCERS OF THE DIGESTIVE TRACT.

STOMACH ACHE. *See* ABDOMINAL PAIN.

STOMACH CANCER

THE INCIDENCE OF STOMACH CANCER in the United States has been steadily decreasing for the last 40 years. This fact is generally related to improvements in food preservation, especially in refrig-

eration, that combat microbial contamination. Another fortunate change in statistics is that in the last 20 years, the mortality rate for stomach cancer has dropped by about 40 percent.

Cancer of the Stomach

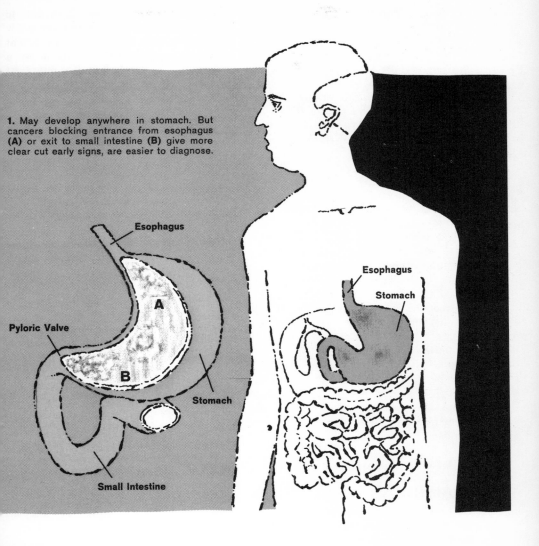

1. May develop anywhere in stomach. But cancers blocking entrance from esophagus **(A)** or exit to small intestine **(B)** give more clear cut early signs, are easier to diagnose.

Esophagus

Pyloric Valve

A

B

Stomach

Small Intestine

Esophagus

Stomach

2. General symptoms: loss of weight, strength, appetite (particularly for meat), fullness and gas after eating, discomfort over abdomen. In later stages fully developed cancer can be felt through abdominal wall.

causes

Research on the causes of stomach cancer has been concentrating on factors *in* the diet as well as factors *absent* from the diet as possible explanations for the world distribution of stomach cancers. Inherited tendency and various environmental factors play a role in family histories of the disease. Worldwide, Japan has the highest incidence of stomach cancer.

symptoms

Unfortunately, early symptoms of stomach cancer are so vague as to be easily confused with chronic indigestion. It is therefore advisable to investigate *all* persistent symptoms of abdominal discomfort, especially when accompanied by vomiting, weight loss and blood in the stools. Early diagnosis is possible through x-rays taken as part of a gastrointestinal checkup involving the ingestion of barium in solution.

treatment

Stomach cancer is treated surgically, with postoperative x-ray and with chemotherapy. Life expectancy is prolonged in about 25 percent of all cases that are treated before metastasis has become rampant.

STOMACH ULCER. *See* PEPTIC ULCER.

STOMATITIS, inflammation of the mucous membrane of the mouth, due to local irritants such as tobacco and spices, a variety of infections, trauma from rough dentistry, or a riboflavin deficiency. *Gingivitis* (inflammation of the gums) and *glossitis* (inflammation of the tongue) are forms of stomatitis. *See also* CANKER SORE; DEFICIENCY DISEASES; GINGIVITIS; GLOSSITIS; MOUTH; RIBOFLAVIN; THRUSH *and* **medigraph** TRENCH MOUTH.

STOOLS. *See* FECES.

STRABISMUS. *See* SQUINT.

STRANGULATION, *asphyxia* due to crushing the neck and air passages, as by choking or hanging. Also, constriction of a structure with loss of circulation, as in a *strangulated hernia*. *See also* ASPHYXIA; HERNIA *and* **medigraph** WHIPLASH INJURY OF THE NECK.

STRAWBERRY MARKS, congenital birthmarks derived from the fetal blood vessels, characterized by their raised, bright red, soft and often lumpy appearance. They are not malignant and cause no trouble except disfigurement. *See also* BIRTHMARK; HEMANGIOMA.

STREP THROAT, the popular designation for an acute and contagious infection of the throat or tonsils by a strain of streptococcus bacteria. Since this species —*Streptococcus pyogenes*—is also responsible for scarlet fever, rheumatic fever and glomerulonephritis, it is of the utmost importance that any incidence of acute sort throat be accurately diagnosed by a laboratory test of throat washings so that antibiotics can be prescribed without delay if the cause is bacterial. This urgency is especially important if the victim is a child because of the potential danger of irreversible heart or kidney damage resulting from unchecked streptococcus invasion. *See also* INFECTION *and* **medigraph** TONSILLITIS.

STREPTOCOCCUS, a dot-shaped germ arranged in a chain like a string of beads. It causes many serious diseases including *tonsillitis, erysipelas, scarlet fever, rheumatic fever, childbirth fever,* and infections of the heart lining and kidneys. The streptococcus is vulnerable to antibiotics. *See also* ANTIBIOTICS; BACTERIA; INFECTION.

STREPTOMYCIN, an antibiotic derived from a fungus that grows in the soil. It is specific for *tuberculosis, tularemia, bubonic plague, undulant fever* and certain other infections. A serious side effect is deafness. Because of its hazards, the use of other broad-spectrum antibiotics is often preferred. *See also* ANTIBIOTICS.

STRESS, a state of high tension or pressure, resulting from an accident or injury or a psychological reaction of heightened emotional response. Certain occupations are particularly stressful, such as acting, advertising, controlling air traffic, politics, investing and gambling. As an effect of stressful emotions such as fear and anger, the blood pressure rises, the pulse beats faster, breathing is accelerated, digestion stops, and the adrenal glands become overactive.

Fear and anxiety are the greatest causes of psychological stress. In modern times people are constantly beset by the threat of calamities. They fear depression and inflation, unemployment, cancer and heart failure, missiles and bombs, and famine. At home they may be confronted with marital incompatibility, quarrels, family illness, or financial troubles.

Many illnesses are caused or aggravated by mental stress, including ulcers, spastic constipation, diarrhea, high blood pressure and migraine headaches. Sometimes latent mental disorders are precipitated by stressful circumstances, as in the case of manic-depressive psychosis, schizophrenia, hysteria and neurasthenia.

When a person is subjected to repeated stresses, he is likely to develop what people call a "nervous breakdown," an unscientific but expressive term. The stress produced by the problems of everyday living has led to the widespread use of tranquilizers, a last resort when there does not seem to be any escape from a difficult situation.

Stress exists in almost every human activity and is not the same as nerve tension. Some stress is beneficial since it may stimulate action.

Psychiatrists at the University of Chicago found that for the avoidance of ex-cessive stress being married is better than being divorced or single; being old is better than being young. The investigators studied 735 individuals in households in Oakland, California, asking them about being confused, feeling tense or keyed up, having outbursts of temper, or feeling blue. The studies showed that the death of a child is the most stressful of any of life's events. Other items included a jail sentence, major financial problems, divorce and the beginning of an extramarital affair. Some of the environmental factors that may be related to stress are the status of health, the social class, and the size of the household. *See also* ANXIETY; FEAR; NERVOUS BREAKDOWN.

STRESS INCONTINENCE. *See* INCONTINENCE.

STRESS TESTING, measurement of the maximum effort a person can expend without overstraining the heart. This is done with tests on a standing bicycle and a treadmill under the supervision of a physician.

Prior to the actual physical exertion, the person's medical history is taken and an electrocardiogram made of the heart action when at rest. With sensors attached to the body to monitor heart rate and the sphygmomanometer's rubber cuff (for blood pressure readings) on the arm, the active testing begins.

The subject first pedals the bicycle at gradually increasing speeds for about 20 minutes. The doctor observes the electrocardiogram for readings of the heart's electrical action in response to the growing stress. Periodically blood pressure readings are taken to monitor the intensified force of the heartbeat and how efficiently it continues to pump the blood through the arteries during strenuous physical activity. The rate of blood flow, the elasticity of the main arteries—which controls steadiness of blood flow, resistance to flow within the arteries, thickness and quantity of blood are all factors influencing blood pressure and thus affecting the heart's stability as the pump of the body's circulatory system.

The same procedure is followed as the subject runs on a treadmill—again at gradually increasing speeds. Steadiness of heart performance under increased blood pressure is carefully noted over a designated period of time. It is not uncommon for the person being tested to be unable to complete the time period of activity on either or both devices. This is especially true of a middle-aged person who does not exercise regularly—either in the form

of calisthenics or participation in a sport. Because of a lack of conditioning, the heart muscle has limited ability to work harder under stress.

Stress testing has value for healthy hearts as well as those recovering from damaging attacks or incapacitated by disease. It is particularly recommended for persons past 40 who may be contemplating taking up a strenuous sport or switching to a line of work that would make unusual or unaccustomed physical demands. Such testing reveals a heart's outermost capacity for normal function, and can reveal conditions likely to pro-

Stress Testing—Three men with sensors attached to their chests ride stationary bicycles in the course of a stress test. Later they will run on a treadmill. At left, the men are being timed, bi-

cycle speed noted, and heart rates monitored. Stress testing establishes reasonable limits of physical activity for healthy hearts as well as those damaged by disease or a heart attack.

Courtesy, American Sterilizer Company

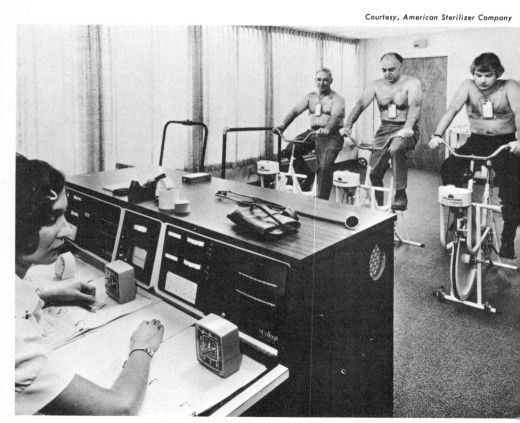

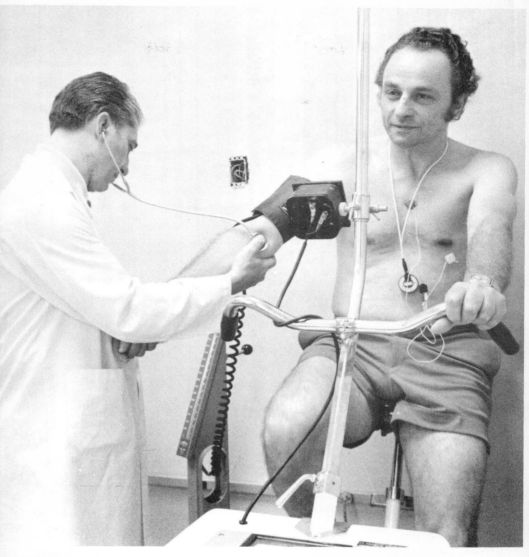

Physical stress tests serve a useful and important function, especially for persons entering middle age. Stress tests are designed to determine how much physical exercise a person can safely undertake without risk to his or her heart. Some of the individuals who take the stress test are actually in excellent health; the results of this test serve to confirm their good condition, but also help to provide guidelines concerning the extent and degree of physical exercises they can reasonably allow themselves. Others who take the test have had a history of heart trouble; again, the purpose is to ascertain the degree and extent of exercise that can be safely undertaken. The test is very useful in establishing the condition of the heart. It is believed to be 85 percent accurate in identifying potential coronary attack victims. Such persons can then take remedial measures to obviate heart attacks that might well have eventually occurred had they never taken a stress test. Above, this man is being given a stress test. There are two basic types of stress test: the bicycle test and the treadmill test. Here he takes a bicycle test. The whole test takes about an hour, the actual bicycling 20 minutes.

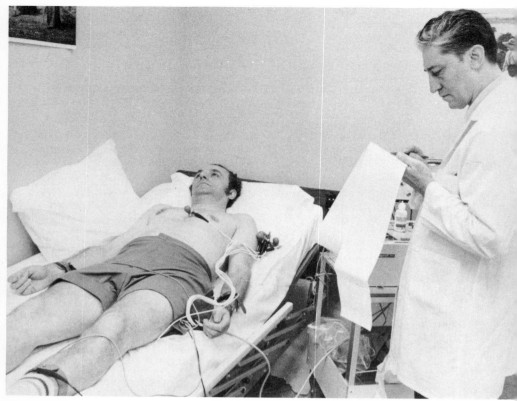

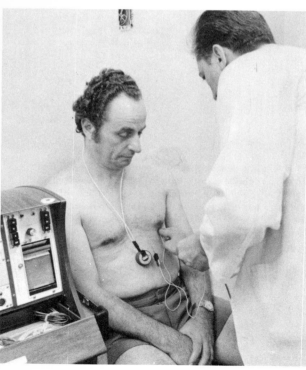

After first conducting an interview to determine the patient's prior medical history, the testing physician administers an electrocardiogram (above). The telemeric electrocardiographic system on the table (left) is the receiver, with an antenna on top; a sender with a battery is attached to the chest of the examinee. Opposite page at top, another view of the bicycle test. The black box in front of the patient's chest is a speedometer. If the patient's condition is poor, the test can be shortened and the speed of the bicycle lowered. Center left, full view of the receiver. The electrocardiograph itself comes out at right. Bottom left, the dial that regulates the treadmill in the treadmill test. The lower right switch changes the elevation of the apparatus. Bottom right, patient on the treadmill. Blood pressure is checked every one to two minutes.

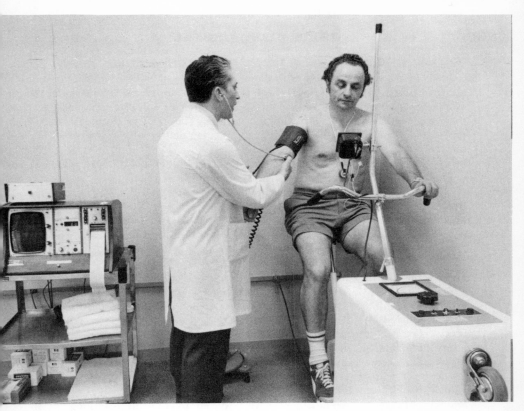

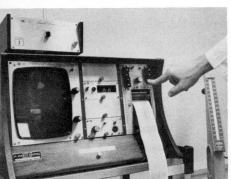

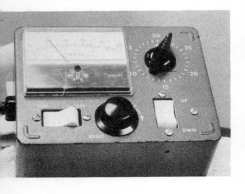

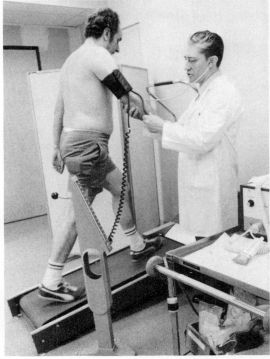

voke a heart attack if abused or left un-treated. In the case of people with dam-aged or diseased hearts, stress testing establishes healthy levels of activity so that they neither overdo and cause fur-ther damage and perhaps a fatal attack, nor will they wrongfully deprive their hearts of any exercise at all out of fear.

Physicians are also using series of grad-uated stress tests to learn the factors that trigger attacks of angina pectoris in in-dividuals. As stress increases, the heart requires more of its own blood supply from the coronary arteries to provide ex-tra oxygen. When these arteries that nourish the heart are obstructed or nar-rowed from fatty buildup, they cannot provide enough blood flow to answer the heart's demand and the pain of angina occurs. For a person with this coronary artery limitation, the degree of stress at which pain occurs during the testing is the level of activity to which the indi-vidual should restrict himself. *See also* ANGINA PECTORIS; EXERCISE; HEART; HEART CARE; PHYSICAL FITNESS *and* **medigraph** MYOCARDIAL INFARCTION.

STRETCH MARKS, sharply defined, white or red, slightly sunken lines on the skin due to overstretching, as in the ap-plication of adhesive tape or tight dress-ings. They may be located over the ab-domen and breasts in pregnancy or over any distended organ, over the abdomen in obesity or fluid in the abdomen, on the neck in goiter, or in the loins in dis-orders affecting the sacroiliac region.

STRICTURE, an abnormal narrowing or closure of a canal, duct or passage due to contraction of scar tissue or a deposit of obstructive material. *Stricture of the urethra* (urinary tube) in the penis re-sults mostly from gonorrhea. It can be stretched by inserting and rotating a *ure-thral sound.* Other strictures may form in the *anus, rectum,* or *ureter* (the tube that carries the urine from the kidney to the bladder).

STRIDOR, a harsh vibrating sound pro-duced by difficult breathing, as in ob-struction of the respiratory passages from any cause. *See also* BREATHING.

STROKE

A STROKE IS AN INTERRUPTION in the normal circulation of blood through the brain leading to a sudden loss of con-sciousness and some degree of paralysis, which may be temporary or permanent depending on the severity of the oxygen deprivation of the brain cells. A popular term for stroke is *apoplexy.* Technically it is known as a *cerebrovascular acci-dent.* It is most common after middle age, but may occur to a younger person who has a vascular disorder of the brain.

causes
Most strokes can be traced to previously existing conditions of atherosclerosis, hy-pertension, or arterial aneurysm. The three immediate causes are: *cerebral*

thrombosis, in which normal circulation through the brain is cut off from a part of it by a clot in an atherosclerotic ar-tery; *cerebral embolism,* in which an embolus of air, fat, or a traveling blood clot settles in one of the cerebral arteries and chokes off the circulation; *cerebral hemorrhage,* in which there is a rupture of a blood vessel within the brain, usu-ally an artery with a thin spot (aneurysm) in its wall. This latter type of stroke may be triggered by overexertion, overeating, unusual emotional stress, or a violent coughing fit.

symptoms
A stroke caused by thrombosis may be preceded by symptoms that occur a few

Stroke (Apoplexy)

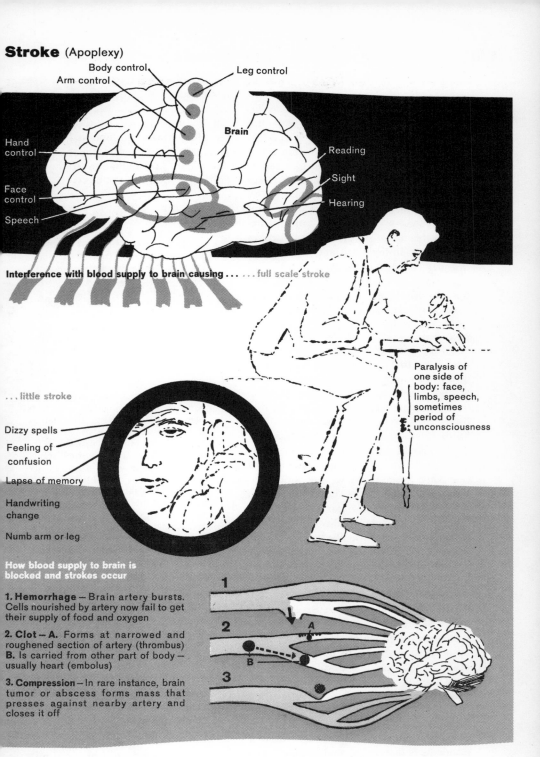

Body control

Arm control

Leg control

Hand control

Brain

Reading

Sight

Face control

Hearing

Speech

Interference with blood supply to brain causing .... full scale stroke

Paralysis of one side of body: face, limbs, speech, sometimes period of unconsciousness

... little stroke

Dizzy spells

Feeling of confusion

Lapse of memory

Handwriting change

Numb arm or leg

How blood supply to brain is blocked and strokes occur

1. Hemorrhage — Brain artery bursts. Cells nourished by artery now fail to get their supply of food and oxygen

2. Clot — A. Forms at narrowed and roughened section of artery (thrombus) **B.** Is carried from other part of body — usually heart (embolus)

3. Compression — In rare instance, brain tumor or abscess forms mass that presses against nearby artery and closes it off

1

2

3

A

B

1365

hours or a few days before: dizziness, loss of balance, slurred speech, or sudden memory loss. When an embolism is involved, onset of the stroke is swift and sudden: paralysis, loss of speech and loss of consciousness may occur within a few minutes of each other. A stroke resulting from cerebral hemorrhage produces symptoms similar to those produced by an embolism, plus acute headache, nausea and loud ringing in the ears just before a blackout occurs. Minor strokes may occur during sleep and on awakening, the victim may be dizzy, disoriented and aware of pains in the arms or legs. Speech distortion and memory disturbance may also occur.

treatment

A stroke is a medical emergency, and a doctor or ambulance should be called at once. In the meanwhile, the victim should be placed in a reclining position with his head turned to one side so that fluids can drain from his mouth. No fluids, and especially no alcoholic beverage, should be given.

All victims of strokes, even minor ones, are hospitalized so that kidney or lung involvement can be avoided and diagnostic procedures can assess the extent of the damage. Physical therapy and rehabilitation usually begin *as soon as possible*. The prognosis for recovery is based on the person's physical and emotional health and the willingness of various members of the family to become involved in therapy. Several striking cases of recovery of speech and movement after major strokes have been accomplished thanks to new methods of rehabilitation and the devoted efforts of close relatives and friends as well as professional physiotherapists.

prevention

Since the incidence of cerebrovascular accidents is directly related to atherosclerosis and hypertension, the most effective means of preventing them is to see a good doctor for a complete checkup once a year and to follow his instructions for the maintenance of good health. Also, the elimination of emotional stress and pressure is a better safeguard in many cases than the elimination of cholesterol. RESEARCH REPORT *follows* APOPLEXY.

RESEARCH REPORT

LONG-TERM REDUCTION OF BLOOD PRESSURE SAFE FOR STROKE PATIENTS

Results of a large-scale study to determine the safety of continuing *antihypertensive* drug therapy for patients who have had a stroke indicate that long-term reduction of blood pressure does not increase the risk of stroke recurrence. The report by NATIONAL INSTITUTE OF NEUROLOGICAL AND COMMUNICATIVE DISEASES AND STROKE (NINCDS) scientists establishes a basis for recommending such ongoing treatment even if the stroke patients have only moderately high blood pressure. Findings also confirm the fact that the risk of congestive heart failure in these patients is reduced by the antihypertensive therapy.

The study, in which ten university medical centers and hospitals participated, was the first to provide this category of information about a large group of stroke survivors with mild to moderate hypertension. Of the total 452 patients observed over a three-year period, half received antihypertensive medicines and the other half placebos. The drugs used were *deserpidine* and *methyclothiazide*.

There were 37 stroke recurrences in the drug-treated group and 42 in the group receiving placebos. Although the difference may not appear to be statistically striking, it demonstrates the safety of the treatment and indicates its benefits.   NIH615

RESEARCH REPORT

SIGNIFICANT ADVANCES IN MEDICAL AND SURGICAL STROKE TREATMENT

An optimistic outlook for *stroke* victims is provided by several recent significant advances in the medical and surgical treatment of *cerebrovascular* disease.

From the MAYO CLINIC for example comes the news that aspirin may soon be used to control the *clotting* mechanism which characterizes a majority of strokes. The chemical action by which aspirin inhibits platelet aggregation is being explored in experiments that separate various blood and blood cell components in order to identify the fraction or fractions that participate in aspirin's effectiveness.

Elsewhere, a new approach to the surgical treatment of cerebral *aneurysms* and other vascular defects caused by stroke involves the use of powerful *magnets.* Laboratory scientists at MASSACHUSETTS GENERAL HOSPITAL have demonstrated that magnets can be used to guide catheters into previously inaccessible branches of damaged cerebral arteries. Aneurysms artificially produced in animals have thus been thrombosed—or plugged —with detachable silver-plated catheter tips. The tips are then held in place magnetically until clotting seals the aneurysm.

These investigators are also attempting a chemical procedure that could replace major brain surgery for some stroke victims. This procedure involves the use of *ferrofluid,* a liquid containing tiny iron compound particles. The ferrofluid, which is fed into aneurysms by catheter, is held there by an external electromagnet until the aneurysm is filled and sealed off by clotting. If successful in humans, this technique promises to increase the chances of patient survival.

A new surgical technique whereby blood is channeled into the brain from the scalp arteries through holes drilled in the skull is being investigated at the NATIONAL NAVAL MEDICAL CENTER. Results with patients in Europe and the United States indicate that these grafts significantly increase cerebral blood flow, and that autoregularity of circulation is maintained despite some instability.   NIH925

STRYCHNINE, the principal alkaloid of *Strychnos nux vomica,* a convulsant poison formerly prescribed as a tonic and stimulant to the nervous system. Its use has been discontinued because of its dangerous effects, especially on the spinal cord. In cases of poisoning, the medical examiner can detect traces of strychnine after death, even in the exhumed body. *See also* FIRST AID.

STUPOR, partial or nearly complete unconsciousness. It may occur after shock, in the late stage of a serious disease, after an epileptic convulsion, or as a symptom of a mental disease such as schizophrenia. *See also* **medigraphs** ALCOHOLISM; ENCEPHALITIS; EPILEPSY; HEROIN ABUSE; HYPOGLYCEMIA.

STUTTERING, sometimes called *stammering,* a speech defect of emotional origin. It is characterized by sudden stops in uttering words and syllables or a rapid repetition of a particular consonant— especially *p, b, m* or *w*—which are sounds made by the lips.

Children usually begin to stutter at about age 3 or 4, the age when the child begins to form complicated sentences. However, a sudden severe fright—as a bite by a dog or beating by a parent— causes the child to tighten the larynx and thereby begin to stutter. Thereafter, the child may stutter every time he wants to talk because of memory of the previous stress. With the larynx tight, the air does not pass through. The child cannot speak even with the vocal cords open, but tries to talk—leading to a struggle. However, stutterers usually do not have difficulty when they sing, shout or whisper. Some stutterers improve when they are taught to keep the larynx relaxed, which can be done when the child is taught to speak in a breathier soft voice.

Stuttering can cause great embarrassment, especially when speaking in public. The defect is an expression of shyness and self-consciousness and is aggravated when the audience reacts to it. While talking to a small group of persons who

Sty

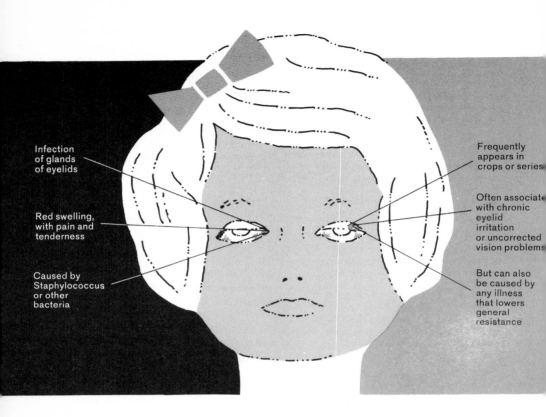

Infection
of glands
of eyelids

Red swelling,
with pain and
tenderness

Caused by
Staphylococcus
or other
bacteria

Frequently
appears in
crops or series

Often associated
with chronic
eyelid
irritation
or uncorrected
vision problems

But can also
be caused by
any illness
that lowers
general
resistance

Course of Development

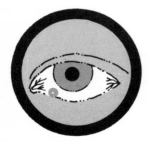

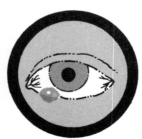

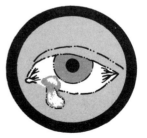

1 Starts as red
swelling with
pain and
tenderness

2 Grows in size,
comes to
yellowish head

3 After day or two,
softens and bursts.
Yellowish pus
is discharged

do not appear to notice the defect, the stutterer may speak normally.

The best cure is to associate with sympathetic and understanding people and enlist the services of a speech therapist.

Children who stutter should never be scolded or ridiculed, a mistake which would exaggerate their emotional stress and the associated speech defect. *See also* SPEECH.

STY

A STY IS A SMALL INFLAMED swelling (abscess) on the rim of the eyelid at the opening of a sebaceous gland. Sties may occur in groups or in series—always on the lid and near the lashes. They are more common among children and younger people than among the middle-aged and elderly.

cause
Sties are caused by bacterial infection—usually *staphylococcus*—when an eyelash blocks the opening of a gland duct on the lid, or when general health is poor and resistance to infection is low.

symptoms
The sty starts as a small red pimple causing mild irritation to the eye. In a day or so, the pimple becomes filled with pus and abscessed, taking on a yellow appearance and becoming slightly more swollen. In many cases, the sty ruptures and drains by itself.

complications
Since staphylococcus bacteria are highly contagious and self-infecting, people with sties are likely to spread them to other members of the family or to reinfect themselves when the pus begins to drain unless they exercise care about contagion.

treatment
A sty is usually treated at home with the application of hot compresses of plain water to the affected eye for ten minutes every two hours. An antibiotic ophthalmic ointment may also be prescribed by the doctor so that infection is prevented

from spreading and recurring. Sties that do not respond to this treatment and refuse to drain but increase in size may have to be lanced by an ophthalmologist.

prevention
Rubbing the eyes with unwashed hands increases the risk of sties. So does the use of other people's mascara brushes. Poor health and cleanliness habits lead to a greater vulnerability to bacterial infection in general, and to "staph" infection in particular.

STYPTIC, an astringent drug that stops bleeding from small cuts as in shaving. *Alum* and *tannic acid* are two common styptics. *See also* ASTRINGENT.

SUBCONSCIOUS, below the conscious level of thought. According to Freud and other psychoanalysts, the subconscious mind contains buried experiences which can be recalled by *hypnosis* or *dream analysis*. Such repressed memories may be responsible for a neurosis or psychoneurosis, which can be treated by psychoanalysis. *See also* DREAMS; HYPNOSIS; MEMORY; PSYCHOANALYSIS; PSYCHONEUROSIS.

SUBCUTANEOUS, beneath the skin. For quick action, drugs are injected subcutaneously through a hypodermic needle. *See also* INJECTION.

SUDDEN INFANT DEATH SYNDROME (SIDS), *crib death,* death of an apparently healthy infant—during sleep, usually at night and frequently during the

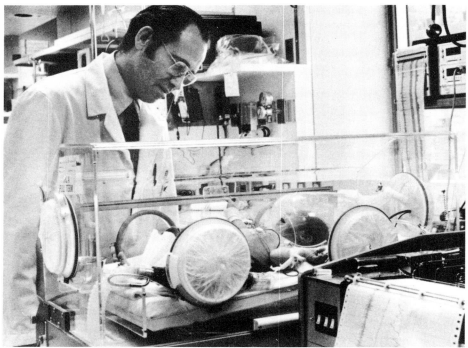

Sudden Infant Death Syndrome—An infant is monitored electronically in an incubator as part of the search for ways to prevent the sudden infant death syndrome. The physician and associates are studying normal full-term and premature infants to assess the effect of full development and sleep on the automatic control of breathing. This may provide a basis for recognizing infants with abnormal breathing mechanisms who may be in danger of developing SIDS.

cold winter months. SIDS is the single greatest cause of death in babies between one week and one year of age, with about 10,000 such deaths occurring yearly in the United States alone.

The precise cause or causes of these tragic deaths have eluded medical science. Theories have pointed to and studies have pursued such possible causes as congenital heart defect, allergy, viral infection and enzyme deficiency. Promising leads having to do with recurrent oxygen deprivation and some abnormality in the automatic control of respiration are under investigation. A recent study has suggested that an inherited abnormality in the electrical signal controlling the heartbeat may be the cause in some cases of crib death. Researchers hope that identification and electronic monitoring of babies at risk of SIDS may eventually become possible.

RESEARCH REPORT

NEW ALARM SYSTEM
MONITORS INFANT BREATHING

An *ultrasonic alarm system* which monitors an infant's breathing without being connected to its body is being developed by UNIVERSITY OF WASHINGTON scientists as a safeguard against the *sudden infant death syndrome*. By tracking the respiration rate of a newborn in an enclosed chamber or an open crib, the device can detect any aberration which approaches a dangerous level of breathing failure. When the period of respiratory failure exceeds a preset standard of about 20 seconds, a light flashes and an alarm sounds. This warning indicates the need for prompt emergency measures to restore the infant's respiration.   NIH824

NEW TEST ALERTS DOCTORS TO POSSIBILITY OF SUDDEN INFANT DEATH

A prenatal test that can predict the likelihood of respiratory distress in newborn babies and thus alert obstetricians and pediatricians to the possible onset of the *sudden infant death syndrome,* has been developed under the sponsorship of the NATIONAL INSTITUTE OF CHILD HEALTH AND HUMAN DEVELOPMENT.

The test, which resulted from studies of the biochemical development of surface-active materials on prenatal lung growth in both animals and humans, uses a sample of the *amniotic fluid* for an assessment of the functional maturity of fetal lungs before delivery. Ongoing studies of the amniotic fluid may reveal why some abnormal pregnancy states stimulate pulmonary maturity while others seem to retard it.

Since the SIDS is believed to result from an aberration in the automatic control of respiration, assessments are also being made of the effects of maturation and sleep on respiratory control in both full-term and prematurely born infants. Information about *normal* regulatory mechanisms during the first month of life should provide the basis for recognizing abnormal variations, thus anticipating the need for protective measures to safeguard the lives of high-risk SIDS newborns.   NIH1124

CONGENITAL CARDIAC IRREGULARITY MAY CAUSE SUDDEN INFANT DEATH SYNDROME

An inherited heart irregularity may be one cause of the *sudden infant death syndrome* (SIDS) or *"crib death"* according to a medical report presented to the AMERICAN HEART ASSOCIATION. This specific congenital abnormality in the electrical signal that makes the heart beat shows up in *electrocardiograms* and has been found to produce fainting spells and even sudden fatalities in children and adults. "Crib death" is the chief single cause of fatalities in newborns between one week and one year of age, taking an annual toll of about 10,000 seemingly healthy infants in the United States. The irregularity now linked to these deaths is called the *prolonged Q-T interval,* deriving its name from an abnormal lengthening of the electrocardiographic line on that portion of the recording tape designated by those letters.

The investigators based their findings on electrocardiograms of 42 sets of parents who had sustained the loss of at least one infant through SIDS. Of these subjects, 26 percent indicated prolonged Q-T intervals, a percentage significantly higher than that observed in the general population. In addition, 40 percent of the living offspring of these parents showed the same abnormality. Also, one infant who had an episode of cardiac arrest at seven weeks of age showed marked Q-T interval prolongation after surviving a possible crib death. NIH116

SUFFOCATION. *See* ASPHYXIA.

SUICIDE, intentionally taking one's own life. The annual toll in the United States, for example, is about 20,000. The rate of suicide is higher in elderly persons, often due to discouragement and hopelessness. The means frequently employed are guns, barbiturates, poisons, carbon monoxide, jumping from a height, and hanging. The usual causes are illness such as terminal cancer, loss of one's mate, financial failure, alcoholism and drug addiction.

Despondency due to *involutional melancholia* or another mental disease often results in suicide or a suicidal attempt. Contrary to a popular belief, depressed persons who threaten suicide are apt to carry it out and must be watched closely. Inquiry about depressive and suicidal states should be made an essential part of every routine medical examination. The use of depressant tranquilizers increases the hazard of suicide.

Depressed persons with suicidal impulses are sometimes confined in a mental hospital for their own protection. The use of *electric convulsive therapy* (ECT) has a calming effect and greatly reduces the number of suicides. Melancholy may be corrected during depressed periods by administration of antidepressant drugs. Pleasant surroundings and psychological and social therapy aid early recovery from depression. *See also* DEPRESSION.

SULFONAMIDE DRUGS, *sulfa drugs,* antibacterial agents derived from *sulfanilamide,* the prototype of the group. Because of their potential toxicity, they have been superseded to a large extent by penicillin and other antibiotics.

The United States Pharmacopeia lists *sulfadiazine, sulfamerazine, sulfamethazine, sulfapyridine, sulfisoxazole,* and *sulfinpyrazone.* Sulfanilamide has been omitted because of its toxicity.

The National Formulary lists *sulfacetamide, sulfadimethoxine, sulfamethizole,* and *sulfamethoxazole.*

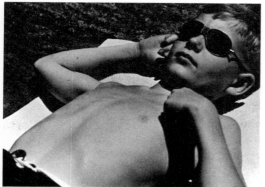

Sunburn—Painful sunburn can be avoided by gradual exposure and using a lotion that screens out the sun's ultraviolet rays. Repeated overexposure to strong sunlight damages the skin. Fairskinned people are especially vulnerable and should restrict their time in the sun.

The sulfonamides have proved useful in a wide range of infections including lobar pneumonia, spinal meningitis, gonorrhea, boils, streptococcus blood poisoning, dysentery, cystitis and mastoiditis. They differ in degree of activity, the antibacterial spectrum, the rate of absorption, pharmacological actions, and their toxic side effects. The principal adverse reactions in sensitive individuals are hives, purpura, skin eruptions, nausea, vomiting, headache, mental depression, fever and destruction of white blood cells. *See also* ANTIBIOTICS; INFECTION.

SULFUR DIOXIDE, SO$_2$, antioxidant pharmaceutical aid, a colorless gas obtained by burning sulfur in oxygen. It is a moderately powerful *germicide* in the presence of moisture. Dry sulfur dioxide is effective in killing mosquitoes, fleas, flies, rats and other vermin. It is toxic when inhaled and causes irritation of the eyes, nose, throat and lungs. *See also* AIR POLLUTION; FUMIGATION.

SUNBURN, *erythema solare,* an inflammation of the skin caused by the actinic ultraviolet rays of the sun, manifested by simple reddening of the skin in mild cases and blisters and blebs after severe exposure. Later the burned skin becomes flaky and peels off in scales. Blonds, infants and persons with red hair are especially sensitive to sunburn, and *heliophobes* are morbidly vulnerable. There is greater penetration of ultraviolet rays near the sea, and the burning effect of bright sunlight is reflected by snow. The constitutional symptoms are headache, dizziness, fever, vomiting, sunstroke, heat exhaustion and shock.

Sunburn can be prevented—at the same time permitting a tan—by application of a lotion containing a sun screen. When present, sunburn should be treated the same as any other burn. If the burn is deep or the area extensive, the victim should be treated for *shock*

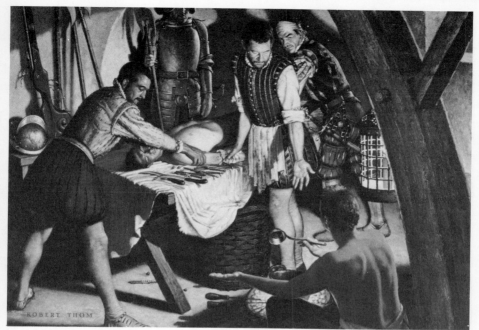

Surgery—Up to the moment depicted here, boiling oil was the treatment for gunshot injuries. The supply of a young French army surgeon, Ambroise Paré, ran out during a battle in 1536. He improvised, discovered that unburned patients healed much better, and never used hot oil again. Paré revolutionized wound treatment, invented surgical instruments and introduced artificial eyes and limbs. He is considered one of the illustrious figures in surgery's history.

and a physician called. For local relief of the burn, various ointments, lotions and creams are available.

Excessive and repeated exposures to strong sunlight are damaging to the skin and may result in skin cancer. *Heliotherapy*—the treatment of certain diseases by exposure to sunlight under medical supervision—is employed at many spas, especially for tuberculosis and arthritis. *See also* BURNS; EXFOLIATION; HELIOPHOBE; HELIOTHERAPY; PABA; PHOTOSENSITIVITY; PIGMENTATION; SKIN *and* **medigraphs** HEAT STROKE; LUPUS ERYTHEMATOSUS; SKIN CANCER.

SUNGLASSES, deeply tinted glasses worn as a protection from strong sunlight. They should not be worn indoors, as they tend to impair vision, or outdoors on dull days, as an accident may result from poor visibility.

SUNSTROKE. *See* HEAT SICKNESS.

SUPPOSITORY, a cone-shaped piece of solid—usually fatty or glycerin—substance, containing medication, adapted for insertion into the vagina, rectum or urethral opening.

SUPPRESSION, a sudden cessation of a normal secretion as of the urine or menstrual fluid.

In psychoanalysis, conscious inhibition, as contrasted with *repression* (which is subconscious).

SUPPURATION, formation of *pus* in an infected area. Pus is a creamy, yellow or greenish thick fluid composed of broken-down white blood cells, serum and germs. The color varies with the infecting germ. *See also* INFECTION; PUS.

SURGEON. *See* DOCTOR.

SURGERY, the treatment of diseases by manual, instrumental and operative pro-

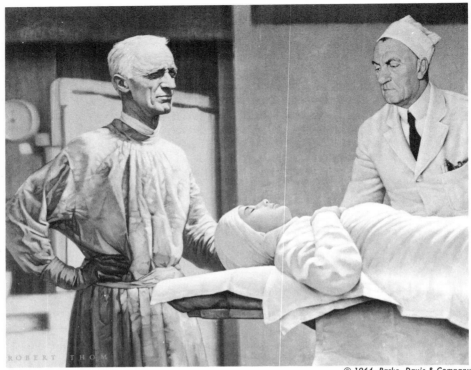

Surgery—Great medical advances of the 19th century included the introduction of ether anesthesia, discovery of x-rays, recognition of infection by microorganisms and measures to prevent it. These made possible such 20th century achievements as surgery on the sensitive tissues of the brain. The man depicted here, Dr. Harvey Cushing, in the early 1900s developed many of the delicate techniques for brain surgery. He became renowned as a brain surgeon and as a teacher.

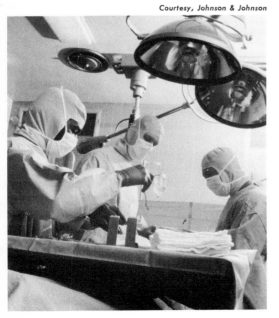

cedures. Modern surgical technique has developed rapidly since the demonstration of *ether* anesthesia at Massachusetts General Hospital in the 1840's, which enabled surgeons to operate freely without causing pain during the operation. Another epochal advance has been the development of *asepsis* (absence of germs) beginning with the use of car-

Surgery—This scene *(left)* in a modern operating room is a far cry from the infection-plagued procedures of little more than a century ago. Here everything is sterile—the air, instruments, bedding and clothing—to keep germs from the point of surgery. Powerful lights leave little chance for oversight. Awkward devices have given way to precisely crafted surgical steel instruments. Today's surgeon also has the special skills of an anesthesiologist and nurses, x-rays before and during surgery, intravenous infusions, antibiotics and an enormous body of knowledge.

bolic acid as an antiseptic by Joseph Lister; progressing to the wearing of sterilized rubber gloves by the surgeon and his assistants; and finally complete sterilization of the whole operative field and the instruments.

The achievements of surgery during the last 50 years have culminated in successful operations on the open heart and the transplanting of living organs from victims of fatal accidents to persons with organs damaged beyond repair. *See also* ADHESION; ANESTHESIA; ANTISEPTICS; CORNEAL TRANSPLANTATION; CRYOSURGERY; EYE BANK; HEART SURGERY; HEART SURGERY, ARTIFICIAL; ORGAN TRANSPLANTS; ORTHOPEDIC SURGERY; PLASTIC SURGERY. Rᴇsᴇᴀʀᴄʜ *follows* HYPOTHERMIA.

SURGERY AND OLDER PEOPLE.

Age is no longer a barrier to successful operations, especially when they are performed *electively* (at the option of the patient), when the patient is best able to withstand the surgical shock, and at a time when resistance to infection has reached its peak. Thorough preparation and especial care are, of course, required. Whenever time is available, a complete and comprehensive medical checkup precedes the operation. *Emergency* operations are avoided or postponed as far as

possible on older patients. *See also* AGING; SURGERY.

SUTURE, in anatomy, a line of junction between two or more bones, as a *cranial suture* in the skull; in surgery, a fine thread to stitch a wound, usually composed of silk or absorbable catgut (actually from the sheep's intestine).

SWAB, a piece of cotton, cloth or sponge on the end of a long stick, used for applying medication to the throat or other part of the body; for cleansing the mouth and teeth; and for obtaining specimens of secretions. Swabs are sterilized and kept in containers ready for use.

SWALLOWING, *deglutition,* the passage of masticated (chewed) food from the mouth through the throat and esophagus (gullet) into the stomach. It is a complicated reflex which begins under the control of the brain by muscular action and then is propelled the rest of the way automatically. The steps of swallowing are as follows:

1. The mouth cavity is shut off by the position of the tongue against the hard palate and by the contractions of the muscles in the upper part of the throat.

Suture—The fine thread closing the wound is called a suture. Catgut sutures dissolve in body fluids and disappear. Other materials used are silk and nylon. After surgery, incisions through different layers of tissue are sewn separately *(left)* until closure is complete *(right).*

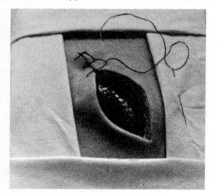
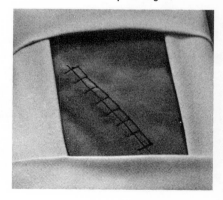

2. The nasal cavity is shut off by elevation of the soft palate against the postnasal openings.
3. The opening into the larynx (voice box) is closed by the vocal cords and the *epiglottis* (trap door of the larynx), to keep the food from getting into the lungs.

Mechanism of Swallowing

1st Phase: Tongue forces Food past the Palatine Arch into Oropharynx
2nd Phase: Food passes through Oropharynx into Esophagus
3rd Phase: Food passes down Esophagus

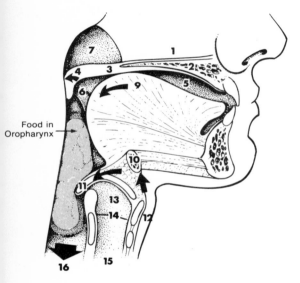

Food in Oropharynx

1. Nasal Cavity	9. Tongue
2. Hard Palate	10. Hyoid Bone
3. Soft Palate	11. Epiglottis
4. Uvula	12. Adam's Apple
5. Oral Cavity	13. Larynx
6. Palatine Arch	14. Vocal Cords
7. Nasopharynx	15. Trachea
8. Oropharynx	16. Esophagus

Swallowing—This act begins with the voluntary muscular action of the tongue and throat. Once food passes from the throat, the involuntary muscles of the esophagus automatically propel it down to the stomach. The illustration shows how food is kept from the nasal passages (7) by the flipping back of the uvula (4), and from the windpipe (13) by movement of the epiglottis (11).

The passage through the gullet is entirely automatic, propelled by the wavelike contractions of its muscles. *See also* APHAGIA; DYSPHAGIA; ESOPHAGUS; MOUTH; THROAT.

SWAY-BACK. *See* LORDOSIS.

SWEAT. *See* PERSPIRATION.

SWELLING, any morbid enlargement, inflation, or abnormal protuberance of the body. *See also* EDEMA; INFLAMMATION; SWOLLEN GLANDS.

SWOLLEN GLANDS. In different areas of the body, swollen glands may be diagnostic of certain conditions. In the neck they suggest *Hodgkin's disease* or *scrofula* (tuberculosis of the lymph glands); in the groins, venereal diseases such as *gonorrhea;* and in the armpit, cancer of the breast. *See also* LYMPHATIC SYSTEM *and* **medigraphs** ANTHRAX; BREAST CANCER; GERMAN MEASLES; GONORRHEA; HODGKIN'S DISEASE; LEUKEMIA; LUPUS ERYTHEMATOSUS; MONONUCLEOSIS, INFECTIOUS; SYPHILIS; TONSILLITIS; TRENCH MOUTH.

SYDENHAM'S CHOREA. *See* CHOREA.

SYMPATHETIC NERVOUS SYSTEM. *See* NERVOUS SYSTEM.

SYMPATHETIC PAIN, pain transmitted indirectly to the brain center via the *sympathetic nervous system.* The sensation may be referred to a distant organ. Sympathetic pain may be felt in shell shock, nervous breakdown and psychosomatic disorders. *See also* PAIN.

SYMPTOM, a complaint by patients which leads them to seek medical advice or one that is elicited by the physician's questions. A *constitutional symptom* is one that is produced by the disease on the whole body; a *pathognomonic symp-*

Synovial Membranes
in the Knee Joint

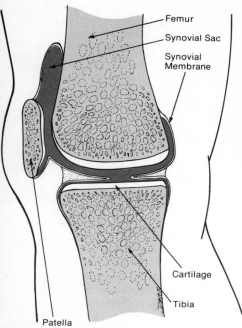

Femur

Synovial Sac

Synovial
Membrane

Cartilage

Tibia

Patella

Synovial Membranes—Synovial membranes surround the ends of the bones forming the knee (patella, femur and tibia). Synovial fluid nourishes the cartilage and keeps bone interaction in the joint cushioned and without friction.

tom, one that in itself indicates the nature of the disease; the *presenting symptom,* that of which the patient complains first and most to the doctor; a *sympathetic symptom,* one that is experienced in a part of the body other than the site of the disease.

SYNCOPE. *See* FAINTING.

SYNDROME, a group of symptoms and signs which, when considered together, is characteristic of a certain disease or disorder.

SYNOVIAL MEMBRANES, the linings of joint capsules concerned with the secretion of clear *synovial fluid* to lubricate the joint surfaces.

Inflammation of these membranes, *synovitis,* is characterized by swelling with clear fluid, fluctuation of the fluid on pressure, pain and restricted mobility. It may be caused by injury or a variety of infections. *Water on the knee,* due to accumulation of fluid in the joint following an injury, is a typical example of synovitis. *See also* JOINT; JOINT DISORDERS *and* **medigraphs** GOUT; RHEUMATIC FEVER; RHEUMATOID ARTHRITIS.

SYPHILIS

SYPHILIS IS A HIGHLY CONTAGIOUS venereal disease, worldwide in incidence, and on the rise once again in spite of earlier indications that it might be eradicated through the use of penicillin. The greatest rate of increase of the disease in the United States is among teenagers and adults of casual sexual habits.

cause

The type of bacteria that cause syphilis are known as spirochetes, specifically *Treponema pallidum.* The infection is transmitted by direct sexual contact through the mucous membranes, or

through a lesion in the skin. The disease is not known to spread through contact with a "contaminated" toilet seat or eating utensils, since the microorganism is quickly killed by a change in temperature or humidity. It is not anaerobic, as formerly assumed. Congenital syphilis is not inherited; it is transmitted during pregnancy by an infected mother to the unborn child and can result in spontaneous abortion, stillbirth, or defects.

symptoms

The disease progresses in three clearly delineated stages, each with its charac-

1377

Syphilis

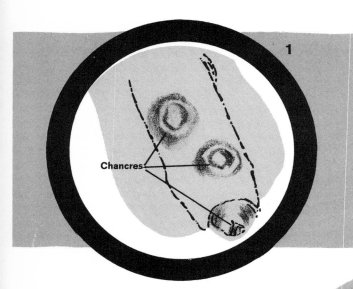

1

Chancres

1. Primary Stage:
Chancre is characteristic symptom of primary stage of syphilis. Usually one but sometimes several chancres appear — generally in genital regions. Occasionally syphilis chancres emerge on lip, tongue, nipples or finger.

1A. Frequently there is accompanying painless swelling of lymph glands near genitals. Chancres too are painless — and generally heal in 3-4 weeks without leaving scars.

1A

Swelling of Lymph Glands

Chancre

2. Secondary Stage:
Mild rash sometimes occurs after chancre disappears. May appear anywhere on body—and has no characteristic appearance.

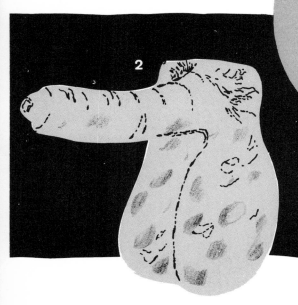

2

teristic symptoms. *Primary syphilis* produces a painless ulceration called *chancre* several weeks (in some cases several months) after infection has occurred. The sore appears on the part of the body that has been in contact with the spirochetes: typically on the penis, vagina, lips, breast, or anus. This sore will disappear within ten days to six weeks without any treatment—it may have been so small or so hidden that it was never noticed in the first place. If the disease has not been treated by a doctor with antibiotics, the second stage occurs within two to six months.

Secondary syphilis, which may last for about two years, begins with a rash that covers the whole body, including the face, hands and feet. The rash may or may not itch. Following the eruption, mucous sores may be visible around the mouth and around the genitalia and rectum. Fever, headache, sore throat and discomfort in the muscles and joints may develop. Some hair may fall out and vision may be affected. This stage of the disease is extremely contagious and may be spread by kissing if there are sores in the mouth. It can be positively identified by blood tests and cured by proper medical attention. However, as in the primary stage, symptoms will once again vanish without treatment, and the disease enters a latency period that may last for as long as five, ten, or fifteen years, or even for a lifetime. During this latency period, there are no symptoms, and the disease does not show up in a blood test. The first two stages are known as *early syphilis.*

The third stage is called *tertiary* or *late syphilis,* and although it is not contagious, it can be extremely damaging to the victim.

complications

Total disablement and death may result when the spirochetes affect the brain and spinal cord (*tabes dorsalis*), or the aorta and the heart. Although any organ may become fatally involved in tertiary syphilis, 90 percent of all deaths are caused by failure of the heart or nervous system.

treatment

Even in its final phases, treatment with antibiotics can halt the progress of the disease. Syphilis at any stage can be completely cured only by an accredited doctor, an accredited hospital, or an accredited public health clinic.

prevention

The increase in syphilis can be halted only if condoms are once again promoted as a contraceptive device that safeguards health. With the rise of the use of the pill or the IUD and the change in sexual mores, the continuing spread of syphilis need not be inevitable, especially if all educational campaigns stress the point that syphilis is a *disease,* not a disgrace.

RESEARCH REPORT

CELLULAR IMMUNITY SUPPRESSION MAY EXPLAIN CLINICAL COURSE OF SYPHILIS

The theory that a general suppression of cellular immunity is the cause of the unusual clinical course of untreated syphilis is supported by recent studies sponsored by the NATIONAL INSTITUTE OF ALLERGY AND INFECTIOUS DISEASES.

It has been suggested that the waxing and waning of the disease over a period of months before it enters a latent stage is the result of a balance between the development of the infection and the suppression of immunity. It has also been observed that antibodies specifically generated by the disease-bearing organism *Treponema pallidum* are present throughout the disease.

Latest information indicates that although the antibodies are present in the lymphocytes of syphilitic patients, they do not respond normally *in vitro* to treponemal or to nontreponemal antigens. Investigators believe that cellular immunity fails to

O   develop or is suppressed for some
    time during the waxing and waning
O   of the disease until the intervention of
    unknown factors which cause the
O   cell-mediated response of the latent
    period.   NIH925

SYRINGE, a medical instrument made
of glass, plastic, metal or rubber used to
inject fluid under the skin or irrigate a
cavity or wound. The *hypodermic syringe*
is used to inject a dissolved drug for
quick effect. Inexpensive sterilized disposable hypodermic syringes with the
needle attached are now available and
highly recommended. The large *irrigat-
ing syringe*—equipped with a rubber bulb
and a nozzle—is used to wash out earwax and cleanse the vagina, the urinary
passage in the penis, and the rectum; it
is also used to irrigate wounds. *See also*
MEDICAL INSTRUMENTATION.

SYSTEM, the body as a whole or a combination of similar or related parts.

In anatomy, the different systems of
the human body are classified under the
headings of *osteology* (bones); *arthrol-
ogy* (joints); *myology* (muscles and their
covering fasciae or membranes and associated tendons or pulleys); the *blood-
vascular system* (including the arteries,
veins and capillaries); the *lymphatic system* (including the lymph glands and
vessels); the *digestive system* (including
the stomach, intestines and liver); the
respiratory system (including the lungs,
bronchi, and larynx); *neurology* (the nervous system, including the brain, spinal
cord and nerves); the *urinary system;*
the male and female *genital systems;* the
organs of the *senses;* the *integument* (the
skin and its appendages); and the *ductless glands* of internal secretion.

T

TABES DORSALIS, *locomotor ataxia,* a chronic, progressive degeneration and hardening of the nerve fibers at the rear of the spinal cord. These fibers transmit sensory muscle messages to the brain. The degeneration is caused by untreated syphilis and begins 10–20 years after the initial disease. It is more common in men than in women. Tabes dorsalis is believed to be due to a special neurotropic strain of the *Treponema* (organism causing syphilis) and occurs in less than 5 percent of untreated syphilitics.

Loss of muscular sense results in awkward movements. The victim walks with a stumbling, unsteady gait, the feet wide apart, and kicks the foot high and forward with each step. When asked to stand with the feet together and eyes closed (*Romberg sign*), the person sways unsteadily. Lightning stabbing pains in the legs and other parts of the body occur in about 75 percent of cases. The pupil is small and does not contract when light is flashed upon it (*Argyll Robertson pupil*). The knee jerk and the ankle jerk reflexes are absent. In most cases the Wassermann reaction is positive in both the blood and the spinal fluid.

Impotence is the most common complication; delayed and difficult urination are also common. Atrophy of the optic nerve resulting in blindness occurs in about 10 percent of cases. The weight-bearing joints (*Charcot's joints*) and adjacent bones are destroyed in 5–10 percent of the victims.

Tabes dorsalis can be prevented by early treatment of syphilis. *See also* ATAXIA; GAIT; KNEE JERK; NERVOUS SYSTEM; PARESIS; SPINAL CORD *and* **medigraph** SYPHILIS.

TACHYCARDIA, an abnormally rapid pulse, one that is faster than 100 beats per minute. It occurs during running and fast walking, in fevers, in certain heart conditions, and in a number of diseases including *exophthalmic goiter*. *See also* HEART; PULSE.

TACHYPHAGIA, a nervous habit of eating rapidly. It occurs normally in persons who have insufficient lunch or dinner periods, who must hurry to keep a date, or who try to cram other activities into the allotted time for meals. Some poor eaters dislike food and try to finish the meal as fast as possible. Sometimes tachyphagia leads to gulping the food while standing. Eating repeatedly at a quick-lunch counter can lead to the habit of tachyphagia.

The cure is to develop a habit of

leisurely eating of a proper diet at regular hours, to learn to sit down and relax during meals, and to avoid shoptalk at mealtimes.

TALIPES, one of a variety of foot deformities such as flatfoot, clubfoot, or abnormal curvatures of the arch of the foot. *See also* CLUBFOOT.

TAMPONS, plugs of cotton, sponge or other material inserted into the vagina for control of menstrual bleeding, into the nose to stop nosebleed, or into the rectum or other openings. Tampons also are applied to fistulas and deep discharging wounds.

TANNIC ACID, *tannin,* an astringent present in tea, used medically to check bleeding and as an astringent. Obtained from the bark and fruit of many plants, tannic acid is also used to clarify wine and beer. *See also* ASTRINGENT.

TAPEWORM

THE VARIOUS TAPEWORMS that infect human beings require an animal or fish host as well as a human one. As their name indicates, these parasites are flatworms that are segmented, and they may grow to 50 feet.

cause
The larvae of tapeworms embedded in beef, pork, or fish, enter the human body by way of the mouth in food that has been insufficiently cooked to destroy them. The larvae then attach themselves to the intestinal walls where they develop to maturity, attaining a length of 6–10 feet if they are pork tapeworms, 15–20 feet if they are beef tapeworms, and 40–50 feet if they are fish tapeworms.

symptoms
A stool sample of an infected person will contain worm eggs and segments of adult worms will emerge through the anus. These segments, called *proglottids,* may be found in the bedding or inside the clothes before any other symptoms appear. In milder cases, general health is rarely affected. When the infestation is chronic or heavy, stomach cramps, dizziness and obstruction of the bowel may occur. The fish tapeworm is particularly insidious since it requires large amounts of vitamin B_{12} for its growth, thus causing pernicious anemia in the human host.

treatment
As soon as accurate diagnosis is made, treatment is simple and effective when supervised by a doctor over a sufficiently long period to make sure that the parasites have been completely eliminated.

prevention
People who eat raw or rare beef, insufficiently cooked pork, or undercooked fish are exposing themselves to the likelihood of tapeworm infestation.

TARTAR, *dental calculus,* a secretion deposited on the teeth and beneath the gums composed of organic matter and minute food particles plus various salts. Unless removed periodically by the dentist, it may cause *gingivitis* and *pyorrhea. See also* DENTAL HYGIENE; GINGIVITIS; PYORRHEA; TEETH.

TASTE, the special sense by which the nerves on the tongue distinguish acid, bitter, salty and sweet foods and liquids. The message is carried from the tongue to the brain center for taste by the *glossopharyngeal* (ninth cranial) *nerve.* The great variety of taste sensations is due to

Tapeworm

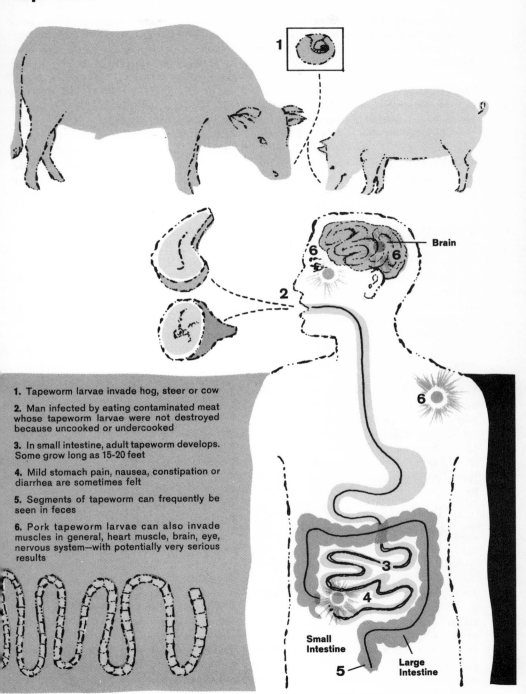

1. Tapeworm larvae invade hog, steer or cow

2. Man infected by eating contaminated meat whose tapeworm larvae were not destroyed because uncooked or undercooked

3. In small intestine, adult tapeworm develops. Some grow long as 15-20 feet

4. Mild stomach pain, nausea, constipation or diarrhea are sometimes felt

5. Segments of tapeworm can frequently be seen in feces

6. Pork tapeworm larvae can also invade muscles in general, heart muscle, brain, eye, nervous system—with potentially very serious results

Brain

Small Intestine

Large Intestine

a combination of the taste and smell perceptions. *See also* NERVOUS SYSTEM; SMELL; TONGUE.

R ESEARCH
  E P O R T   *follows* INFANT.

TATTOO, artificial coloration of the skin by introducing various insoluble dyes such as *carmine, cinnabar, indigo* and *carbon* beneath the surface layers by special needles. Various pictures and designs are portrayed according to the wishes of the recipient. Infectious diseases including *syphilis, viral hepatitis,* *tuberculosis* and *erysipelas* have been transmitted by tattooing.

In many Western societies the practice of tattooing has neither social nor medical acceptance. It is of Polynesian origin, was employed by the Maori and Tahitian peoples as a mark of distinction, and is still a ritual in some African countries.

Since the coloration is indelible, removal of tattoos is difficult and dangerous. The procedure involves peeling the skin with a caustic substance or special motor-powered burrs and emery wheels.

TAY-SACHS DISEASE

Tay-sachs disease is one of several inherited and incurable lipid storage disorders found almost entirely among Ashkenazic Jews. In these disorders, there is an abnormal accumulation of fatty materials in various organs, especially in the brain cells. Children born with Tay-Sachs disease rarely live beyond the age of five.

Tay-Sachs Disease—A scientist studies methods of enzyme replacement as a possible treatment for Tay-Sachs disease. Absence of a crucial enzyme causes this incurable inherited disease in which fatty substances accumulate in cells of various organs—especially those of the brain. This interferes with function and causes progressive blindness, brain damage and early death.

cause
The disease is caused by a congenital metabolic disorder in which there is an absence of the enzyme *hex-A* (*hexosaminidase A*) which normally breaks down waste materials within the cells so that they can function properly. The offspring of two parents who are carriers of the Tay-Sachs gene have a one in four chance of having the disease and a 50–50 chance of being a carrier. It is assumed that approximately one out of every 30 Jews of middle European origin is a carrier.

symptoms
A Tay-Sachs infant will seem normal at birth, but within five or six months, its development ceases, regression sets in, and as the nervous system is increasingly destroyed, convulsions, paralysis and blindness occur.

treatment
At present, there is no treatment for this genetic killer, but scientists are ex-

Tay-Sachs Disease

Disease caused by abnormal accumulation of fatty substances in the Brain

Brain of

Normal Infant   **Tay-Sachs Victim**

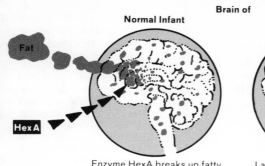

Enzyme HexA breaks up fatty substances so that they can be utilized by Brain and other organs

Lack of HexA enzyme means abnormal deposit of fatty substances in Brain—gradually stopping it from functioning

Course of Tay-Sachs Disease

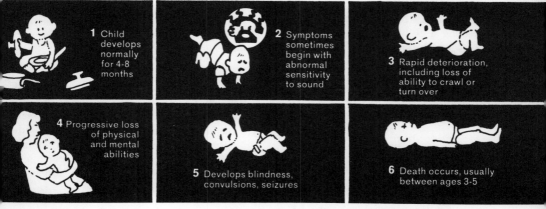

1 Child develops normally for 4-8 months

2 Symptoms sometimes begin with abnormal sensitivity to sound

3 Rapid deterioration, including loss of ability to crawl or turn over

4 Progressive loss of physical and mental abilities

5 Develops blindness, convulsions, seizures

6 Death occurs, usually between ages 3-5

Chance of Inheriting Tay-Sachs Disease if Parents are Carriers

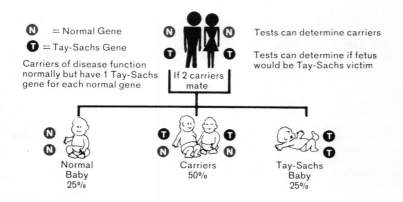

N = Normal Gene

T = Tay-Sachs Gene

Carriers of disease function normally but have 1 Tay-Sachs gene for each normal gene

If 2 carriers mate

Tests can determine carriers

Tests can determine if fetus would be Tay-Sachs victim

Normal Baby 25%

Carriers 50%

Tay-Sachs Baby 25%

ploring the possibility of replacement therapy of the missing enzyme. Tay-Sachs disease is one of the disorders being researched by the National Foundation for Jewish Genetic Diseases. The organization is also a clearing house for information about genetic counseling, special pediatric hospital facilities and other matters of interest to families concerned with the disease.

prevention

Since there is a 1 in 900 risk that a marriage uniting two Ashkenazic Jews would bring two Tay-Sachs carriers together, it is considered advisable for all potential parents within this group to take screening tests that can identify them. If following the genetic counseling, two carriers of the disease decide to risk having a child, a prenatal determination can be made to ascertain whether the child will have the disease. If the fetus is discovered to have Tay-Sachs, a therapeutic abortion can be performed.

R ESEARCH
  EPORT

○   "FEEDING" TAY-SACHS CELLS   ○
        WITH ENZYME MAY ADVANCE
○   TREATMENT OF THE DISEASE   ○
           The possibility of treating *Tay-*
○   *Sachs disease* by enzyme replacement   ○
        has been advanced by a team of NEW
○   YORK UNIVERSITY scientists who suc-   ○
        cessfully "fed" the missing enzyme,
○   *hexosaminidase A* (hex A) to pa-   ○
        tients' white blood cells in test tubes.
○   The enzyme was contained in micro-   ○
        scopic capsules of fatty material
○   called *liposomes.*   ○
           Tay-Sachs disease, which causes
○   progressive brain damage and early   ○
        death, is one of the congenital *meta-*
○   *bolic* disorders resulting from the ab-   ○
        sence of various *enzymes* in the cells'
○   own digestive system. These enzymes,   ○
        called *lysosomes,* normally break
○   down waste materials. If the lyso-   ○
        somes are absent, the undigested ma-
○   terials that accumulate inside the cells   ○
        eventually interfere with normal cell
○   function.   ○

○   Past efforts to supply the necessary   ○
        enzymes by injection were unsuccess-
○   ful because the purified enzymes   ○
        were destroyed or inactivated in the
○   blood or other tissues before they   ○
        could reach the central nervous sys-
○   tem where they are most needed.   ○
           In the current experiments, the
○   liposomes containing the essential en-   ○
        zyme were coated with antibodies
○   that would attract the white cells   ○
        which, as part of their scavenger
○   function, readily engulf antibody-   ○
        coated microbes and other foreign
○   matter. This technique caused the   ○
        Tay-Sachs cells in the test tube to
○   devour the liposomes and their en-   ○
        zyme content.
○   The experimenters hope to dupli-   ○
        cate this reaction inside the body.
○   The risks of injecting antibody-   ○
        coated liposomes into the human pa-
○   tient and the eventual effectiveness of   ○
        such a procedure have yet to be
○   assessed. In the case of Tay-Sachs   ○
        disease, it is not yet known whether
○   postnatal treatment can halt the dis-   ○
        order.   MDSN216

TEAR GAS, vapor containing a chemical which causes irritation of the mucous membranes of the eyes and nose, and shedding of tears with temporary blindness but without any permanent injury. It is used by police and military personnel to disperse mobs and to force suspected criminals to surrender.

TEAR GLANDS. *See* LACRIMAL GLANDS.

TEETH, two sets of hard bonelike structures implanted in the sockets of the jaws and used to tear and grind food into pieces small enough to be easily swallowed and digested. They consist of an inside sensitive *pulp* carrying blood and nerve supplies, surrounded by *dentin*—ivory-like tissues which forms the major part of the teeth, and an outer layer of *enamel.* The composition is largely of mineral salts, chiefly *calcium* and *phosphorus,* but also smaller amounts of *magnesium* and *fluorine.* The deposit of

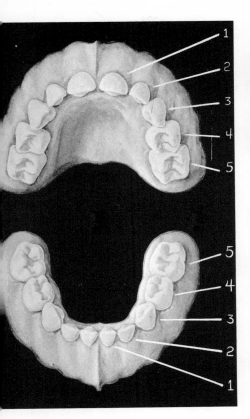

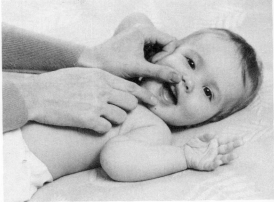

Teeth—The baby seems as pleased with his first tooth as his parents undoubtedly are. There is no rigid time pattern for the growth of teeth, but the first usually emerges when an infant is several months old. Occasionally a baby is born with a tooth already erupted.

Teeth—These are the first teeth, called deciduous —subject to being shed. They number 20, as opposed to 32 in the second and final set. In the upper and lower jaws the central incisor (1), lateral incisor (2), canine (3) and first and second molars (4, 5) are duplicated on the other side of the jaw. The first of these teeth to be replaced are usually the central incisors.

these minerals in the teeth requires vitamin D, without which teeth become soft and subject to decay.

The tooth consists of a *crown,* a *neck,* and one or more *roots* in the jawbones. The root of the tooth is covered by cement resembling bone. It carries blood vessels and nerves, and its central canal is delicate, sometimes requiring special root canal surgery. The *periodontal membrane* holds the tooth within the jawbone, and the surrounding gums further support the teeth.

Two successive sets of teeth occur in life: the 20 *deciduous* (milk) teeth and the 32 *permanent* teeth. The milk teeth, which are formed and in place at the age of three years, are smaller than the permanent teeth and consist of two sets, upper and lower, of four incisors (cutters), two canines (tearers), and four molars (grinders). The permanent teeth—which gradually replace the milk teeth between the ages of six and 12—consist of (above and below on each side) two *incisors* (front teeth), one *canine* (biting tooth), two *bicuspids* located in front of the molars, and three *molars* (grinding teeth). The back molars (wisdom teeth) are the last to come.

In recent years some communities have added small amounts of *fluorine* to the drinking water to prevent dental decay in children and adolescents. It has proved successful, but excessive amounts may cause mottling and discoloration and are also theoretically harmful to older persons. A balanced diet, providing adequate amounts of vitamin C and D in particular but also calcium and phosphorus, is needed to nourish the teeth. Calcium and

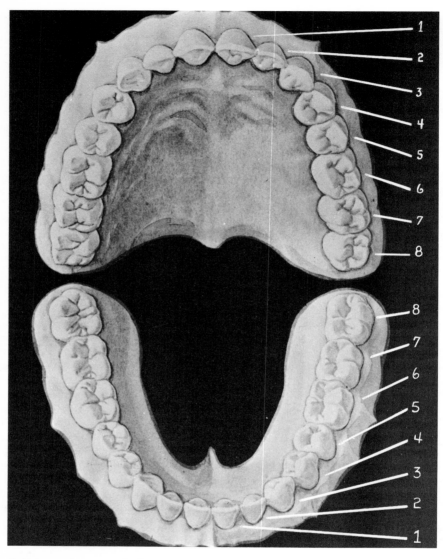

Teeth—Between the ages of about 6–12, the baby teeth are gradually replaced by these 32 larger permanent teeth. Duplicated on the other side of the upper and lower jaws are the central and lateral incisors (1, 2), canine (3), first and second bicuspids (4, 5) and the three molars (6,7,8). The four rear molars, the wisdom teeth, are last to appear—sometimes not until the mid-20s. Occasionally they cannot grow properly for lack of space and are removed surgically.

phosphorus are especially important and are contained abundantly in milk, fish, leafy green vegetables and whole-grain cereals. Rough foods that require chewing are beneficial and massage the gums in the process. Sugar, candy, sweet foods and nondietetic carbonated drinks are harmful and too much of them can lead to dental decay.

Children should be taught to brush

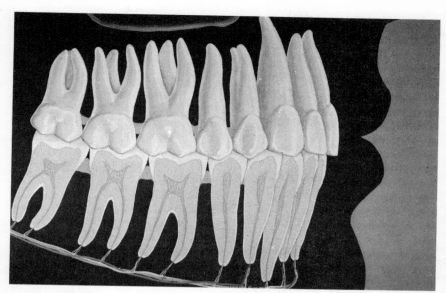

Teeth—Note the precise contact between closed upper and lower teeth when occlusion is correct. The cut-away lower teeth show the roots imbedded in the jawbone. Within them are the darker canals containing blood vessels and nerves. The roots of the upper teeth are similarly supplied. These root canals require delicate surgery if there is damage from decay or injury.

Teeth—The life-long effort to maintain healthy teeth is given a head start with early care by a dentist. He also trains children to brush correctly and stresses wise eating habits. This youngster is evidence of another advantage of early dental visits—she is cheerful, not apprehensive.

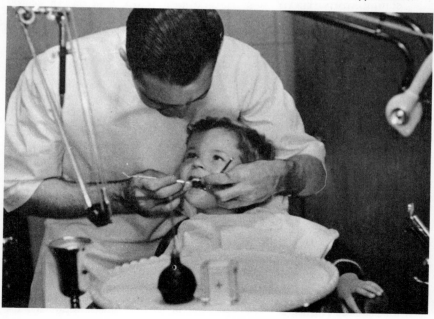

their teeth properly after each meal or snack, preferably away from the gum line. Periodical visits to a dentist can lead to detection of cavities and *pyorrhea* just beginning and may prevent future loss of teeth and *gingivitis*. Regular use of dental floss removes particles of food from between the teeth and thus avoids a prolific source of decay.

The teeth may be darkened and stained by tobacco, coffee, tea and iron medications. When teeth are lost, dentists can provide natural-looking artificial dentures. *See also* BICUSPID; DENTAL CARIES; DENTAL HYGIENE; DENTAL RESEARCH; DENTIFRICE; DENTIN; DENTIST; DENTISTRY; DENTURE; ENAMEL; FLUORIDATION; GINGIVITIS; GUMS; JAW; OCCLUSION; ORTHODONTIA; PYORRHEA; TARTAR *and* **medigraphs** LEUKOPLAKIA; RICKETS; SCURVY; TRENCH MOUTH.

R<small>ESEARCH</small> R<small>EPORT</small> *follows* DENTAL CARIES; DENTAL RESEARCH; FLUORIDATION; PERIODONTAL DISEASE; VACCINATION.

RESEARCH REPORT

SCHOOL-ADMINISTERED FLUORIDE TABLETS LOWER TOOTH DECAY

Children who chewed two *fluoride* tablets each school day over a five-year period had about one-third as many cavities as those children who did not receive the tablets. These results are reported by the NATIONAL INSTITUTE OF DENTAL RESEARCH which, since 1969, has been sponsoring a study of 1000 elementary schoolchildren in Wayne County, North Carolina where the drinking water contains insignificant fluoride levels. The protection afforded by the tablets has been found to be more effective for teeth that erupted during the test period than for teeth already erupted when the tablet administration was begun.

Investigators point out that this method of tooth protection is inexpensive and takes little time. The fact that it can be routinely supervised by the classroom teacher is an advantage over a home-based program in which tablets are likely to be forgotten or taken haphazardly. It was emphasized, however, that even though the tablets provide a safeguard against the spread of cavities, continual exposure to fluoridated drinking water remains the best available public health measure for preventing tooth decay.   NIH525

RESEARCH REPORT

FLUORIDE MUST BE INGESTED FROM INFANCY FOR MAXIMUM BENEFIT TO CHILDREN'S TEETH

Children who receive *fluoride* from *infancy* either in drinking water or in supplements have *healthier* teeth than those who begin fluoride supplements at age four. These findings are the result of a 10-year NATIONAL INSTITUTE OF DENTAL RESEARCH study of 1500 youngsters living in two non-fluoridated areas: Oneida, New York, and a suburb of Kalamazoo, Michigan. Children who did not receive fluoride served as controls; others, who did not receive fluoride supplements but who live in Kalamazoo proper which does have fluoridated water, were also studied. Accumulated data covered the extent of decay in both first and permanent teeth, percentage of children without decay, and prevalence of decay in six-year molars. Results also revealed that breast-fed infants receive practically no fluoride by way of their mothers' milk even if the mothers drink fluoridated water.

The children who began fluoride supplements at age four had the same amount of decay in their primary teeth as those children who got no supplementary fluoride at all; however, their *permanent* teeth were protected as effectively as those of the children who had been drinking fluoridated water from birth.

The survey of permanent teeth in the 7–10 age group of children given fluoride supplements from birth showed the highest percentage of sound teeth and the *lowest* average number of newly decayed and filled teeth.

Six-year molars were especially investigated since they are the first permanent molars to appear, the first to be lost through decay, and the most important for an efficient adult bite. Since the outermost enamel layer on these teeth is formed at age four just before eruption, it might have been anticipated that fluoride supplements begun at age four would protect them. This was not the case. According to these studies, such protection is afforded *only* when the fluoride supplement begins at birth.

All the youngsters involved in the study were given vitamins to avoid any possible variations in fluoride retention. It is known that less fluoride is excreted in the urine when the fluoride dose is consumed with a vitamin supplement.

Since dentists rarely see children before age three, the researchers stress prescribing fluoride from infancy in non-fluoride areas, and for breast-fed babies no matter what the local water content.   NIH1215

TELANGIECTASES, dark red wartlike growths on the skin formed by dilated groups of blood capillaries. They are usually harmless though disfiguring and are best left alone, but they may be destroyed by freezing or by the electric needle.

TELEMETRY, the taking of measurements at a distance from a person, the evidence of the signs under investigation being transmitted by radio signals. In medical treatment, it is employed in association with *electrocardiography* and *electroencephalography. See also* SPACE MEDICINE.

RESEARCH **R**EPORT

NEW TELEMETRY TECHNIQUES SIMPLIFY PATIENT MONITORING

In recent years, increasing use is being made of new *telemetry techniques* for the measurement and long-distance transmission of such medically important information as a

Telemetry—A patient has vital signs monitored by telemetry during open heart surgery. This is a method of measuring blood pressure, temperature, heartbeat and brain waves that transmits the information by radio waves rather than direct connection to a machine. It allows complete isolation of the patient from the recording apparatus for greater protection from contamination.

Courtesy, National Institutes of Health

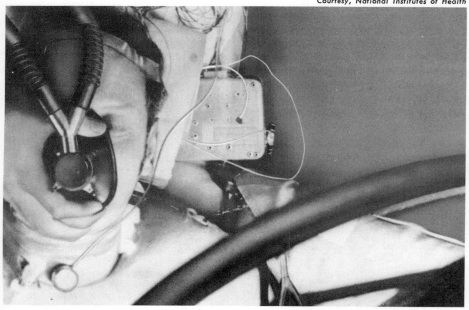

patient's blood pressure, temperature and heart condition. Scientists at the UNIVERSITY OF CALIFORNIA AT LOS ANGELES now report that instead of connecting *epilepsy* patients by wires to a machine that indicates their brain wave patterns, this electroencephalographic data is being transmitted by radio waves. Since the transmitter is not cumbersome to wear, the monitored patient can move about freely and thus tolerate much longer recording periods. The wireless device is also being used by the University's BRAIN RESEARCH INSTITUTE doctors for monitoring the brain wave patterns of *autistic* children whose hyperactivity had made other types of EEG recordings virtually impossible.

The California scientists have also developed a telemetry device that automatically records a patient's medical intake. It is called the *Medication Chronolog* and was designed to monitor the regularity with which *glaucoma* outpatients were using prescribed eyedrops. The Chronolog, which is no larger than a package of cigarettes, is activated when the patient opens it to take his medication. It contains a bottle of eyedrops and an electronic system that compiles data for a three-week period. The oscillographic data can then be checked at a glance to determine whether the patient has used the drops at the precise intervals prescribed by the doctor.   NIH1014

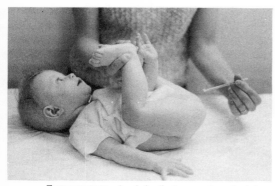

Temperature—An infant's temperature is taken by insertion of a special clinical thermometer into the rectum. Another, even less disturbing, way is to place a thermometer in a baby's armpit. The degree of fever will give immediate indication of whether or not the baby's upset is serious.

TEMPERATURE, the heat level of the body as measured by a calibrated mercury thermometer. The average normal temperature of the human body is 98.6° F. (37° C.), ranging from 97° in the early morning hours to 99° in the evening. The temperature is usually taken by placing the thermometer under the tongue of an adult. A child's temperature is usually taken by rectum.

Normally the body maintains a balance between heat production and heat dissipation. Heat is produced by muscular contractions and the physiological processes of the body and especially by exercise. It is dissipated chiefly through the air and vapor from the lungs and sweat which evaporates on the skin.

When one feels hot or cold, the sensation is not necessarily due to a change in the body temperature but sometimes to a change in the temperature of the skin to which the body responds automatically.

A rise of temperature above 101° F. is due to a fever for which a doctor should be called. The pulse rate is usually increased ten beats per minute for each degree that the temperature goes up, and breathing also becomes faster in a ratio of 1:4 as compared with the pulse. Fevers ranging from 101° to 105° F. are common in many infections; fever above 105° F. is ominous. A temperature below 96° F. may indicate shock and collapse. In recovery from a fever, the morning temperature may be subnormal, a good sign. In severe illnesses, shortly before death, the temperature may register as high as 107° to 109° F. In many instances the fever is preceded by a chill, during which the person feels cold and shivers. A *sustained fever* is one in which the temperature stays high throughout the 24 hours; an *intermittent fever* falls daily to normal or below and then rises again; a *remittent fever* rises and falls daily without returning to normal; and a *relapsing fever* returns after being normal for several days.

Tendons

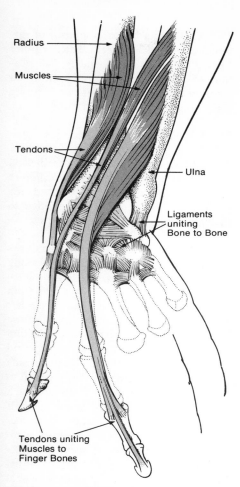

Radius

Muscles

Tendons

Ulna

Ligaments uniting Bone to Bone

Tendons uniting Muscles to Finger Bones

Tendon—The skeletal muscles end in strong bands called tendons. This fibrous tissue fuses with the connective tissue covering bones, thereby attaching muscles to the bones they move. Though subject to inflammation, the tough tendons are seldom torn, even by severe injury.

Chilling of the body lowers resistance to infection, especially in elderly persons. The response may be congestion in the nose, with symptoms similar to those of a cold. Some people are more susceptible to excessive cold or heat than others, reacting to such exposure with symptoms of an allergy.

The treatment of a fever depends upon its specific cause. Often the proper antibiotic for the condition will stop the fever rapidly. As a general measure, sponge or tub baths and the application of cold compresses or an ice cap to the head are helpful. To control high temperature *antipyretic* drugs such as aspirin may be used. They do not alter the course of the illness but simply reduce the fever. *See also* ANTIPYRETIC; FEVER; FROSTBITE; HAZARDS OF COLD; HUMIDITY; PERSPIRATION; THERMOMETER.

TEMPERATURE INVERSION, an atmospheric phenomenon in which the temperature of the air rises with increasing altitude (instead of falling, as is normally the case). When this combines with a lack of wind over an urban or industrialized area, man-made pollutants become trapped in the colder surface air which cannot escape to higher levels. If this trapped air pollution is combined with fog, the result is *smog. See also* AIR POLLUTION.

TENDON, *sinew,* a band of dense fibrous tissue at the end of a muscle, attached to a bone to act as a lever. Inflammation of a tendon is called *tenositis. See also* ACHILLES TENDON; MUSCLE *and* **medigraph** BURSITIS.

TENESMUS, straining, especially the painful straining to empty the bowels or bladder without result, a common symptom of spastic constipation or enlargement of the prostate.

TENNIS ELBOW, a painful stiffness of the elbow joint, common in tennis players, caused by an acute or chronic *synovitis* (inflammation of connective tissue) at the juncture of the lower part of the arm bone and the upper part of the rotary bone of the forearm. Some tennis professionals attribute the condition to a faulty playing of the backhand stroke—namely,

Tennis Elbow

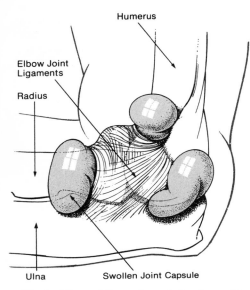

Humerus

Elbow Joint Ligaments

Radius

Ulna   Swollen Joint Capsule

Tennis Elbow—Inflammation of the tissue surrounding the bone ends at the elbow can be extremely painful and disabling. Playing tennis (hence the name "tennis elbow") or repeated carrying of a heavy suitcase are among the chief causes of the condition.

a lifting drive which puts a strain on the elbow joint. *See also* ELBOW *and* **medigraph** BURSITIS.

TENSION, the state of being stretched or strained, usually applied to high blood pressure or excessive irritability of the nerves. *See also* ANXIETY; PREMENSTRUAL TENSION *and* **medigraph** HIGH BLOOD PRESSURE.

TENSION STRIPES. *See* STRETCH MARKS.

TERATOGENS, certain drugs or other agents that cause the production of physical defects in the developing embryo, as in the case of the deformed babies whose mothers took *thalidomide* during the early months of pregnancy. Other drugs are suspected teratogens. *See also* BIRTH DE-

FECT; GENETIC COUNSELING; THALIDOMIDE.

TERATOMA, a tumor composed of different tissues such as teeth, hair, or other foreign materials not found in the location of the tumor. It results from an embryonic misplacement of tissue during early pregnancy. *See also* TUMOR.

TERRAMYCIN, trade name for *oxytetracycline,* a broad-spectrum antibiotic derived from fermentation of specific soil bacteria. It is effective in many different infections and is often substituted for penicillin when patients are sensitive to that antibiotic. *See also* ANTIBIOTICS.

TESTICLES, *testes,* the two male sex glands which hang outside the body proper in a thin skin sac called the *scrotum,* so as to protect the sperm cells from the higher heat of the body. The left testicle hangs lower than the right because the spermatic cord which suspends it from the abdomen is longer. At an early period of fetal life, the testicles are located inside the abdomen, from which they descend to the scrotum before birth. The testicle is a soft oval gland weighing about one-half ounce. The testicles manufacture *spermatozoa* (sperm cells) in enormous numbers, so that millions of them are ejaculated into the vagina during sexual intercourse. Each testicle contains several hundred twisted tubules (*seminiferous tubules*) which manufacture the spermatozoa, separated by bands of fibrous tissue nesting the *Leydig cells* of internal secretion that manufacture the male sex hormone (*testosterone*). The developed spermatozoa pass through the *epididymis* and *vas deferens* tubes to the *seminal vesicle* located near the bladder, from which they are ejaculated during sexual intercourse.

The secretion of testosterone begins at puberty and is responsible for the masculine attributes of heavier bones, stronger muscles, deep voice, beard, heavy growth of hair on the body, and aggressiveness.

A *eunuch* is a man whose testicles have been removed. *Eunuchoidism* is a condition of impaired masculinity with feminine traits due to failure of the testicles to descend into the scrotum or insufficient secretion of the male sex hormone. Sexual impotence is not due to eunuchoidism but is more often of psychological origin. Testosterone may produce descent in cases of undescended testicles but surgery may be required.

Mumps in male adults may migrate to the testicles and cause swelling, pain and inflammation. Typhoid and undulant fever may also affect the testicles. Primary cancer of the testicles is rare but metastases may come from distant organs. *See also* ANDROGENS; CASTRATION; ENDOCRINE GLANDS; EPIDIDYMIS; GLANDS; REPRODUCTIVE SYSTEM; SCROTUM; SEMEN; TESTICULAR TUMORS; TESTOSTERONE; VAS DEFERENS *and* **medigraphs** ORCHITIS; UNDESCENDED TESTICLES; VARICOCELE.

TESTICULAR TUMORS. Primary cancer of the testicle is rare but other tumors may occur as metastases from distant organs. Any hard painless mass in the scrotum which does not recede within a few days is suspected of being a tumor. The most common growths are *adrenal rests chorionepithelioma,* a form of cancer. *See also* CANCER; TESTICLES; TUMOR.

TESTOSTERONE, the male sex hormone (secreted by the *Leydig cells* in the testicles) which controls the secondary sexual attributes. Testosterone is used in the treatment of eunuchism, eunuchoidism, and as a palliative for breast cancer, but not for impotence as it may cause enlargement of the prostate. *See also* HORMONES; REPRODUCTIVE SYSTEM; TESTICLES.

TESTS. Most tests are performed by the doctor as part of a physical examination,

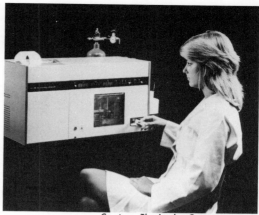

Courtesy, The London Company

Tests—Laboratory testing has reached high levels of speed and accuracy, thanks to the sophisticated devices of modern technology. The automatic analyzer (*above*) prints out data on blood gas/acid-base balance of a blood sample in just a couple of minutes. The serum separation tubes (*below*) provide better serum samples faster and more cheaply.

Courtesy, Becton, Dickinson and Company

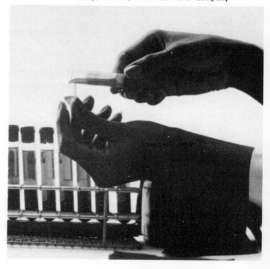

including measurement of the blood pressure, the pulse and breathing rates, and the tendon reflexes. Analytical chemists and testing laboratories are equipped to perform various chemical and laboratory tests as ordered by the doctor. The re-

REPRESENTATIVE LABORATORY TESTS

Test	Method and Specimen Used	Testing For:
AFP	Analysis of amniotic fluid for the presence of abnormally high levels of AFP (alpha fetoprotein)	Defects of the central nervous system, such as spina bifida
Amniocentesis	Microscopic analysis of amniotic fluid aspirated from a pregnant uterus by needle through the abdomen	Certain birth defects; sex of fetus in cases involving carriers of certain inherited diseases
Amylase	Reaction of blood sample to mixture with enzyme amylase	Acute pancreatitis
Aschheim-Zondek	Urine injected into test animal	Pregnancy
Barium Enema	X-rays of the large intestine after injection of barium into emptied rectum as a contrast medium	Diseases of the colon
Basal Metabolism (BMR)	Breathing through a mask to establish an individual's rate of oxygen intake and consumption	Thyroid and other glandular functions
Biopsy	Microscopic examination of a tissue sample	Any suspected malignancy; liver cirrhosis
BSP	Analysis of blood after injection of dye sulfobromophthalein in the vein of a fasting person	Liver function to detect cancer or cirrhosis
Blood Urea Nitrogen (BUN)	Measurement of urea and nitrogen compound in blood (normally excreted by kidneys)	Kidney function
CEA	Analysis of blood sample to determine levels of carcino-embryonic antigen	Useful in diagnosing several types of cancer; also serves to evaluate affect of various cancer treatments
Complete Blood Count (CBC)	Determination of total units of each type of circulating ,blood cell in a blood sample	infections, anemias, leukemias, bone marrow failure, adverse drug reaction; basic screening procedure
Coombs	Antigen-antibody reactions in blood serum	Certain anemias; crossmatching for transfusions; Rh incompatibility in pregnancy
CPK	Blood serum sample is subjected to chemical analysis to measure the level of CPK (creatine phosphokinase) enzyme	Duchenne muscular dystrophy. Also detects carriers of this type of MD
CSF Analysis	Cell counts, bacterial smears and cultures of cerebrospinal fluid sample taken in spinal puncture	Infections, tumors and hemorrhage of the brain; multiple sclerosis
Frei	Skin reaction to injection of the heated virus responsible	Lymphogranuloma venereum (a venereal disease)
GI Series	X-rays of stomach and intestine after a fasting person swallows barium as a contrast medium	Ulcer or cancer of the stomach or duodenum
Glucose Tolerance	Blood and urine tests after swallowing prescribed amount of glucose on an empty stomach	Early diabetes mellitus, hypoglycemia, other metabolic disorders

REPRESENTATIVE LABORATORY TESTS (Continued)

Test	Method and Specimen Used	Testing For:
Hanger's	Blood serum reaction to mixture with emulsion of cholesterol, cephalin and water as a reagent	Liver function to determine the cause of jaundice
KUB	Urinary tract x-rays after administration of a special dye	Cancer and other diseases of the kidneys and bladder
Latex Fixation	Blood serum reaction to latex particles that have been coated with gammaglobulin	Rheumatoid arthritis
Lead	Determination of lead levels in blood and urine	Lead poisoning
Mantoux	Injection into the skin of an extract of tubercle bacilli culture	Tuberculosis
Nonprotein Nitrogen (NPN)	Measurement of nonprotein nitrogen content in blood (normally excreted by kidneys)	Kidney function; circulatory disease impairing the kidney blood supply
Papanicolaou (Pap Test)	Microscopic examination of smear of fluid from the vagina	Cancer of the uterus and cervix
Paul-Bunnell	Blood serum test to determine the presence in an individual's blood of antibodies for the red blood cells of sheep	Infectious mononucleosis
PKU	Blood and urine testing of infant 3–6 days old to detect excessive accumulation of amino acid phenylalanine	Phenylketonuria (lack of phenylalanine metabolism, causing mental retardation)
Protein-Bound-Iodine (PBI)	Measurement of protein-bound iodine in blood sample	Thyroid function as an indication of abnormality, disease or therapy reaction
Sedimentation Rate (ESR)	Determination of settling rate of red blood cells out of unclotted blood in one hour	General screening procedure
Serum Enzyme	Blood serum analysis to determine measurement of various muscle enzymes	Certain muscle enzymes are abnormally increased very early in the course of dystrophy
Sweat	Chemical analysis of sweat	Cystic fibrosis
Thayer-Martin	Microscopic examination of suitably cultured specimen of a discharge from penis or vagina, cervix and rectum	Gonorrhea
Thorn	Microscopic analysis of blood after hormone injection	Adrenal gland function
Urinalysis	Chemical, microscopic and visual examination of urine	Diabetes mellitus, kidney disease or abnormality, infections, other diseases
Venereal Disease Research Laboratory (VDRL)	Blood serum reaction to a certain strain of Treponema pallidum, the organism responsible for syphilis	Syphilis
Widal	Blood sample reaction to mixture with typhoid bacilli	Typhoid and paratyphoid fevers

ports of such tests may aid materially in making a correct diagnosis when considered in conjunction with the patient's history and physical examination, and also in determining the proper treatment and the patient's susceptibility to various diseases. The accompanying chart lists the more common laboratory tests. Since the normal values are dependent upon the laboratory, they are not included. *See also* AMNIOCENTESIS; BINET-SIMON TEST; BIRTH DEFECT; DIABETIC TESTS; DIAGNOSIS; DICK TEST; GENETIC COUNSELING; KAHN TEST; KIDNEY FUNCTION TESTS; PAP SMEAR TEST; PREGNANCY TESTS; RINNE TEST; RORSCHACH TEST; SCHICK TEST; SEDIMENTATION RATE; SMEARS; THYROID TESTS; WASSERMANN TEST.

TETANUS

TETANUS IS AN ACUTE DISEASE of the nervous system that was once a major killer, especially in the rural areas. Each year it strikes fewer than 500 persons in the United States, thanks to widespread and early immunization against it. The early detection of symptoms and inoculation with neutralizing antitoxins have also contributed to the decrease in fatalities. Tetanus is frequently called *lockjaw* because one of the early symptoms is a paralyzing spasm of the muscles involved in opening the mouth.

causes
Tetanus is caused by the toxin of the microorganism *Clostridium tetani,* found in the soil and dust, and in the intestines of horses, cows and man. The infection is spread by contaminated animal and human feces. The germs may enter the body through any break in the skin, such as might result from a puncture wound, an insect sting, an animal bite, or a gunshot wound.

symptoms
In some cases, the infected wound site may heal, but usually, the area becomes sore and inflamed. Within about three weeks, the victim becomes irritable and restless, experiencing stiffness in the neck and difficulty in swallowing. Severe muscular spasms occur in the abdomen, back and face. Slight disturbances, such as a creaking door or a sudden draft, will trigger painful convulsions.

complications
If convulsions are sufficiently severe, respiration may fail, leading to fatal asphyxiation.

treatment
A doctor should be consulted promptly if there is even a remote possibility that a wound has been contaminated by the tetanus bacillus. This might occur when walking barefooted in a barn and picking up a splinter or stepping on a nail; falling in a pasture and getting deep scratches contaminated with dry cow droppings; and the like. The doctor takes into account the date of the victim's last dose of antitoxin or booster shot of tetanus toxoid. When passive immunization is indicated, human antitetanus globulin is preferred to horse serum if it is available. Antibiotics are also given, and if a tetanus attack should occur, anticonvulsants and sedatives are administered. Where emergency hospitalization is essential, the victim may be placed in a hyperbaric chamber to combat the risk of respiratory failure.

prevention
Immunization against tetanus is one of the routine procedures of infant care. At six months, a baby has usually received

Tetanus (Lockjaw)

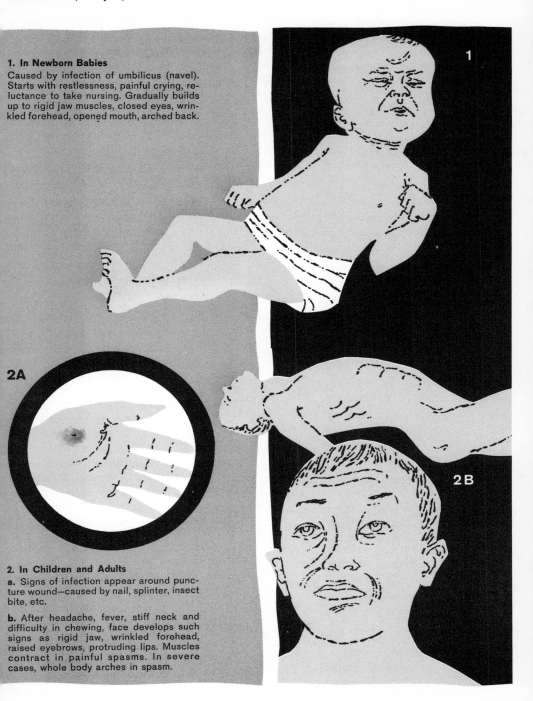

1. In Newborn Babies
Caused by infection of umbilicus (navel).
Starts with restlessness, painful crying, reluctance to take nursing. Gradually builds
up to rigid jaw muscles, closed eyes, wrinkled forehead, opened mouth, arched back.

2A

2B

2. In Children and Adults
a. Signs of infection appear around puncture wound—caused by nail, splinter, insect
bite, etc.

b. After headache, fever, stiff neck and
difficulty in chewing, face develops such
signs as rigid jaw, wrinkled forehead,
raised eyebrows, protruding lips. Muscles
contract in painful spasms. In severe
cases, whole body arches in spasm.

1399

a series of three shots containing toxoids against diphtheria, pertussis (whooping cough), and tetanus. Booster shots are administered at suitable intervals. Adults who have not had a booster shot within a five-year period should be especially alert to the dangers of infection, especially on farms and in stables.

TETANY. *See* PARATHYROID GLANDS.

TETRACYCLINE, a broad-spectrum antibiotic, a biosynthetic product derived from soil, effective for a wide range of bacteria and rickettsiae and used as a substitute for penicillin in people who are sensitive to it. *See also* ANTIBIOTICS.

TETRAHYDROCANNABINOL, is a mood-stimulating drug derived from *cannabis* (marijuana) with similar properties. Cannabis produces mental elation and a sensation of heightened consciousness. It has no recognized medical uses. *See also* **medigraph** MARIJUANA ABUSE.

TETRALOGY OF FALLOT, a combination of heart defects: narrowing of the opening between the pulmonary artery and the right ventricle (chamber), a defect in the partition between the two ventricles, enlargement of the right ventricle, and a displacement of the aorta (main artery) to the right so that it overrides the partition between the two ventricles and receives both venous and arterial blood. *See also* BLUE BABY; HEART *and* **medigraph** CONGENITAL HEART DISEASE.

THALASSEMIA, the term for a group of *genetically determined* blood disorders in which the body produces red blood cells with insufficient *hemoglobin,* a substance that enables the red cells to carry oxygen. The most common of these disorders is *Cooley's anemia,* also known as *Mediterranean anemia (thalassemia major),* in which the red blood cells are extremely thin and fragile. Another type is called *thalassemia minor* which may present no symptoms at all.

Normal red blood cells have a life span of 3–4 months and as they die they are continuously replaced by new cells. In Cooley's anemia, the red blood cells cannot survive for more than a few weeks resulting in anemia. This condition appears shortly after birth and becomes progressively worse as time passes.

Both parents must carry and transmit the trait for the child to develop Cooley's

Tetralogy of Fallot
(Shown in cross-section of Heart)

4 Components in Tetralogy
1. Disproportion and Displacement of Aorta and Pulmonary Artery
2. Narrowing of Pulmonary Artery
3. Interventricular Septal Defect
4. Enlarged Right Ventricle

Tetralogy of Fallot—One of the signs of this condition is cyanosis—bluish discoloration due to poorly oxygenated blood. Open-heart surgery is the most successful treatment in most cases.

anemia. It is most likely to be inherited by persons whose ancestors lived in the countries surrounding the Mediterranean Sea (particularly Greece and Italy). One out of every 1000 American children of Mediterranean descent will inherit the disease.

Symptoms are similar to those of other anemias—pallor, listlessness, loss of energy and appetite, and irritability. However, a physician's examination often reveals an enlarged liver and spleen, pallor of the skin and mucous membrane and sometimes a slight yellow coloration (jaundice) in the whites of the eyes. A blood test will show the changes in the shape and number of red blood cells that distinguish Cooley's from most other anemias.

Children with the disease are usually small for their age because bone growth is poor. Their bones are sometimes so fragile that fractures occur almost spontaneously.

The only way to maintain a blood count sufficient for survival is to administer periodic blood transfusions. Sometimes, the victims of Cooley's anemia must undergo surgical removal of the spleen. Because of an increased susceptibility to infection, they also may endure unpredictable complications of the disease.

The hundreds of pints of transfused blood create a buildup of iron which becomes deposited in the victim's body and vital organs—including the heart. Once iron has been deposited in these tissues, it cannot be removed by any normal life process. Chemical agents that can remove this excess iron are too toxic for widespread use. The resulting iron overload can cause the development of heart and liver failure, kidney failure, diabetes and hepatitis—any of which can eventually lead to death.

Ongoing research is providing a better understanding of Cooley's anemia, and improved management of its complica-

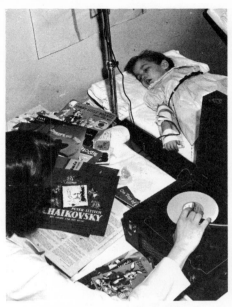

Thalassemia—Transfusions are a way of life for this victim of thalassemia, also called Cooley's anemia. Her fragile red blood cells are short-lived, causing severe anemia. Regular transfusions are needed to maintain enough hemoglobin in her system for survival.

tions will enable the victims to live longer with less pain and disability.

Children who inherit the trait from only one parent will develop thalassemia minor which can present itself as a mild form of anemia, or there may be no symptoms at all. Since this condition never worsens or converts to thalassemia major, individuals have a normal life span and normal health. *See also* ANEMIA; BIRTH DEFECT; BLOOD CONDITIONS; GENETIC COUNSELING; HEMOGLOBIN; RED BLOOD CELLS, DISEASES OF.

RESEARCH REPORT

COOLEY'S ANEMIA DIAGNOSABLE IN FETUS USING ASPIRATION TECHNIQUE

Scientists at the UNIVERSITY OF CALIFORNIA have been using the transabdominal aspiration technique which samples fetal cells in utero to analyze the cells for *Cooley's anemia (thal- assemia*) and to establish a correct diagnosis of a normal fetus. Fetal blood can be obtained with this method aided by *ultrasonography* from women pregnant for 18–22 weeks.

A couple whose first child had Cooley's anemia and therefore required monthly blood transfusions, requested prenatal diagnosis during the second pregnancy. Applying the new diagnostic method at the 20th week of gestation, investigators localized the mother's placenta posteriorly by ultrasound and aspirated it with a 20-gauge needle to obtain fetal red blood cells. The sample was then studied for globin-chain synthesis.

Analysis indicated that although the fetus was a high risk for the disease, it was normal or at worst a carrier of the disease and that a planned abortion was unnecessary. The infant was born at term and showed no signs of imbalance in blood synthesis.

With additional experience in fetal blood acquisition, prenatal diagnosis is rapidly becoming a reality for families whose offspring are potential risks for Cooley's anemia or sickle cell anemia.   NIH925

THALIDOMIDE, a drug which was marketed extensively as a sleep-inducer in Germany and England after animal and clinical tests had established its apparent safety. Because of the vigilance of the U.S. Food and Drug Administration, thalidomide was never cleared for use in the United States. Scientists later discovered that women who took the drug during the second month of pregnancy gave birth to deformed infants with short fin-like arms and legs and other deformities. With this information, the manufacturers of thalidomide withdrew the drug from German, British and other markets. The tragic history of thalidomide led to an amendment of the U.S. Federal Food, Drug, and Cosmetic Act in 1962 with stricter provisions for the clinical testing of new drugs on human beings. *See also* BIRTH DEFECT; TERATOGENS.

THERMAL POLLUTION, pollution of the air or waters by incinerators, heating plants, and the use of heating devices in industry. *See also* POLLUTION.

THERMOGRAPHY, a non-invasive diagnostic technique that measures the temperature of the skin surface by the use of photographic film sensitive to infrared radiation. The resulting measurement, called a *thermogram,* can alert the physician to the possible presence of a breast tumor, since such a growth is one of the causes of a rise in the temperature of the tissues surrounding it. *See also* **medigraph** BREAST CANCER.

THERMOMETER, a calibrated glass tube containing a column of mercury used as an instrument to take the temperature of the body. The heat of the body expands the mercury, so that it rises proportionately to the temperature. In the United States, Canada and Great Britain the Fahrenheit scale has been in general use, calibrated from 94° to 108°. The normal body temperature of 98.6° F. (37° C.) is sometimes indicated by an arrow. In Europe and most other countries the Centigrade (Celsius) scale is used and the United States is converting to this system as well.

In adults, the thermometer is usually inserted into the mouth; in children, it is inserted into the rectum, where it registers a fraction of a degree higher. Before use, the thermometer is shaken down below the normal mark. In general, it should remain under the tongue for three minutes and the person should not have a hot or cold drink before having the temperature taken; also the person must not roll the thermometer under the tongue. After each use the instrument is thoroughly washed and not used for another person (until it is sterilized), as it can transmit infection.

A thermometer should be in every home for immediate use when a fever is suspected. A temperature ranging from 100°–102° F. (37.7°–38.8° C.) is a warning to stay home; above 102°, a warning to call a physician. *See also* FEVER; MEDICAL INSTRUMENTATION; TEMPERATURE.

THIAMIN, water-soluble vitamin B_1—*thiamin hydrochloride*—needed in carbohydrate metabolism, abundantly present in many foods including whole-grain cereals, peas, beans, pork, lean meats, yeast and nuts, and in rice husks. It is destroyed by heat and cooking. The chief symptoms of thiamin *deficiency* are poor appetite, nerve paralyses, heart symptoms, and ultimately the disease *beriberi* —causing paralysis of the legs and arms. Alcoholics often suffer from thiamin deficiency because they get their calories from alcohol instead of vitamin-rich foods; people whose diet is low in proteins and high in starches also suffer from thiamin deficiency. *See also* DEFICIENCY DISEASES; NUTRITION; VITAMIN DEFICIENCIES; VITAMINS *and* **medigraph** BERIBERI.

THIRST, a craving for water produced by exercise, heat and sweating. Usually it is caused by a loss of both water and salt, so that salt should be added to the drinking water. In fevers thirst is strong and should be relieved by drinking plenty of water.

THORACENTESIS, removal of fluid from the chest cavity, usually because of fluid or pus in the pleural sac. Excessive accumulations in the area can cause breathing difficulties as well as being an indication of disease.

Thoracentesis is performed with the person sitting up, with arms and head resting on a table over the bed. If there is only a small amount of fluid, it is most easily and safely obtained with the person lying on the affected side on an examining table. After injection of a local anesthetic, a special hollow needle

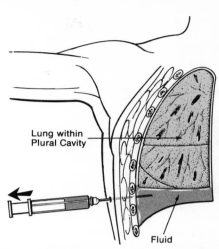

Thoracentesis
(Shown on cross-section of Chest)

Lung within Plural Cavity

Fluid

Thoracentesis—After injection of a local anesthetic, a hollow needle is pushed through the chest wall between two ribs. The syringe's plunger is then slowly withdrawn by the physician. The resulting suction draws off fluid from the chest.

is inserted through the chest wall between two ribs. The suction action of a syringe attached to the needle then draws off the fluid.

When the procedure is completed, the wound is sealed and dressed and must be monitored carefully in order to detect any leakage which may occur. The person must also be observed for excessive coughing, bloody sputum, and color or respiratory changes. Often a chest x-ray is made in order to check for any remaining fluid and for the possible introduction of air into the cavity.

Aspiration of chest fluid by thoracentesis is performed both for relief and for testing to aid in diagnosis of infections or growths in the lungs or the pleural cavity.

THORACOPLASTY, plastic surgery of the thorax, especially removal of several ribs to collapse the lung in *pulmonary tuberculosis*.

THORAX, the bony chest cage containing the heart and lungs, composed of 12 vertebrae, 24 ribs, and the breastbone. *See also* CHEST.

THREE-DAY FEVER. *See* SANDFLY FEVER.

THROAT, *pharynx,* the passage between the back of the mouth, the larynx (voice box) and the gullet. It is a conical-shaped tube, upside down, composed of muscles and membranes lined by a mucous surface, about five inches long, and the portal of entry for many germs, irritants and infections. On the sides are the *fauces* (passages of the throat) lodging the *tonsils* and bounded above by the *soft palate* and below by the back of the tongue.

The throat is the site of many diseases including pharyngitis, due to tobacco smoke or colds; septic sore throat, due to streptococcus infection; diphtheria, scarlet fever and measles; influenza; postnasal drip; and cancer. The treatment of these diseases depends upon the specific cause: a soothing gargle for minor pharyngitis; antibiotics for septic sore throat; antitoxin for diphtheria and scarlet fever, nasal douches for postnasal drip; and surgery for cancer.

Direct application of an antiseptic on a swab is useful for throat infections and an ice pack around the neck may relieve the pain. The primary purpose of a mouth- or throat-wash is to cleanse and soothe the throat. A household remedy is salt solution, made by adding one-fourth teaspoonful of bicarbonate of soda to one-half glass of warm water. *See also* LARYNGITIS; LARYNX; PALATE; PHARYNX; QUINSY; SWALLOWING; TONGUE; TONSILS *and* **medigraphs** DIPHTHERIA; FLU; GERMAN MEASLES; MERCURY POISONING; MONONUCLEOSIS, INFECTIOUS; SCARLET FEVER; TONSILLITIS; TRENCH MOUTH.

THROMBOANGIITIS OBLITERANS. *See* BUERGER'S DISEASE.

THROMBOCYTOPENIA, a deficiency in the number of *blood platelets* attributed to the presence in the blood plasma of an unidentified anti-platelet substance. The platelets are needed for normal blood clotting. The onset of an acute attack may be precipitated by an infection or temporarily by use of certain drugs. Bleeding and bruising from slight injuries and the appearance on the skin of scattered red purpuric spots are the main symptoms. The suspected causes are overactivity of the spleen or an involvement of the bone marrow. The diagnosis is established by a blood count showing a greatly reduced number of platelets.

Remissions (absence of symptoms) may be produced by certain steroid drugs. Splenectomy (removal of the spleen) puts an end to the bleeding and the blood platelet count returns to normal. About 75 percent of victims of this disorder have a prompt response to splenectomy, three-fourths of whom have remissions lasting more than ten years. *See also* BLOOD CONDITIONS; COAGULATION; PURPURA; SPLEEN.

THROMBOPHLEBITIS. *See* PHLEBITIS.

THROMBOSIS, formation of a clot inside a blood vessel most often a vein, due to a slowing of the circulation or the blood's increased tendency to clot, accompanied by an injury. The long *saphenous vein* inside the thigh—especially when it is varicose—is commonly affected. *Milk leg* is due to a *thrombus* (clot) in the *femoral vein,* with painful swelling in the thigh and leg, usually following childbirth or an attack of typhoid fever. The main symptoms of thrombosis are local swelling and pain. The complication to be feared is detachment of a piece of the clot to form an *embolus* which may be carried by the circulation to various parts of the body, especially the lung. When thrombosis is treated with anticoagulants, *pulmonary* *embolism* occurs in only 2 percent of cases.

The treatment of thrombosis in the thigh or leg is complete bed rest for about a week, with a cradle over the foot of the bed to remove the weight of the bed-clothes, and cold applications to relieve the pain. To overcome the clotting tendency, anticoagulant drugs are often prescribed, but the victim must be watched carefully because of the possibility of excessive bleeding. *See also* APOPLEXY; ATHEROSCLEROSIS; CLOT; COAGULATION; CORONARY THROMBOSIS; EMBOLISM; HEPARIN; INFARCTION *and* **medigraphs** ARTERIOSCLEROSIS; BUERGER'S DISEASE; MYOCARDIAL INFARCTION; PHLEBITIS; STROKE.

THRUSH, a fungus infection of the mouth due to *Candida albicans,* (a yeast-like parasite that may also infect other parts of the body including the groins, buttocks and vagina). It is common in infants and sometimes affects elderly persons. The disease causes a crop of white, slightly raised, adherent patches resembling milk curds, beginning on the tongue and inside the mouth and spreading to the palate, gums, tonsils, throat, larynx and elsewhere. An effective treatment is with fungicidal antibiotic mouth washes. *See also* FUNGUS; MONILIASIS.

THUMB, the short and thick first digit of the human hand, differing from the other fingers in having only two instead of three digital bones and greater freedom of movement. Ability to place the thumb in contact with the other fingers accounts largely for human manual skill. *See also* FINGER; HAND.

THUMB-SUCKING, an instinctive habit of infancy related to suckling the mother's breast. In moderation, it is harmless and the baby outgrows the habit. Excessive and persistent thumb-sucking may deform the jaws and cause forward protrusion of the upper front teeth as the lower

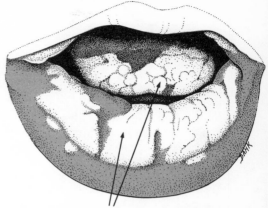

Thrush
Seen in Front View of Tongue and Mouth with Lower Lip everted

Velvety white Lesions resembling coagulated Milk commonly occur on the Edges of the Tongue and Inner Surfaces of the Lips and Cheeks

Thrush—The yeastlike parasite Candida albicans causes this fungus infection. The white patches on the tongue spread all over the mouth and throat. Repeated use of an antifungal antibiotic mouth wash is the best treatment.

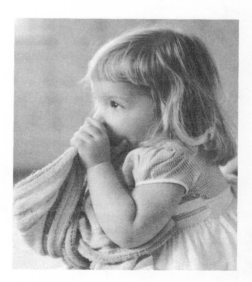

Thumb-Sucking—For some babies, thumb-sucking alone seems not to be enough. They find added comfort fondling a blanket and sucking that, too. Most children outgrow both blanket and thumb as they become more independent.

The Thymus Gland

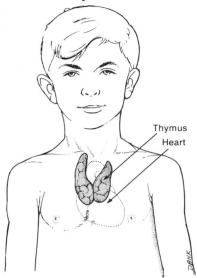

Thymus

Heart

Thymus Gland—The thymus is largest during the first several months of life. Subsequently it shrinks and is very small in the adult. This gland is essential in the development of the body's defense system against infection. Enlargement of the gland in infancy can cause sudden death by cutting off breathing and circulation.

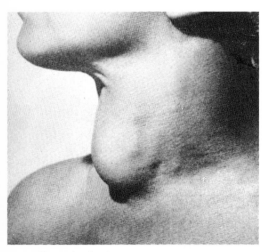

Thyroid Gland—When enlargement of the thyroid gland is this great, it is called a goiter. It can be caused by a deficiency of iodine in the diet, or by excessive or diminished activity of the thyroid gland in producing its hormone.

back teeth are tipped backward. One way to try to correct the habit is to wrap adhesive tape lightly around the thumb. *See also* CHILD CARE.

THYMUS GLAND, a temporary organ of childhood located in the front of the neck and the upper part of the thorax (chest cage). It is largest during the first eight or nine months of life and after the second year normally shrinks almost to the point of disappearance. The functions of the thymus are related to the metabolism of calcium, the development of the skeleton and sex glands, and to the body's disease-fighting mechanism.

The most important disease of the thymus is *hypertrophy* (abnormally large growth) with serious results, including involvement of the lymphoid tissues. Male adults whose thymus has failed to shrink are apt to have a soft complexion, no beard, a boyish appearance, lack of body hair, low blood pressure and they tire easily.

A persistent thymus may cause sudden death in infancy, when the gland enlarges instead of shrinking and interferes with the circulation and breathing because of its nearness to the heart and windpipe. *See also* ENDOCRINE GLANDS; GLANDS; SUDDEN INFANT DEATH SYNDROME *and* **medigraph** MYASTHENIA GRAVIS. R_{ESEARCH} *follows* BIRTH DEFECT.

THYROID GLAND, a ductless gland of internal secretion, containing many blood vessels, situated at the front and sides of the neck in front of the windpipe, with right and left lobes connected across the middle by a narrow portion called the *isthmus.* It weighs about an ounce and is heavier in females, becoming enlarged during menstruation and pregnancy.

The internal secretion of the thyroid gland, *thyroxin,* is characterized by its iodine content. This hormone regulates metabolism, controls the consumption of oxygen, and monitors the pulse. *Hyper-*

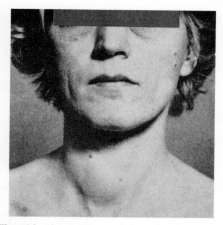 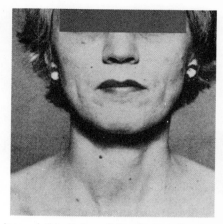

Thyroid Gland—The two-lobed thyroid in the neck is one of the most important endocrine glands. It manufactures a hormone vital to regulating metabolism—the body's physical and chemical processes and reactions. Insufficient thyroid hormone production causes a disruptive slowing down of this body activity. Oversupply of the hormone speeds up metabolism, causing such symptoms as nervousness. The enlargement of the woman's thyroid (*left*) is another sign of these conditions. Prompt treatment to regulate thyroid activity reduced the swelling (*right*).

thyroidism (excessive thyroxin secretion) is the cause of *exophthalmic goiter*, which is indicated by nervousness, rapid pulse, bulging eyes, high basal metabolism, and loss of weight. *Hypothyroidism* (deficient thyroxin secretion) causes *myxedema*, a condition of mental and physical sluggishness, an enlarged gland in the neck, puffiness of the face and hands, a harsh croaking voice, and low basal metabolism. *Cretinism* is a form of infantile myxedema resulting from a lack of iodine in the drinking water. Myxedema and cretinism respond to medication with thyroid. *See also* BASAL METABOLISM; ENDOCRINE GLANDS; EXOPHTHALMIC GOITER; GLANDS; GOITER; HYPOTHYROIDISM; INFANTILISM; IODINE; NUCLEAR MEDICINE; THYROID TESTS; THYROPTOSIS; THYROTOXICOSIS *and* **medigraphs** CRETINISM AND MYXEDEMA; HYPERTHYROIDISM; THYROID HEART DISEASE.

THYROID HEART DISEASE

THYROID HEART DISEASE is a condition that develops as a result of the speeded-up metabolism associated with *hyperthyroidism*, a disorder more common among women than men, and typically associated with the years between 40 and 50.

causes
When the thyroid gland is overactive, the excessive amount of the hormone *thyroxin* secreted into the bloodstream causes an abnormal quickening in the rate at which energy is produced, and the result can be compared to a car whose motor is always racing. The stress placed on the heart because of the glandular disturbance causes it to work harder and faster, and in many cases to become enlarged.

symptoms
The chief manifestations of thyroid heart disease are the enlargement of the heart accompanied by symptoms of congestive heart failure.

Thyroid Heart Disease

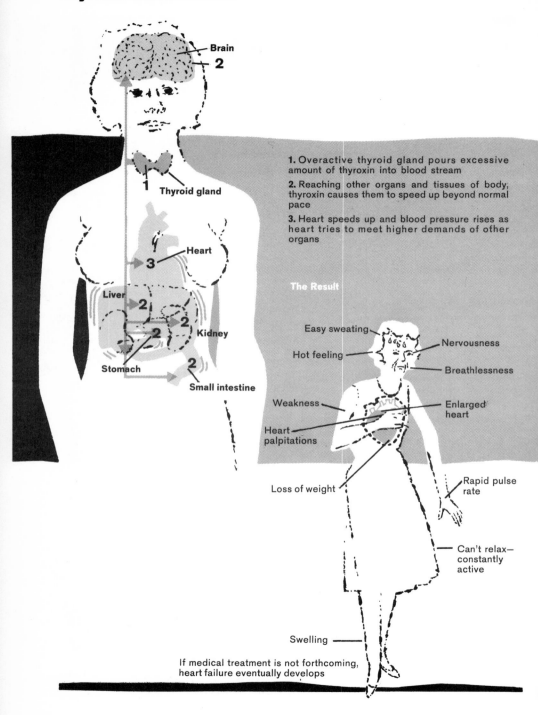

1. Overactive thyroid gland pours excessive amount of thyroxin into blood stream

2. Reaching other organs and tissues of body, thyroxin causes them to speed up beyond normal pace

3. Heart speeds up and blood pressure rises as heart tries to meet higher demands of other organs

The Result

Brain

2

Thyroid gland

Heart

Liver

Kidney

Stomach

Small intestine

Easy sweating

Nervousness

Hot feeling

Breathlessness

Weakness

Enlarged heart

Heart palpitations

Loss of weight

Rapid pulse rate

Can't relax— constantly active

Swelling

If medical treatment is not forthcoming, heart failure eventually develops

treatment

Thyroid heart disease is treated by correcting the hyperthyroid condition that causes it. Accurate diagnosis of overactivity of the thyroid gland is based on a laboratory procedure known as the *protein-bound iodine test*. Since there are several different causes for this overactivity—including tumor, disturbance of the pituitary gland, or an inherited predisposition to the disorder—therapy is based on the doctor's evaluation of each individual case.

THYROIDITIS, inflammation of the thyroid gland usually caused by infection. Many victims respond to the applicable antibiotic. *See also* THYROID GLAND.

THYROID TESTS. Many laboratory tests are available to determine the functional activity of the thyroid gland. The *basal metabolic rate* may indicate excessive or deficient thyroid activity. The se-

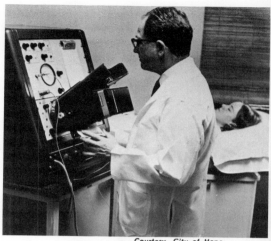

Courtesy, City of Hope

Thyroid Heart Disease—Overactivity of the thyroid gland can provoke heart disease, but this cause must be ascertained before effective treatment can be given. This device, a sphygmorecorder, uses pulse measurements to aid in heart diagnosis. The technique furnishes clues to thyroid disorders as well as heart ailments, thereby detecting any relationship between the two.

Thyroid Tests—Thyroid function tests provide data enabling physicians to diagnose and treat a wide variety of thyroid diseases or disfunction involved in other disorders. Today's advanced products have vastly improved such testing procedures. Accurate results are now often available

in a matter of hours rather than weeks, as was the case in the past when they were not even always reliable. The group shown here includes kits and automated devices to detect the presence, quantity and activity of proteins, hormones and cells that are involved in thyroid function.

Courtesy, Miles Laboratories

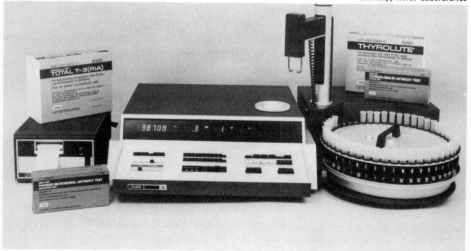

rum *protein-bound iodine test* (PBI) is a reliable index of thyroid function. The normal range is 3.5–7.5 micrograms per 10 cubic centimeters. A higher range indicates *hyperthyroidism;* a lower range, *hypothyroidism.* Tests employing *radioactive iodine* are now available, the most common being the thyroid uptake after an oral dose. The serum cholesterol is usually low in people with hyperthyroidism and high in those with hypothyroidism. Another test is measured by the response to therapeutic doses of the iodides. *See also* BASAL METABOLISM; TESTS; THYROID GLAND.

THYROPTOSIS, a condition in which a goitrous thyroid gland has dropped from the neck into the thorax. *See also* GOITER; THYROID GLAND.

THYROTOXICOSIS, hyperthyroidism with accompanying symptoms, as in *exophthalmic goiter. See also* THYROID GLAND.

TIC. *See* HABIT SPASM.

TIC DOULOUREUX, *trigeminal neuralgia,* brief attacks of sudden severe stabbing facial pain along the course of the *trigeminal* (fifth cranial) *nerve,* usually in people around the age of 50 and more often in women. The stabbing pain is momentary but may recur over periods lasting about 20 seconds, triggered by touching, a slight draft or application of cold water on the sensitive spot. Attacks are influenced by seasonal changes and occur mostly in the spring or autumn months, gradually increasing in frequency and severity. Remissions (absence of symptoms) last weeks or months. The cause of the disorder is not known and the trigeminal nerve shows no pathological change.

Analgesics such as aspirin give only temporary relief, as does niacin. Favorable results following injections of vita-

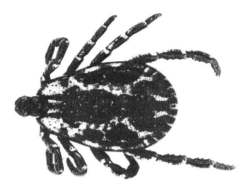

Courtesy, National Institutes of Health

Ticks—The wood tick is one of the hard-shell parasites that can be a carrier of the organism causing Rocky Mountain spotted fever. If ticks are removed from the skin as soon as possible, before they start sucking blood, there is less chance of disease being transmitted.

min B_{12} have been reported. Other treatments also are used. When the pain is excruciating, injection of the branches of the trigeminal nerve with alcohol may abolish it for as long as 18 months but recurrence is the rule. As a last resort, permanent relief can be obtained by cutting the sensory root of the nerve close to its ganglion (knot of nerve cells). *See also* AGUE; NEURALGIA; NEUROLOGICAL AND NEUROMUSCULAR DISORDERS.

TICKS, blood-sucking spiderlike parasites which attach themselves to the skin and often carry the rickettsiae that cause *Rocky Mountain spotted fever* and other infectious disorders. *See also* INSECT BITES; RELAPSING FEVER; RICKETTSIAL DISEASES *and* **medigraph** ROCKY MOUNTAIN SPOTTED FEVER.

TINEA, *ringworm,* affecting the scalp (*tinea capitis*), the beard (*tinea barbae*), the perineum (*tinea cruris*), the feet and toes (*athlete's foot*), or the skin of the body (*tinea corporis*). The disease is caused by a fungus—of which there are several different types—which burrows into the skin. Antifungal ointments rubbed thoroughly into the skin are highly effective in treating tinea. *See also* BARBER'S ITCH; FUNGUS; RINGWORM *and* **medigraph** FUNGUS INFECTIONS OF THE SKIN.

TINNITUS. *See* RINGING IN THE EARS.

TIPPED UTERUS, a forward or backward direction of the neck of the womb. In *anteflexion,* the body of the uterus is bent excessively forward on the cervix (neck). In *anteversion,* the uterus is tilted and displaced forward. In *retroflexion,* the uterus is bent backward upon itself; in *retroversion,* it is tilted backward. Tipped uterus is a common disorder after childbirth and may require manual or surgical correction. *See also* UTERUS.

TOBACCO, the dried and cured leaves of the tobacco plant. It is ignited and its smoke is inhaled, or it is chewed.

Inhalation of cigarette smoke is the leading cause of *cancer of the lung,* due to a cancer-producing tar. Cigar- and pipe-smoking share this danger but to a lesser degree because of the lower temperature at which the tobacco is smoked. Other diseases for which cigarettes are blamed include *emphysema, cancer of the larynx* (voice box), *coronary heart disease,* and *Buerger's disease* (in which the arteries of the legs are thickened and obstructed, leading to gangrene affecting the feet and toes).

Cancer of the lung may occur in non-smokers who are compelled to work or live in smoke-filled rooms. The dangers are so great that in the United States cigarette advertising on television is forbidden and every package must carry a warning that smoking may be hazardous to one's health. In spite of this warning, cigarette-smoking continues and authorities predict that by the year 2000 there will be 630,000 deaths from lung cancer annually. The habit of smoking can be broken by will power, psychological aver-

Displacements of Uterus

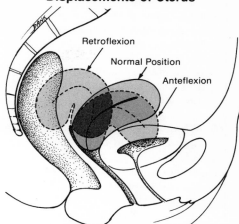

Shown in Female Pelvis Cross-section

Tipped Uterus—These are the types of displacement of the uterus that can exist. The defect can be present from birth or be caused by a tumor on a Fallopian tube or ovary. Most instances of displacement are the result of injuries sustained during childbirth.

sive conditioning, or the substitution of a bitter lozenge for a cigarette to curb the desire to smoke. *See also* ADDICTION; CANCER; CANCER PREVENTION; DRUG WITHDRAWAL; SMOKING AND LUNG CANCER *and* **medigraphs** BUERGER'S DISEASE; EMPHYSEMA; LEUKOPLAKIA; LUNG CANCER; MYOCARDIAL INFARCTION. R_{E P O R T}ᴱˢᴱᴬᴿᶜᴴ *follows* CAFFEINE.

TOENAILS. *See* NAILS.

TOES, the five digits of the foot, each containing three *phalanges* (toe bones) except the big toe, which contains only two. The pressure of tight or narrow shoes causes corns on and between the toes, and a short shoe with pointed toe may cause a bunion of the big toe. *See also* BUNION; CORNS AND CALLUSES; FEET; HAMMERTOE; PIGEON-TOED.

TOILET TRAINING, the training of the young infant in the care of the bowel and bladder movements at regular times and in a clean manner. The establishment of normal bowel and bladder habits should begin in early childhood, so as to avoid later toilet accidents in the kindergarten or primary school. Working mothers especially must be systematic in setting the time for toilet training. *See also* BED WETTING; CHILD CARE.

TONGUE, the organ of taste and speech which also assists in mastication (chewing) and swallowing of food. It is situated in the floor of the mouth within the curve of the lower jawbone. The tongue is composed mostly of muscles covered by mucous membrane. It is attached to the *hyoid bone* in the back of the throat and tapers forward to end loosely at the tip.

Most of the tongue is freely movable but the bottom is attached to the floor of the mouth by a membranous bridle which limits its movements. When the bridle is too short, speech may be tongue-tied, a defect that is easily remedied by cutting the bridle. The taste buds are located on the rear one-third of the back of the tongue whence the impulses travel via the *glossopharyngeal* (ninth cranial) *nerve* to the taste center in the brain.

The tongue is apt to be coated brown if a person is constipated, has stomach disorders, or is feverish. Some children have the nervous habit of biting the tongue so as to cause pain and bleeding. The tongue may be irritated and red-

dened by hot drinks, pepper and spices, and by rubbing it against sharp rough teeth. A deficiency of vitamin B₂ (*riboflavin*) causes inflammation of the tongue, among other symptoms. In advanced syphilis, ulcers of the tongue are common. *Geographic tongue* is characterized by a thickening of the membrane with deep furrows, producing the appearance of a map. Cancer of the tongue afflicts heavy smokers and people who chew tobacco. *See also* BLACK HAIRY TONGUE; GEOGRAPHIC TONGUE; GLOSSITIS; GLOSSOPHARYNGEAL NEURALGIA; MOUTH; SPEECH; STUTTERING; TASTE; THROAT; VITAMIN DEFICIENCIES *and* **medigraphs** HISTOPLASMOSIS; PERNICIOUS ANEMIA; SCARLET FEVER; TONSILLITIS; TRENCH MOUTH; TYPHOID FEVER; WHOOPING COUGH.

RESEARCH REPORT *follows* INFANT.

TONIC, an agent or drug that is supposed to improve the normal tone of an organ or function or of the person generally. Formerly many drugs were called tonics in the mistaken belief that they improved general health and resistance. The term *tonic* is now used in relation to the specific function which it aids. For example, one bitter medicine is termed "a 'tonic to the appetite." *See also* QUININE.

TONSILLECTOMY, surgical removal of the tonsils. *See also* TONSILS.

TONSILLITIS

THE TONSILS, WHICH ARE collections of spongy lymphoid tissue located on each side of the back of the throat, frequently become enlarged or inflamed —especially in childhood—in the process of filtering out mild infections. Acute tonsillitis, however, is almost always a serious condition requiring prompt medical attention.

causes
Although various agents are responsible for tonsillitis, the infection in its acute form is typically caused by streptococcus pyogenes inhaled through the nose or mouth. When the tonsils have already been removed, the equivalent inflammation of the pharynx or the back of the throat is known as a strep throat.

Acute Tonsillitis (Strep Throat)

A. Red, swollen tonsils, pharynx, soft palate. Patches of yellow, gray or white membrane covers inflamed area. Tongue has heavy gray coating.

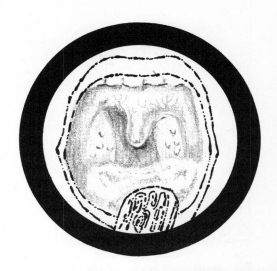

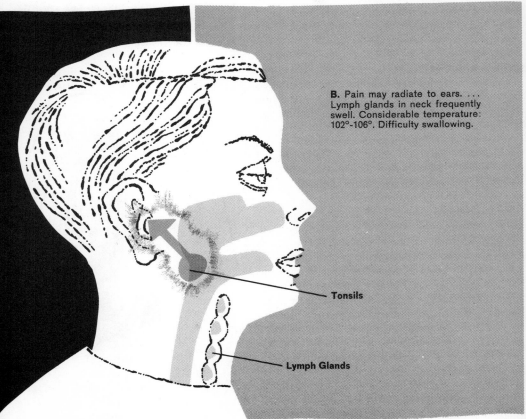

B. Pain may radiate to ears. .... Lymph glands in neck frequently swell. Considerable temperature: 102°-106°. Difficulty swallowing.

Tonsils

Lymph Glands

1413

symptoms

Onset of the infection is usually sudden and severe, with fever reaching 105° F. (40.5° C.), extreme discomfort when swallowing, chills, headache and pain in the lymph glands in the neck.

complications

The chief complications of any respiratory infection with streptococcus bacteria are secondary involvement of the heart in rheumatic fever and of the kidneys in glomerulonephritis. These complications may occur several weeks after the original infection appears to have subsided. Children are especially vulnerable to these involvements as well as to infections of the middle ear and scarlet fever. The formation of an abscess adjacent to the tonsils may result in the condition known as quinsy. Surgical drainage of the pus in the abscess may be necessary if it does not rupture naturally.

treatment

Antibiotics are administered as soon as diagnosis based on laboratory inspection of throat smears establishes streptococci as the cause of the infection. Although the tonsillitis may be self-limiting and the symptoms may subside within a week, antibiotic therapy is considered essential to prevent complications.

prevention

Removal of tonsils is not recommended, except in recurring cases of ear infection or chronic enlargement that interferes with hearing, since streptococcus invasion can occur even after a tonsillectomy. In circumstances where an epidemic occurs because of contaminated milk or poor hygienic conditions involving close contact with a carrier, preventive medication is usually prescribed for those exposed to infection.

TONSILS, disc-shaped masses of spongy lymphoid tissue, located at the sides of the throat and readily seen and examined when the person opens the mouth widely and says "Ah." The tonsils form part of a circular band of lymphoid tissue that guards the entrances to the digestive and respiratory passages.

The function of the tonsils, if any, is not known. At one time they were considered dangerous sources of infection and were removed by *tonsillectomy* almost routinely. Nowadays the tonsils are removed only for specific circumstances.

Tonsillitis frequently accompanies *septic sore throat*. The illness begins suddenly with a chill and high fever, sore throat, swelling and enlargement in the throat, and prostration. The most serious complications of this disease are *rheumatic fever, endocarditis* affecting the

Tonsils—The tonsils are imbedded on either side at the back of the throat. Part of the body's lymphatic system, they help filter out germs that enter the body through the nose and mouth.

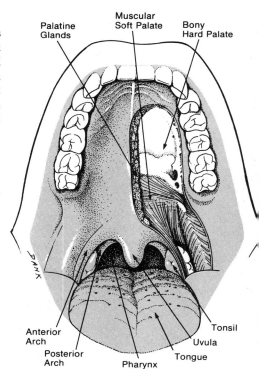

lining membrane of the heart and valves, and *acute nephritis* (inflammation of the kidneys). Depending on the identity of the germ that causes the infection, a specific antibiotic may be curative. Analgesics such as aspirin are given to relieve the pain and lower the temperature. *See also* ADENOIDS; DYSPHAGIA; EAR; LYMPHATIC SYSTEM; PHARYNX; QUINSY; THROAT; TONSILLECTOMY *and* **medigraphs** FLU; TONSILLITIS.

TOOTHACHE, caused by a cavity, exposed dentin, inflammation of the dental pulp, or an abscess. Sometimes the toothache is caused by a disorder in a distant area of the body. A dentist should be consulted as soon as possible. For painful cavities, the emergency treatment is to cleanse the cavity so as to remove food debris and then to apply *oil of cloves.* The dentist may apply *silver nitrate* to the area of exposed dentin; an abscess of the pulp may require opening and drainage or, in extreme cases, extraction of the tooth. *See also* DENTAL CARIES; DENTAL HYGIENE; DENTIN *and* **medigraphs** SINUSITIS; TRENCH MOUTH.

TORPOR, a condition of sluggishness. *Intestinal torpor* is constipation, and *retinal torpor* is visual sluggishness requiring stronger light.

TORTICOLLIS. *See* WRYNECK.

TOURNIQUET, a device to control bleeding. It is wrapped around a bleeding limb tightly enough to compress the artery. It may be in the form of a rubber tube or band or simply a handkerchief in emergencies. Once the bleeding has been controlled, the tourniquet should be loosened. If it is too tight or left in place too long, the lack of blood may cause gangrene. *See also* FIRST AID; HEMORRHAGE *and* **medigraph** SNAKEBITES.

TOXEMIA, the presence of poisonous substances in the blood, produced either by the body itself or by germs. The poisons may arise from a localized infection, from ptomaines (decomposed protein food or dead animal matter), or from toxic drugs. Some bacterial poisons —such as diptheria toxin—can be neutralized by injection of the specific antitoxin. *See also* BACTERIA *and* **medigraph** ECLAMPSIA AND PREECLAMPSIA.

TOXEMIA OF PREGNANCY. *See* ECLAMPSIA AND PREECLAMPSIA.

TOXINS, poisonous substances formed by bacteria or other organisms, such as *diptheria toxin,* or by the body itself, such as *fatigue toxin. See also* ANTITOXIN.

TOXOPLASMOSIS

TOXOPLASMOSIS IS A PARASITIC infection. It is assumed that one out of every four adults in the United States has had contact with toxoplasmosis, thus being immunized against it by naturally created antibodies. It is often undiagnosed because it may produce no immediate symptoms, or the symptoms may be confused with those of influenza or infectious mononucleosis. *Congenital toxoplasmosis* is a much more serious aspect of the disease that occurs when the infectious organisms are transmitted from the mother to the fetus during pregnancy.

causes

The infectious agent is the form of the toxoplasma parasite known as the *oocyst* which is transmitted in the feces of cats who became contaminated by eating mice, birds and other previously infected creatures. It is known that the oocysts can transmit the disease even after the

Toxoplasmosis

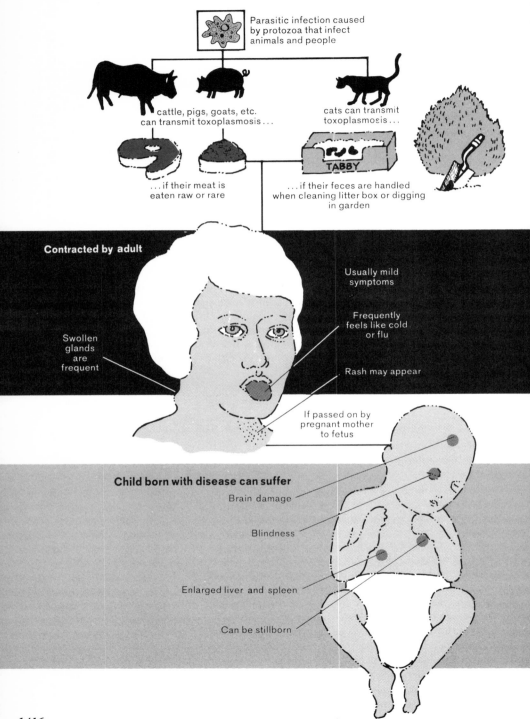

Parasitic infection caused by protozoa that infect animals and people

cattle, pigs, goats, etc. can transmit toxoplasmosis...

cats can transmit toxoplasmosis...

...if their meat is eaten raw or rare

...if their feces are handled when cleaning litter box or digging in garden

TABBY

Contracted by adult

Usually mild symptoms

Frequently feels like cold or flu

Swollen glands are frequent

Rash may appear

If passed on by pregnant mother to fetus

Child born with disease can suffer

Brain damage

Blindness

Enlarged liver and spleen

Can be stillborn

cat feces containing them has been buried in the soil for as long as a year.

symptoms

In a healthy adult, a mild case of toxoplasmosis may produce no symptoms other than a slight fever, or a sore throat and swollen glands. If resistance is low, or a person is undergoing certain types of chemotherapy or treatment with hormones, the infectious agent (which may have lain dormant in the body) will be triggered into attacking the liver, heart, or lungs.

complications

Of the several thousand cases of congenital toxoplasmosis that occur in the United States each year, about 25 percent of the infants are born with irreversible defects: brain damage, blindness and enlarged liver and spleen. In some cases, the babies are stillborn.

treatment

Medicines used to treat toxoplasmosis may produce negative side effects and are used only when symptoms are acute.

prevention

Since the test for the presence of toxoplasmosis antibodies in the blood is not easily available, pregnant women might take the precaution of avoiding contact with cats, refraining from eating raw or rare meats, and assigning the task of cleaning out a cat's litter box to some other member of the household.

RESEARCH REPORT

TRACERS DETECT LENGTHY SURVIVAL OF TOXOPLASMA OOCYSTS IN SOIL

The infectious agent in cat feces that causes *toxoplasmosis* has been shown to be capable of transmitting the disease even after being buried in the soil for more than a year, according to studies sponsored by the NATIONAL INSTITUTE OF INFECTIOUS DISEASES.

Using radioactive tracers, the researchers evaluated the infective potential of *toxoplasma oocysts* by determining their survival rates under varied soil conditions. After being in the soil in Costa Rica for a year, and for 18 months in Kansas, the dried oocysts were still infectious.

Since children playing in the dirt are likely candidates for toxoplasmosis, this finding may explain the high incidence of the disease in youngsters under the age of five in some Central American areas.   NIH725

RESEARCH REPORT

PREGNANT WOMEN ALERTED TO DANGER OF TOXOPLASMOSIS EXPOSURE

The dangers of exposure to *toxoplasmosis,* especially to pregnant women, are stressed in a recent report from the NATIONAL INSTITUTE OF ALLERGY AND INFECTIOUS DISEASES. It is now estimated that 30–50 percent of all adult Americans become infected by the "toxo" parasite at some time during their lives. In some cases symptoms are negligible; in others, the illness runs a course resembling *infectious mononucleosis* or a common cold. The infection may also produce *retinitis,* inflammation of the retina.

When contracted by a pregnant woman, however, toxoplasmosis may severely and irreversibly *damage* the unborn child. Symptoms usually bypass the mother, but infants infected before birth may suffer eye and brain damage and death is not uncommon.

The process by which the disease-bearing agent *toxoplasma gondii* invades the fetus is the following: prenatal infection is spread initially throughout the mother and the unborn child who shares her protective antibodies. But the fetal brain does not receive the same share of antibody protection as the rest of its body does. Thus, the parasites continue to live in the developing brain tissue, causing significant prenatal harm.

Since *cats* have been identified as the chief source of human infection and since it has also been indicated that many other animals harbor the parasite without themselves showing symptoms of the disease, the Institute

○ researchers suggest that precautionary measures should be taken for avoidance of exposure. A pregnant woman should *not* be in charge of cleaning out a cat's litter box which may harbor the *oocysts* contained in an infected animal's fecal droppings. Cats free of infection should not be fed table scraps of undercooked meat, nor should raw meat be part of their regular diet. Household cats should be prevented from hunting rats or mice which might carry the disease.

A woman planning a pregnancy or already pregnant who has been in close daily contact with a free-roaming cat should have the animal checked for any evidence of the infectious oocysts in its stools. NIH1125

TRACE ELEMENTS, essential minerals present in extremely small amounts. These trace elements include *chromium, manganese, cobalt, copper, fluorine, zinc,* *iodine, molybdenum* and *selenium.* The value to life of some of these elements has not been determined. *See also* DEFICIENCY DISEASES; NUTRITION.

TRACHEA, *windpipe,* the breathing tube about four-and-a-half inches long and one-inch wide, larger in men, which extends from the larynx (voice box) to the two large bronchial tubes in the upper part of the chest cavity. It carries fresh oxygenated air to the lungs and expels carbon dioxide. It is composed mostly of rings of cartilage and is lined by mucous membrane.

The trachea is subject to the same infections as the bronchial tubes, manifested by a hacking cough that is worse at night, pain in the lower part of the neck and behind the breastbone, and spitting of mucus and pus. A culture of the sputum indicates the specific bacterial cause of the disturbance. A specific antibiotic may combat certain causes, but others (such as viral infections) must be fought by other means. A vaporizer may give a measure of relief by moistening the inhaled air and providing a soothing medication. In obstruction of the trachea by a chunk of swallowed meat, strangling, or diphtheritic membrane, the surgical operation of *tracheostomy* (opening the trachea and inserting a breathing tube) is an emergency measure. *See also* RESPIRATORY SYSTEM; TRACHEOSTOMY.

TRACHEOSTOMY, the emergency surgical operation for obstruction of the trachea or larynx, by opening the trachea and inserting a breathing tube. An incision is made through the front of the neck and the trachea is opened for insertion of a tube to permit the passage of air to and from the lungs. In cases of obstruction due to a chunk of swallowed meat, strangling, or a diphtheritic membrane, tracheostomy may save the victim's life. It is a very important first aid measure. *See also* CHOKING; TRACHEA.

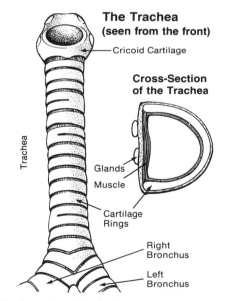

The Trachea
(seen from the front)

Cricoid Cartilage

Cross-Section of the Trachea

Trachea

Glands

Muscle

Cartilage Rings

Right Bronchus

Left Bronchus

Trachea—The fibroelastic windpipe descends from the larynx to the two main bronchi that carry air in and out of the lungs. Stabilizing rings of cartilage maintain its uniform tube shape. Blockage of this vital air passage is fatal unless the obstruction can be forced out or an incision is made through the neck and a breathing tube inserted into the trachea.

TRACHOMA, *granular conjunctivitis,* a chronic, highly contagious infection of the insides of the eyelids that afflicts possibly 400–500 million people in the world. It is widespread in northern Africa and southern Asia, and is probably the greatest single cause of preventable loss of eyesight and even total blindness. It is caused by the microorganism *Chlamydia trachomatis* and is transmitted by direct contact, unclean water, improper sanitation and flies.

The illness begins about one week after contact. The insides of the eyelids become congested and swollen, the eyes are sensitive to light, tears flow profusely, and after 1–4 weeks small granules form and irritate the eyes. The conjunctivae (eyelid linings) contract to form scars. The diagnosis is established by microscopic examination of scrapings from the insides of the eyelids.

Complications include ulceration of the cornea (front of the eyeball) causing loss of its ability to transmit light, loss of vision, and blindness in neglected cases. Some people may recover with little or no traces left. Other people get infected over and over again and many may develop special sensitivity to the infection. Ultimately each case should be seen by either a physician or a well-trained public health worker who can confirm the diagnosis, define the area involved and direct the infected person to proper treatment.

Fortunately, sulfonamide and antibiotic drugs have had specific effects in controlling trachoma. When severe scarring changes have occurred in the eyes, surgical correction may be necessary. Attempts have been made to prepare suitable vaccines of the Chlamydia, but these are still experimental. *See also* EYE; OPHTHALMIA *and* **medigraph** CONJUNCTIVITIS.

TRANCE, a semiconscious dreamlike state, in which sensation is suspended

Trachoma

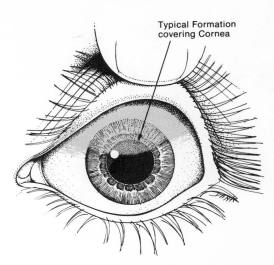

Typical Formation covering Cornea

Trachoma—This chronic contagious infection attacks the inner eyelids. Redness and swelling are followed by the formation of granules. Left untreated, it ulcerates the cornea. Resulting scar tissue, as shown, blocks vision and may cause total sight loss if unchecked. Early antibiotic treatment effectively controls trachoma, which is still widespread in many areas, especially where sanitation is primitive.

and breathing is almost imperceptible. The onset of a trance and the awakening are both sudden. The condition occurs in certain mental and psychological disorders and may be induced by hypnosis. *See also* HYPNOSIS; HYSTERIA.

TRANQUILIZERS, drugs which calm the nerves and relieve anxiety without causing undue depression or clouding the mind. In the United States, they are classified as controlled drugs and require a special prescription. Most tranquilizers have side effects and they should not be taken except on medical instruction. *See also* ANXIETY; RELAXANTS; RESERPINE.

TRANSFUSION, blood, the direct transfer of blood from a donor to the recipient, or indirectly with stored blood or plasma obtained from a blood bank.

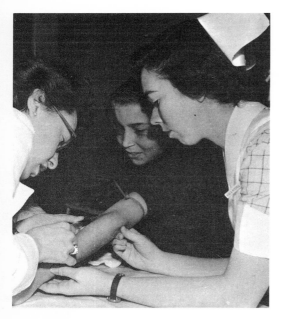

Transfusion, Blood—A nurse assists as the doctor prepares a woman for a blood transfusion. Indirect transfusion, in which donor blood is stored and later fed into a recipient, is most common. Discovery of the four main blood types in 1900 made transfusions safe and effective.

The extensive use of blood transfusions proves that they are lifesaving in many emergencies including battle injuries, stab and gunshot wounds, surgical shock, pre- and postoperative routines, loss of blood in childbirth, hemorrhages from ruptured peptic ulcers or varicose veins of the gullet, bleeding due to accidents, radiation burns, severe anemias, hemophilia, ulcerative colitis, debilitating diseases, purpura hemorrhagica (low-platelet-caused bleeding into tissues), and for babies inheriting the Rh factor. If one-third of a person's blood is lost suddenly, the victim may die immediately unless the loss is replaced by a transfusion. Every hospital is equipped with the necessary facilities to perform a blood transfusion.

Until discovery in 1900 of the four main blood types, transfusions were of-ten fatal due to the reaction of incompatible bloods. Today correct typing and crossmatching of blood are stressed.

Formerly, many transfusions were performed by connecting both the donor and the recipient to an apparatus that was switched from one to the other as the blood was transferred. Today, the usual procedure is to match the recipient's blood with that obtained from a volunteer donor or with the plasma or serum obtained from a blood bank. The substance is then injected into the recipient's vein separately. The blood is kept from clotting after withdrawal by addition of *sodium citrate*. The injection of a pint or quart of blood is accomplished slowly, over a period of about two hours, by gravity from a large glass or plastic container suspended on a stand. Strict surgical *asepsis* (absence of disease-causing organisms) is maintained at all times since infections are common and serious. The recipient must be attended constantly by a nurse and observed for possible reactions shown by chills, fever, restlessness, shortness of breath and rapid pulse. These are signals to stop the transfusion.

The favorable results of a blood transfusion are immediate and often spectacular. The replaced blood restores the circulating blood volume and also the red blood cells which carry oxygen and nutritive elements to the tissues. The improvement is shown by greater vitality and a healthier color. The transfusions are repeated at intervals according to the result and the condition treated.

All blood donors must be examined closely for good general health, and for freedom from any communicable or venereal disease or malarial parasites in their blood. They should not have any anemia, and should show no evidence of viral hepatitis. Many cases of viral hepatitis following blood transfusions have been reported and this condition presents special problems. It is due to two different viruses and is transmitted exclusively through the blood by blood transfusions or the hypodermic needle. Many apparently healthy persons carry the virus without showing any symptoms and thus transmit it to anyone who receives their blood. About 30,000 cases of viral hepatitis occur every year, although few of them are ever reported. The disease has increased due to infected blood in blood banks and the use of insufficiently sterilized needles and syringes. *See also* ANEMIA; BLOOD; BLOOD BANK; BLOOD CONDITIONS; BLOOD TYPES; CROSSMATCHING OF BLOOD; ERYTHROBLASTOSIS FOETALIS; HEMORRHAGE; THALASSEMIA *and* **medigraphs** HEMOPHILIA; HEPATITIS; LEUKEMIA.

R ESEARCH
EPORT

COMPUTERIZED DONOR LISTS FACILITATE TRANSFUSIONS OF VITAL BLOOD COMPONENT

The lives of patients with leukemia, aplastic anemia, and certain other malignant diseases may be extended through he use of a relatively new technique that permits the transfusion of the blood component essential for clotting. The procedure, known as *plateletpheresis,* involves drawing blood from a healthy person, removing the *platelets,* and immediately returning the remainder—the white and red blood cells and plasma—to the donor. This process, which is repeated four times in each case, takes from two to three hours and involves no risks to the donor, since a healthy individual's platelets are automatically replaced within 36–48 hours. The patients who receive the platelet transfusions are thereby less threatened with the occurrence of severe hemorrhage or fatal bleeding episodes.

In the first six months after the NATIONAL INSTITUTES OF HEALTH initiated a community-wide effort to supply matched platelets to needy patients, nearly 500 donors were used and 1350 plateletpheresis procedures were performed. With NIH funding, a growing number of major medical centers are participating in a platelet exchange pool based on matched donor lists coordinated by computer.

It is much more difficult to achieve platelet-matching compatibility than red blood type compatibility. Since the odds of finding a perfect match between unrelated donor and recipient are about one in 4725, once a suitable combination is found, the same donor is likely to be called upon several times for the requirement of a particular patient. NIH315

TRANSILLUMINATION of the skull, the passage of light through the skull, particularly the sinuses, to determine the density of the parts under examination and possible darkening because of congestion or thickening.

TRANSMISSIBLE DISEASES, diseases that may be transmitted from one person to another by direct contact (*contagion*), through discharges, by sprayed droplets (such as *colds* and *influenza*), or by contaminated instruments (such as *viral hepatitis*). Some diseases may be carried by various vehicles, such as *typhoid fever* in water, *undulant fever* in milk, and *trichinosis* in pork. Mosquitoes carry *malaria* and *yellow fever,* and ticks carry the rickettsiae of *Rocky Mountain spotted fever*. Protection of the public from transmissible diseases is one of the important duties of the Public Health Service. *See also* INFECTIOUS DISEASES.

TRANSPLANTS. *See* ORGAN TRANSPLANTS.

TRANSVESTITE, a man or woman who wears the clothes of, and prefers to be accepted as a member of the opposite sex. *See also* BISEXUAL; SEXUAL ABNORMALITIES.

TRAUMA, physical or psychological injury. Physical traumas include those resulting from automobile and industrial accidents and from war wounds, for example. Psychological trauma is typified by an emotional shock that makes a lasting impression on the subconscious mind.

TREMORS, involuntary trembling or quivering, most often of the outstretched hands. A *fine tremor* is one in which the movements are rapid; a *coarse tremor,* in which they are slow. A *continuous tremor* is typical of Parkinson's disease. An *intention tremor* is one that is intensified by voluntary movements. Tremors of the tongue occur in alcoholism, typhoid fever, and general paresis (syphilitic brain disease). *See also* DRUG ABUSE; NERVOUS SYSTEM *and* **medigraphs** ALCOHOLISM; CEREBRAL PALSY; HYPERTHYROIDISM; MERCURY POISONING; MULTIPLE SCLEROSIS; PARKINSON'S DISEASE; TYPHOID FEVER.

TRENCH FEVER, a mild acute rickettsial infection (prevalent in the trenches during World War I) transmitted by the bite of the body louse. Inability to change underwear frequently and lack of toilet facilities in World War I led to such extensive infestation of the men with lice that delousing stations were set up for their use when off duty.

The fever lasts for several days and is accompanied by headache, dizziness, and pains in the back, legs and eyes. An eruption of red spots characteristically breaks out on the chest and abdomen at the beginning of the illness, later spreading to the whole trunk. In the treatment, broad-spectrum antibiotics yield excellent results. As sanitary measures, all contaminated household articles should be sterilized to prevent transmission of the disease. *See also* RICKETTSIAL DISEASES *and* **medigraph** LICE AND SCABIES.

TRENCH FOOT, a common disturbance of soldiers in the trenches during World War I, resembling frostbite. It was caused by prolonged immersion of the feet in the cold water at the bottom of the trench, combined with disturbed circulation resulting from exposure to cold and lack of movement of the feet.

TRENCH MOUTH

VINCENT'S ANGINA IS AN INFECTION of the mouth and gums that occurs when resistance is low, nutrition is inadequate, health habits are poor and teeth are neglected. Heavy smokers are also susceptible. Because the infection was common among soldiers during World War I, it was named *trench mouth* at that time, and the name has stuck.

cause
The infection is caused by the spirochete *Borrelia vincentii,* named after the French physician who identified it. This microorganism is present in the mouth at all times, but when resistance is poor, it combines with other bacteria and attacks the mucous membranes.

symptoms
Painful ulcers, which may bleed, appear on the gums. Sore throat, fever and swollen glands may also occur, and the breath becomes malodorous. Symptoms are aggravated by smoking and alcoholic intake.

complications
If untreated and chronic, the condition can cause *gingivitis* and pyorrhea, leading to eventual loosening and loss of teeth.

treatment
Antibiotics will cure the infection, but if the underlying conditions remain uncorrected, the infection will eventually recur.

Trench Mouth (Vincent's Angina)

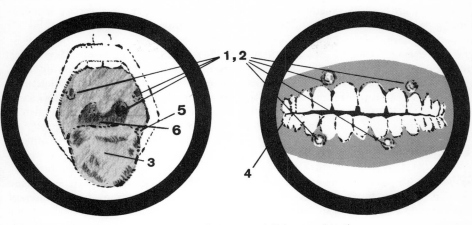

1. Sores (ulcers) appear on gums, throat, or lining of cheeks
2. Gray membrane covers sores
3. Swollen, furry tongue

4. Pain around teeth
5. Metallic taste
6. Foul breath

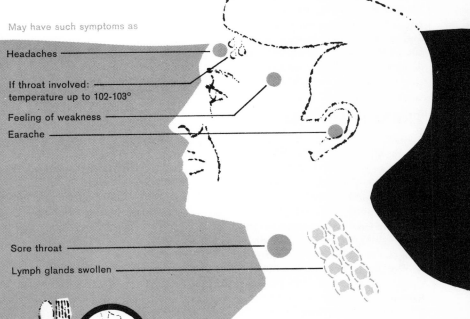

May have such symptoms as

Headaches

If throat involved: temperature up to 102-103°

Feeling of weakness

Earache

Sore throat

Lymph glands swollen

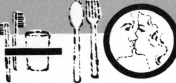

Spread by spirochete—bacillus via toilet articles, silverware, kissing, other contact with infected areas

prevention

Trench mouth is prevented by maintaining good health and visiting the dentist regularly for tooth-cleaning and general checkup. Where the infection does exist and other members of the family might be vulnerable to it because of lowered resistance during another illness or old age, care should be exercised to prevent the infection from spreading by the use of paper plates, plastic cutlery and disposable tissues.

TRICHIASIS, a condition of ingrowing eyelashes, due to distortion resulting from inflammation of the eyelids, which irritate the eyeball by friction. *See also* EYE; EYELIDS.

TRICHINOSIS

TRICHINOSIS IS A PARASITIC disease that is difficult to diagnose and is rarely fatal. It is caused by the roundworm *Trichinella spiralis* found in uncooked pork. Trichinosis may be so mild that the victim is unaware of the infection. It is assumed to have existed in over 15 percent of the adult population of the United States at one time or another. It is practically unknown in the tropics or in countries where swine are fed on root vegetables. Cases in the United States have diminished with the more rigid enforcement of laws requiring that all garbage be cooked before it is fed to animals.

causes

The larvae of the trichinella are encapsulated in cysts in the muscle tissue of contaminated pigs and hogs. When the contaminated pork is eaten undercooked, the human digestive juices liberate the larvae when they enter the intestines where they mature and mate, discharging fresh larvae into the bloodstream. In their progress through the body, natural defenses can destroy them, but when they move into striated muscle tissue, they can become encapsulated in cysts that remain intact over many years—in some cases, for a lifetime.

symptoms

The manifestations of trichinosis depend on the extent and the site of infestation.

When the larvae are maturing in the intestinal tract, they cause cramps, diarrhea and nausea. As the larvae travel through the system, swelling produced by edema becomes apparent in the eyelids, and the eyes may become extremely light-sensitive. Fever, chills, acute muscle pains and profuse sweating follow the gastrointestinal symptoms. As the larvae become encysted in the muscles, there is a gradual abatement of symptoms.

treatment

Diagnostic procedures such as skin tests, examination of muscle samples and chest x-rays may be necessary for the differentiation of trichinosis from other diseases. Once accurately identified, various medicines are available for alleviating muscular discomfort and other symptoms. Although the disease itself rarely results in any permanent disability, victims may need to be protected with antibiotics against bacterial infections such as pneumonia.

prevention

All fresh pork products should be properly cooked and should be grayish rather than white or pink when brought to the table. Ground pork products such as sausages should *never* be sampled raw. The incidence of trichinosis in Alaska is higher than elsewhere in the United States since bear meat is often infected and improperly cooked by hunters.

Trichinosis

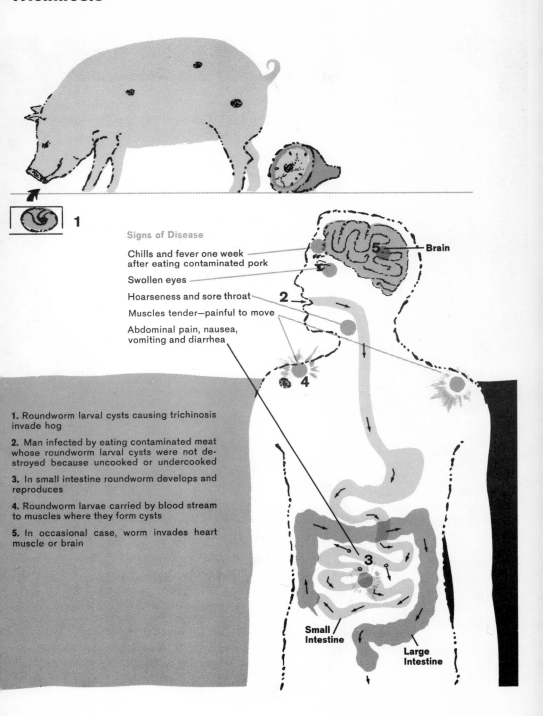

Signs of Disease

Chills and fever one week after eating contaminated pork

Swollen eyes

Hoarseness and sore throat

Muscles tender—painful to move

Abdominal pain, nausea, vomiting and diarrhea

Brain

Small Intestine

Large Intestine

1. Roundworm larval cysts causing trichinosis invade hog

2. Man infected by eating contaminated meat whose roundworm larval cysts were not destroyed because uncooked or undercooked

3. In small intestine roundworm develops and reproduces

4. Roundworm larvae carried by blood stream to muscles where they form cysts

5. In occasional case, worm invades heart muscle or brain

Trichomonas

Infectious disease of the genital organs, spread by protozoan parasite. Occurs much more commonly among women than men.

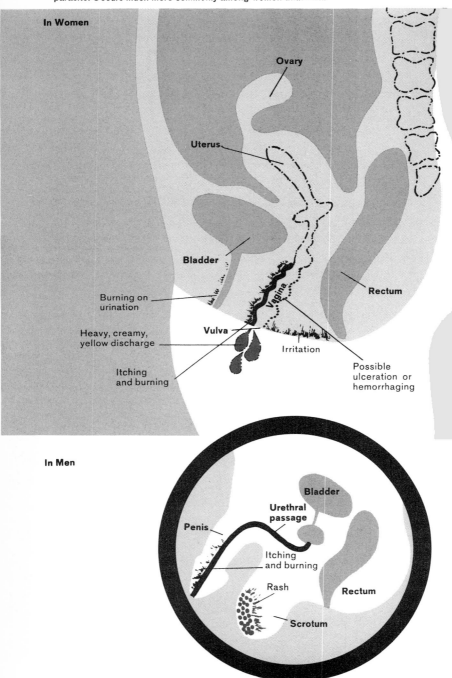

In Women

Ovary

Uterus

Bladder

Burning on urination

Heavy, creamy, yellow discharge

Vulva

Itching and burning

Irritation

Vagina

Rectum

Possible ulceration or hemorrhaging

In Men

Bladder

Urethral passage

Penis

Itching and burning

Rash

Scrotum

Rectum

TRICHOMONAS

A SPECIES OF PROTOZOAL PARASITE, *Trichomonas vaginalis*, causes inflammation of the vagina in the female and of the urethra in the male. The symptomatic disorder known as *trichomoniasis* is more common among women.

causes
The parasite is transmitted during sexual intercourse by the male. The organisms are found in the accumulated smegma under the foreskin of the noncircumcised male, as well as in the semen. The trichomonas is probably the only cause of a genitourinary infection that *can* be picked up from a toilet seat. It may also invade the genitalia because of improper anal hygiene. Trichomoniasis is an infection, but it is not a venereal infection.

symptoms
In women, the infection causes a heavy whitish vaginal discharge (*leukorrhea*) accompanied by localized itching (*pruritis*). If the inflammation is extensive, it will result in a burning sensation during urination and some ulceration of the mucous membranes in adjacent areas. In men, symptoms include itching and burning of the scrotum and penis. A rash may also erupt on the scrotum.

complications
If the vaginitis becomes chronic, there may be some erosion of the membranes, making the area more vulnerable to secondary infection by fungi.

treatment
The infection should be treated by a doctor, and husband and wife should be treated simultaneously even if only one of them has symptoms, since the infectious organism may be passed back and forth between them. An oral medication usually eradicates the parasite within a short time.

prevention
This disorder is more troublesome than serious. Personal hygiene involving soap and water rather than chemical douches and sprays is the best way to keep such omnipresent infectious germs at bay. Some men who are prone to infection by this parasite have chosen to be circumcised as a way of preventing its appearance under the foreskin.

TRICHOTILLOMANIA, an uncontrollable impulse to pull out one's hair. *See also* MANIA.

TRIGEMINAL NEURALGIA. *See* TIC DOULOUREUX.

TRIGLYCERIDES, a group of *lipids* (fats) which, together with cholesterol, are essential components of living cells.

Fats that are eaten pass through the digestive process during which they are broken down into *fatty acids* and *glycerol*. From these, triglycerides—also known as *neutral fats*—are formed during absorption from the small intestine. They may then be turned into energy or they may be carried in the blood for storage in the body's various fat deposits.

Considerably more is known about the role of *cholesterol* in body processes than about the triglycerides. Cholesterol, for example, is known to be the material from which the *bile acids* and the *steroids* (sex hormones and hormones of the adrenal glands) are produced. It is also one of the chief components of gallstones.

Heavy deposits of cholesterol and triglycerides in the walls of the arteries are considered to be a leading cause of *atherosclerosis*. Only recently, however, have simple methods been devised for measuring triglyceride blood levels, and there is less information about how these levels are affected. Elevated cholesterol levels can occur without similarly elevated triglyceride levels.

Abnormally high triglyceride blood levels can be caused by excessive carbohydrate intake, alcoholism, diabetes, thyriod gland malfunction and, in some women, the use of estrogens that are found in oral contraceptives. People suffering from coronary disturbances are thought to be more likely to have higher triglyceride levels than cholesterol levels. *See also* ATHEROSCLEROSIS; CHOLESTEROL; HEART; LIPIDS *and* **medigraph** ARTERIOSCLEROSIS.

TRIMESTER, a stage or time period of three months.

TRIPLETS. *See* MULTIPLE BIRTH.

TRISOMY, presence of an additional chromosome in a cell. This can result in conditions such as *Down's Syndrome.* *See also* BIRTH DEFECT; CHROMOSOMES; DNA; DOWN'S SYNDROME; GENETIC COUNSELING; HEREDITY.

TRUSS, a mechanical device for holding a correctible hernia in place. Special trusses are manufactured for *inguinal hernias* in the groin and *femoral hernias* in the upper inside part of the thigh. The truss should be put on snugly to put pressure over the canal through which the hernia may protrude unless supported. *See also* ABDOMINAL SUPPORTS; HERNIA *and* **medigraph** INGUINAL HERNIA.

TRYPANOSOMIASIS, infection with trypanosomes (parasitic protozoa). These protozoa are the cause of *Chagas' disease* and *African sleeping sickness.* *See also* PARASITES; PROTOZOA *and* **medigraph** CHAGAS' DISEASE.

TSUTSUGAMUSHI FEVER. *See* SCRUB TYPHUS.

TUBAL LIGATION, the operation of tying the two Fallopian tubes for permanent contraception by preventing the union of the female egg with the male sperm cell. This simple operation does not lessen the woman's enjoyment of sexual intercourse. *See also* BIRTH CONTROL; STERILIZATION.

TUBAL PREGNANCY. *See* ECTOPIC PREGNANCY.

TUBERCLE, a small nodule or rounded prominence, particularly one of the multiple tubercles present in the lungs in tuberculosis, where the body attempts to wall off the tubercle bacilli. *See also* LUPUS VULGARIS *and* **medigraphs** OVARIAN INFECTION; TUBERCULOSIS.

TUBERCULOSIS

ONE HUNDRED YEARS AGO, tuberculosis was the chief cause of death throughout the world, and in spite of medical progress, it remains the Number One killer among infectious diseases. Associated with cities since ancient times, it was not considered contagious until Dr. Robert Koch isolated its cause. He also developed the tuberculin test that makes it possible to detect past and present infection.

causes
Pulmonary tuberculosis is caused by breathing in the specific organism *tubercle bacillus.* These organisms are spread by the cough of a person suffering from an advanced stage of the disease. On the basis of widespread tests, authorities assume that at least 35 million Americans have been infected at one time or another, but that they are in sufficiently good health to resist the disease

Pulmonary Tuberculosis

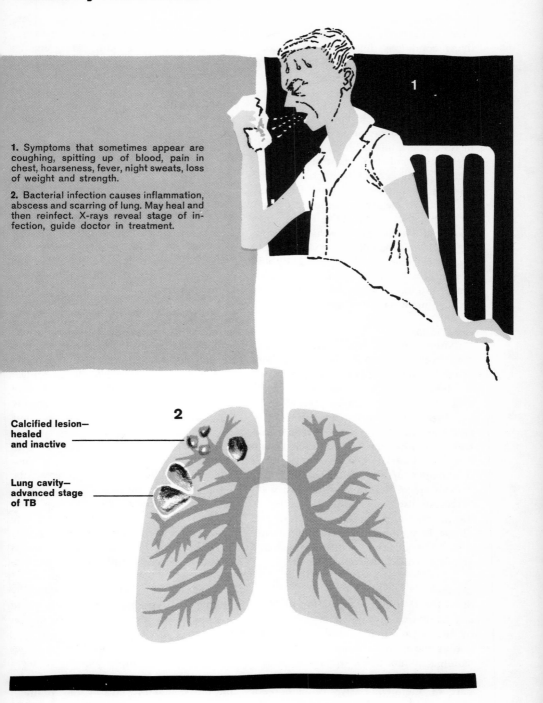

1. Symptoms that sometimes appear are coughing, spitting up of blood, pain in chest, hoarseness, fever, night sweats, loss of weight and strength.

2. Bacterial infection causes inflammation, abscess and scarring of lung. May heal and then reinfect. X-rays reveal stage of infection, guide doctor in treatment.

1

2

Calcified lesion—
healed
and inactive

Lung cavity—
advanced stage
of TB

and keep it at a standstill. Another prime cause of tuberculosis is poverty: crowded living conditions, inadequate diet, questionable habits of personal hygiene and primitive sanitation.

symptoms
Many healthy people have unknowingly sustained a tuberculosis infection, dismissing it as a minor illness with a cough, slight fever and some chest pain. The affected lung area often heals, hardens and remains inactive for a lifetime. Especially in the 20–40 age group, the infection may be reactivated, or the active disease may take hold without previous history, causing a chronic cough, blood in the sputum, chest pain, breathing difficulty and loss of appetite. In women, menstruation ceases. In both sexes, weight loss and profuse night sweating are typical.

complications
Children infected with tubercle bacilli are especially vulnerable to complications of meningitis as the germs spread beyond the lungs to the brain and spinal cord. When the nervous system is thus affected, the disease is called *miliary tuberculosis.* Other possible sites of the spread of infection in adults include the kidneys and bladder. Bone tuberculosis may result in collapse of the vertebrae and permanent spinal deformity. Pulmonary tuberculosis itself may lead to pleurisy; if the infected area spreads to a large part of the lung, tuberculous pneumonia results. Tuberculosis that affects the adrenal glands is called *Addison's disease.*

treatment
Since the 1940's, a combination of drugs effectively treated pulmonary tuberculosis by keeping it in check and all but eliminating the need for lung surgery. Medication is administered over a long period, with regular checkups as a mandatory part of therapy. Early recognition of symptoms has a direct bearing on the effectiveness of treatment. Mass screening of schoolchildren and factory workers by routine tuberculin testing enables health authorities to provide prophylactic treatment for those cases that show evidence of previous infection. One year of therapy with the drug *isoniazid (INH)* has prevented the further development of the disease in a significant number of cases.

prevention
A partially effective immunization vaccine is not routinely used in the United States. It has been successful in controlling the spread of tuberculosis in those parts of the world where—because of mass poverty, primitive sanitation and urban crowding—the disease continues to be endemic.

TULAREMIA, *rabbit fever,* an infectious disease transmitted to people who handle sick rabbits. The germs are also carried by rodents and ticks. The origin of the disease is traced to direct contact with infected wild rabbits in 90 percent of cases. The persons most commonly infected are hunters, butchers, farmers and laboratory workers.

Two to four days after contact with the sick rabbit, the illness begins suddenly with chills, fever, drenching sweats, headache, joint and muscular pains, nausea and weakness. An ulcerous sore breaks out at the location where the germs entered the skin. Recovery begins in 3–4 weeks, but the mortality rate is about 6 percent. Epidemics have occurred with a death rate as high as 85 percent. The diagnosis is confirmed by finding the specific germ (*Pasteurella tularensis*) in the discharge from the sore.

Complications can include enlargement of the lymph glands, atypical pneumonia, and involvement of the lungs, intestines, and the cornea and conjunctiva of the eye. *Pericarditis* (inflamma-

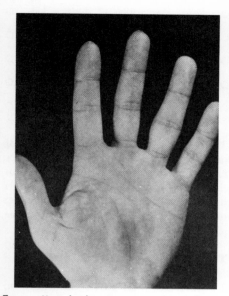
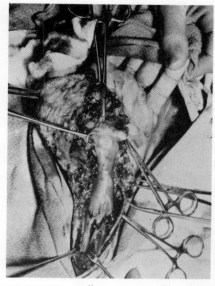

Tumor—Most benign tumors need not be removed. They do not invade neighboring tissue so are not potentially life threatening. But in a small area such as the hand (*left*), a growth can press on nerve endings, compress blood vessels and limit use of the hand. Surgery will bring relief. The photograph at right shows the exposed interior of the palm as the tumor is being excised.

tion of the heart sac) and *meningitis* are distinctive but unusual complications.

All persons who handle rabbits should protect their hands with rubber gloves or wash them in a mild antiseptic solution after contact. Touching the rabbit flesh when the hand has a cut, scratch, scrape, hangnail, or sore must be avoided, and the wrapping paper containing the animal must be burned. Rabbit meat, thoroughly cooked, is safe, since the germs of tularemia are killed by a temperature of 130° F. (54.4° Celsius).

Certain antibiotics are effective for the cure of tularemia. In cases complicated by pneumonia, hospitalization, intravenous feeding, oxygen and blood transfusions may be needed. *See also* INDUSTRIAL HEALTH; INFECTIOUS DISEASES.

TUMOR, *neoplasm,* a new growth of tissue in a limited area, with abnormal structure or location. Tumors are classified in two main groups: malignant and benign. A *malignant tumor* invades neighboring tissue, recurs after removal, and *metastasizes* (travels) to distant organs via the lymphatic or blood system. A *benign tumor* has none of these malignant properties. *Carcinoma* metastasizes via the lymphatic channels; *sarcoma,* via the bloodstream; and *leukemia,* via both channels.

Tumors are also classified according to the nature of the tissue from which they grow. Thus carcinoma arises from cells of the *ectoderm* (outer embryonic layer of tissue or the associated glands); sarcoma from the *mesoderm* (middle layer consisting of connective tissue, muscles, and the urinary and vascular systems); and leukemia from the lymph cells, bone marrow, or spleen. Other tumors are: *glioma* (brain tumor) arising from the supporting tissues of the central nervous system; *angioma* from blood vessels; *fibroma* from fibrous connective tissue; *myoma* from muscle; *os-*

teoma from bone; *chondroma* from cartilage; *adenoma* from glands; *lipoma* from fat, and so forth.

Any lump—particularly in the breast —should be brought to a doctor's attention for early recognition of possible malignancy. If it should prove to be malignant, surgical removal is the best remedy. Most benign tumors do not require surgery unless they cause pressure. *See also* ADENOMA; ANGIOMA; BREAST TUMORS; CANCER; CHONDROMA; CHORIO-CARCINOMA; FIBROADENOMA; FIBROMA; GLIOMA; HYPERNEPHROMA; KELOID; LI-POMA; MALIGNANCY; METASTASIS; MY-ELOMA; MYOMA; NEUROBLASTOMA; OVARIAN TUMORS; POLYP; SARCOMA; TERATOMA; TESTICULAR TUMORS; WILMS' TUMOR; XANTHOMA *and* **medigraphs** AD-ENOMA, BRONCHIAL; BRAIN TUMOR; BREAST CANCER; CANCER OF THE CERVIX AND UTERUS; FIBROID TUMOR; LUNG CAN-CER; PANCREATIC CANCER; PROSTATE GLAND ENLARGEMENT; SKIN CANCER; URI-NARY TRACT PROBLEMS.

R**ESEARCH**
R**E P O R T**

○   VISUAL TECHNIQUE REPLACES
               SURGERY IN DIAGNOSIS   ○
○   OF KIDNEY TUMORS

               A new technique that may eliminate   ○
○   the need for surgical diagnosis of pa-
       tients suspected of having *kidney*   ○
○   *tumors* has been developed by urolo-
       gists at the DELTA REGIONAL PRIMATE   ○
○   RESEARCH CENTER in Louisiana. The
       procedure has already been used for   ○

○   visual examination of diseased kid-   ○
       neys in monkeys and is expected to
○   provide accurate information about   ○
       the presence of malignant tumors in
○   humans.   ○
               The diagnosis is based on *visual*
○   inspection through an *endoscope* of   ○
       a tissue sample extracted by needle
○   from the kidney cyst. The procedure   ○
       is called *renal cystoscopy.* NIH1214

TURNER'S SYNDROME, a group of deformities caused by ovarian deficiency characterized by short stature, webbing of the neck, a decreased carrying angle of the arm, compression and narrowing of the aorta, and other birth defects. *See also* BIRTH DEFECT.

TWINS. *See* MULTIPLE BIRTH.

TYMPANIC MEMBRANE, *eardrum,* separating the external and middle ear cavities. It is attached to the chain of three *ossicles* (small bones of the middle ear by which the sound waves are carried to the organ of hearing in the internal ear and thence to the brain to be interpreted as speech, music or other sound). *Perforations* of the eardrum may follow middle ear infections, diving, or loud noise such as a nearby explosion. *See also* EAR.

TYMPANOPLASTY, surgical reconstruction of the hearing mechanism of the middle ear with restoration of a damaged eardrum. *See also* EAR.

TYPHOID FEVER

TYPHOID FEVER—also called *enteric fever*—is a highly contagious disease whose incidence is directly related to the contamination of water, milk and food by sewage. Together with cholera and dysentery, the disease is endemic in those parts of the world where public sanitation and public health measures continue to be dangerously primitive.

causes

The microorganism that causes typhoid fever is *Salmonella typhi,* and it is eliminated in the urine and feces of those infected with it. The disease can be transmitted by a carrier who is himself immune but who has the bacteria in his gallbladder and eliminates them in his excreta. Carriers who handle, prepare

Typhoid Fever

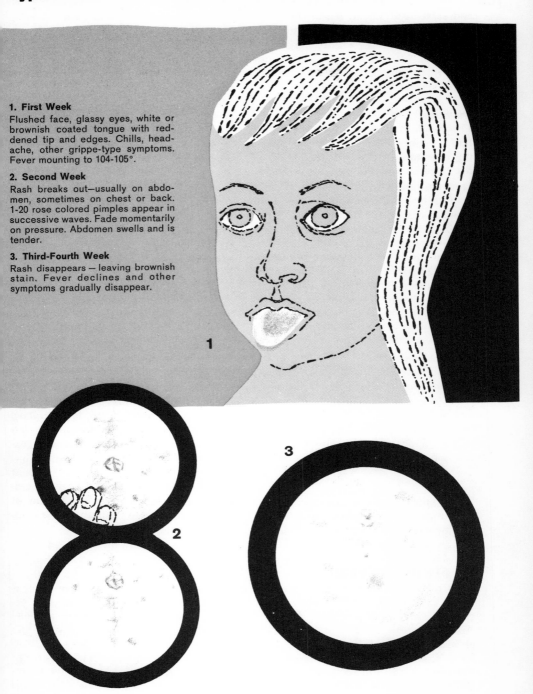

1. First Week
Flushed face, glassy eyes, white or brownish coated tongue with reddened tip and edges. Chills, headache, other grippe-type symptoms. Fever mounting to 104-105°.

2. Second Week
Rash breaks out—usually on abdomen, sometimes on chest or back. 1-20 rose colored pimples appear in successive waves. Fade momentarily on pressure. Abdomen swells and is tender.

3. Third-Fourth Week
Rash disappears — leaving brownish stain. Fever declines and other symptoms gradually disappear.

and serve food spread the disease when they fail to wash their hands after defecating or urinating. The bacteria enter the victims' bodies by way of the intestines when they eat or drink a contaminated substance.

symptoms

The incubation period following infection is approximately two weeks. When the typhoid bacilli begin to multiply in the bloodstream, the victim experiences headache, dizziness and sore throat, plus a fever that rises each day, peaking in about a week to 105°F. (40.5°C.). Nosebleeds, diarrhea and vomiting occur, and the fever may alternate with periods of sweating and chills. In about two weeks, a characteristic rash appears on the chest, abdomen and back. In milder cases, symptoms begin to subside spontaneously during the third or fourth week.

complications

A severe case of typhoid fever will cause delirium, during which highly infectious loose stools are eliminated. Ulceration and perforation of the intestines may be fatal. Even in milder cases, the susceptibility to pneumonia or liver infection can lead to death.

treatment

Since typhoid fever is an extremely debilitating disease in many instances, expert nursing care is essential, in addition to the antibiotics and other medicines that are part of therapy. Hospitalization may be recommended so that the victim's daily regimen of diet, exercise, possible blood transfusions and laboratory tests can be rigorously supervised.

prevention

Large-scale public health measures are necessary if the disease is to be wiped out in primitive areas. An immunizing vaccine is available for travelers to those parts of Asia, Africa and Latin America where typhoid fever remains a problem. Three successive shots are required over a three-week period, and booster shots are necessary every three years. Unvaccinated tourists who find themselves in places where there may be a typhoid fever threat can take the precaution of drinking only bottled water and avoiding uncooked fruit and vegetables, as well as shellfish. Milk presumed to have been pasteurized should be boiled unless it is available in sealed containers.

Local health departments require the registration of known carriers of the disease who are forbidden to handle food. Carriers are also advised that they need not continue to be a health menace; antibiotic cures, and in some cases other medical treatments are available.

TYPHUS, *typhus fever,* an acute epidemic louse-borne or flea-carried infection caused by a specific *rickettsia*—which is an organism intermediate in size between a bacterium and a virus.

There are separate forms of typhus, which differ only in severity and mortality rates: *epidemic louse-borne typhus, Brill's disease,* and *flea-borne typhus* on rats or mice. Typhus is prevalent wherever people live close together under unsanitary conditions that make frequent bathing and changes of underwear inconvenient or impossible, as in jails, detention camps, asylums, holds of ships, slum tenements and cheap lodging houses.

After an incubation of 10–14 days, the illness begins most often abruptly with severe headache and generalized pains and aches all over the body. A skin rash erupts later. In two or three days, the temperature rises to about 104° F. (40° Celsius) and remains high for 10–14 days, gradually subsiding in three or four days in most cases. The death rate is about 20 percent.

Complications can include kidney insufficiency, bronchitis, pneumonia, a fall of blood pressure and gangrene of the skin.

The best preventive measures are to avoid contact with unclean persons and to destroy body lice and rats. During World War I, when typhus was prevalent among the troops, delousing stations were established with facilities for bathing and a change of underwear. During World War II the insecticide *chlorophenothane* (DDT) was sprayed exten- sively to protect the armed forces in the South Pacific, but the use of this agent in the United States was banned in 1972 by the Environmental Protection Agency because of its polluting effects on soil and water. Some antibiotics are highly effective against typhus if used early and in adequate dosage. *See also* FLEAS; PARASITES; RAT CONTROL; RICKETTSIAL DISEASES; SCRUB TYPHUS *and* **medigraph** LICE AND SCABIES.

U

ULCER, any open sore, other than a wound, with an inflamed base. Such a lesion usually occurs in the skin or mucous membrane of some internal organ. They may result from infection, injury to the blood supply, damage to nerves, or from a wide variety of other causes. Ulcers require the attention of a physician who will not only endeavor to learn the specific cause but will plan the treatment accordingly. *See also* ABDOMINAL PAIN; BARIUM SULFATE; BEDSORES; DIET IN DIGESTIVE DISORDERS; LEG ULCERS; PEPTIC ULCER; X-RAYS *and* **medigraphs** TRENCH MOUTH; ULCERATIVE COLITIS; ULCERS OF THE DIGESTIVE TRACT.

ULCERATIVE COLITIS

ULCERATIVE COLITIS IS A CHRONIC inflammation and ulceration of the colon (large bowel). In some cases, the rectum is also involved. It is a progressive disease that is resistant to treatment. Although it may occur in childhood or in old age, it characteristically develops in young people, with 75 percent of all cases beginning before age 40. More women are affected than men, and there is some indication that it is a family disorder.

causes
The exact cause is not known. In individual medical histories, the condition has been related to neurosis, to food sensitivity, or to severe infections of other kinds. Current research is attempting to establish a causal relationship between this disease and an aberration in the autoimmune process in which the body's defense mechanisms are somehow triggered into attacking the body's own tissues rather than a foreign invader.

symptoms
Since ulcerative colitis varies in intensity from person to person and from time to time in the same person, accurate diagnosis must be based on meticulous and detailed evidence so that other conditions are ruled out. Typical manifestations include diarrhea and bleeding which may alternate with constipation in the early stages of the illness. Diarrhea in time becomes the main symptom. The victim may have as many as 20 bowel move-

Ulcerative Colitis

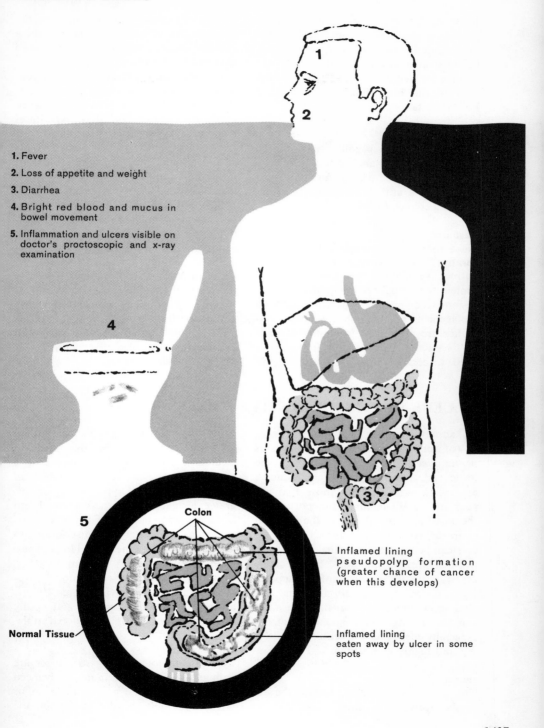

1. Fever
2. Loss of appetite and weight
3. Diarrhea
4. Bright red blood and mucus in bowel movement
5. Inflammation and ulcers visible on doctor's proctoscopic and x-ray examination

Colon

Normal Tissue

Inflamed lining pseudopolyp formation (greater chance of cancer when this develops)

Inflamed lining eaten away by ulcer in some spots

1437

ments in 24 hours, involving sleep interruption and consequent fatigue. Abdominal tenderness, cramps, weight loss, eventual anemia and dehydration severe enough to require intravenous replacement of vital body fluids may necessitate hospitalization.

complications

Untreated ulcerative colitis may lead to hemorrhoids and anal fistulas. Persons who had the disease for more than ten years are at 5–10 percent risk of developing colonic cancer.

treatment

Since there is no complete cure for ulcerative colitis, therapy is designed to correct symptoms. Bed rest, a high-protein low-roughage diet, blood transfusions when anemia is present, and fluid replacement are basic procedures. Antibiotics are prescribed to control secondary bacterial infection. Many victims need a certain amount of psychiatric therapy to sustain them through the depression that is often associated with a chronic disease suffered during one's most productive years.

In some cases, retention enemas containing corticosteroids have proved helpful. These drugs may also be given orally or by injection; however, doses large enough to be therapeutically effective frequently cause negative side effects. Administration in the form of suppositories appears to control the symptoms with the least side effects.

Surgical removal of the affected part of the bowel is advised in extreme cases that appear to be precancerous. This procedure involves an *ileostomy* in which an artificial opening is created between the ileum and the exterior, necessitated by the removal of the colon and rectum. It is generally agreed by persons who have undergone this operation that it is much easier to live with an ileostomy than with chronic or acute ulcerative colitis.

R<small>ESEARCH</small> R<small>EPORT</small> *follows* ILEITIS.

ULCERS OF THE DIGESTIVE TRACT

E RODED AREAS OF THE MUCOUS lining of the digestive tract are known as *peptic ulcers.* Those that occur in the lower end of the esophagus and stomach are called *gastric ulcers;* those that appear in the duodenum—the portion of the small intestine closest to the stomach —are called *duodenal ulcers.* Peptic ulcers can be induced in animals by putting them in stressful situations. Peptic ulcers are widespread among humans, appearing in three out of every thousand, including children over ten; they are more common among men than among women, especially men who are tense, hard-driving and highly competitive.

causes

The immediate cause of ulcers is the excessive secretion of gastric acid that literally "eats up" the digestive tract lining. Why this overproduction that leads to ulceration should be the response of a particular individual to stress—which in others might cause hypertension or migraine headaches—is not known. There is an accumulation of evidence indicating some hereditary predisposition to ulcers, especially among O blood types. Once the ulcer begins to form, any factor that increases the secretion of hydrochloric acid will aggravate the condition: alcohol, spicy food, irregular and hastily eaten meals, and chronic emotional strain.

symptoms

Typical symptoms of a gastric ulcer are pain and vomiting, and in more advanced cases, bleeding. The pain is likely to be felt to the left of the center of the

Ulcers Of The Digestive Tract

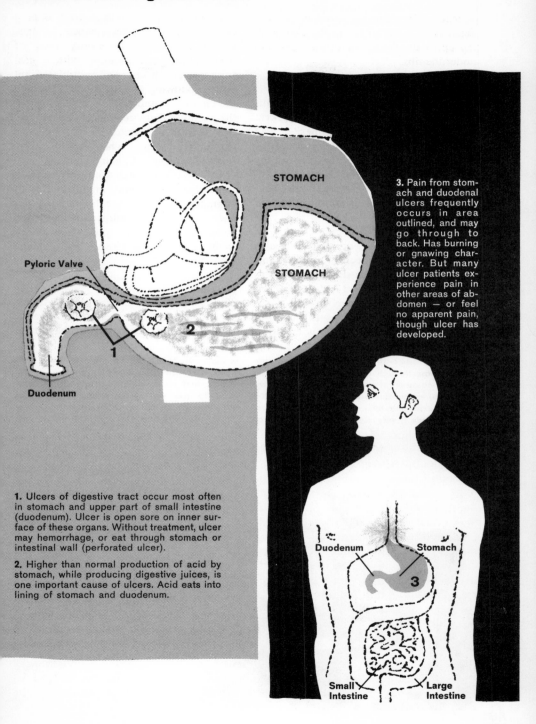

STOMACH

STOMACH

Pyloric Valve

1

2

Duodenum

3. Pain from stomach and duodenal ulcers frequently occurs in area outlined, and may go through to back. Has burning or gnawing character. But many ulcer patients experience pain in other areas of abdomen — or feel no apparent pain, though ulcer has developed.

Duodenum **Stomach**

3

Small Intestine **Large Intestine**

1. Ulcers of digestive tract occur most often in stomach and upper part of small intestine (duodenum). Ulcer is open sore on inner surface of these organs. Without treatment, ulcer may hemorrhage, or eat through stomach or intestinal wall (perforated ulcer).

2. Higher than normal production of acid by stomach, while producing digestive juices, is one important cause of ulcers. Acid eats into lining of stomach and duodenum.

stomach. The pain produced by a duodenal ulcer is felt either in the middle of the upper duodenum or to the right and under the ribs.

complications

When untreated ulcers bleed, the vomitus appears brownish and the stools blacken. Loss of blood over a long period may lead to anemia. If the hemorrhage is sudden or severe, or if perforation occurs in which food from the stomach or intestines escapes into the abdominal cavity, emergency hospitalization is essential.

treatment

Chronic or intermittent stomach pains should always be checked by a doctor. Anyone who dismisses such symptoms as chronic indigestion and refuses to get professional diagnosis may have an ulcer that suddenly worsens and requires emergency attention. Diagnosis to differ-

entiate peptic ulcer from gastritis, disease of the liver or pancreas, cancer, or hernia, is based on laboratory tests of stomach acid, examination with a gastroscope, and a series of gastrointestinal x-rays following barium intake. Therapy for ulcers is based on various changes in the victim's daily regimen: dietary recommendations, medications, supportive psychotherapy, and when essential, corrective surgery. A bland diet of soft creamy foods is eaten frequently and in small quantities, and augmented with vitamins to compensate for lacking nutrients. Antacids, antispasmodics and tranquilizers may be prescribed. Spicy foods, alcoholic beverages and caffeine are eliminated.

prevention

The "go-getters" who get ulcers are advised to learn how to relax and to make fewer impossible demands on themselves

Ultrasonography—Ultra high sound waves are able to pass through body tissue and give an accurate indication of what goes on inside. Ultrasound causes no damage, shows areas of the body not detectable by x-ray and is cheaper, too. This has made it very useful in obstetrics and as

a diagnostic tool. A further use is pictured here. Using ultrasound plus computer graphics, a specialist plans tumor radiation treatment. He positions the scan unit on the patient's body, while the physician at left traces the tumor and pertinent body structure with a sonic pen.

Courtesy, National Institutes of Health

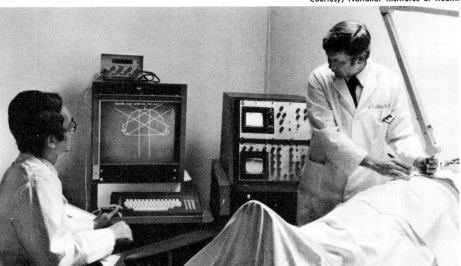

and others. Anyone who is ulcer-prone should avoid smoking, alcohol, highly seasoned food, rushed meals and tensions at the table. Participation in a therapeutic group can be helpful in achieving beneficial behavior modification. In the long run, this change in attitude is a better preventive than dependence on tranquilizers.

ULTRASONOGRAPHY, the recording of ultrasounds having a frequency above that of audible sounds—that is, above 20,000 cycles per second (cps). Ultrasonic waves of moderate intensity have been used in dermatology, neurology and genetics. *See also* BIRTH DEFECT; DETECTING TWINS; MEDICAL INSTRUMENTATION *and* **medigraph** BREAST CANCER.

ULTRAVIOLET KERATITIS, inflammation of the cornea of the eye caused by excessive exposure to the ultraviolet rays of the sun or a sunlamp. *See also* CORNEA; EYE; SNOW BLINDNESS.

UMBILICAL CORD, the flexible tube which connects the unborn infant with the placenta and which carries oxygen and nutrition via the umbilical arteries, and removes carbon dioxide and fetal waste via the umbilical vein. By about two weeks after conception, it is sufficiently developed to function.

In the newborn, the umbilical cord measures about two feet in length and one-half inch in diameter. Soon after birth, it is clamped or tied and then cut. The length that is still in the uterus is expelled with the placenta; the stump that remains attached to the baby's abdomen falls off naturally after a few days.

Torsion (twisting) of the umbilical cord during childbirth may shut off fetal circulation and kill the infant by asphyxiation. *See also* AFTERBIRTH.

UMBILICUS. *See* NAVEL.

Umbilical Cord
(Shown in 12-week Fetus)

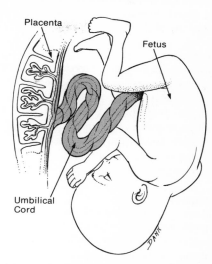

Placenta
Fetus
Umbilical Cord

Umbilical Cord—During pregnancy, fetal blood passes through the umbilical cord to the placenta. There the blood gives off waste products, receives nutrients and oxygen from the mother's blood and flows back through the cord to nourish the fetus. When the newborn infant breathes on its own, the umbilical cord becomes unnecessary.

UNCONSCIOUSNESS, a state of suspended animation during which the subject is unaware of his existence or surroundings, the basal metabolic rate is lowered, and vital functions such as breathing and the heartbeat ebb. *See also* BRAIN CONCUSSION; COMA; ELECTRICAL INJURIES; FAINTING; HEAD INJURIES; SHOCK; STUPOR *and* **medigraphs** ALCOHOLISM; DIABETES; EPILEPSY; STROKE.

UNDERWEIGHT PROBLEMS. The human appetite is fickle and largely subject to habit and prejudices. Some persons eat too much and become overweight; others eat too little and become underweight. Both extremes are damaging to health. In addition to appetite, some people are obsessed with the notion that fat is a reserve source of strength in case of future illness; others, that fat is dangerous per se and must be avoided at all costs. The only food reserve that is needed is *protein,* which is supplied abundantly in many foods.

The best guides are the weight scale and the calorie charts. Life insurance companies provide tables which give the most favorable weight in terms of age, sex and height. The ideal weight is usually considered to be 10 percent less than the statistical average. Provided he is not suffering from a serious disease, the underweight person can achieve his most favorable weight with nutritionally balanced meals at regular hours. In some cases—particularly with young people—results may not show for several years. Candy and sweets shortly before meals should be avoided, as they depress the appetite. Appetite may be stimulated by a beverage *sipped* at the beginning of a meal, such as beer, ale or stout. It should not be quaffed all at once, as this fills the stomach and reduces appetite.

When a person whose weight previously was normal (or who was overweight) loses a lot of weight suddenly, the cause may be serious and the person should consult a physician. Many people think of their weight in terms of fashion and appearance instead of the more important consideration of health. Older underweight women complain more of wrinkles and sagging skin (cosmetic defects which are especially common with crash diets) than those who are plump.

Statistics show that underweight persons live longer than the overweights. This conception is true with respect to dietary control of weight, but underweight due to an undiagnosed chronic illness must also be considered. The one disease to which underweight persons are particularly susceptible is *tuberculosis. Anemia* is also a common complication.

Underweight people should take daily a vitamin and mineral supplement supplying the recommended daily allowances of all essential vitamins and minerals, especially iron. Healthy persons, whether overweight or underweight, can attain any desired reading on the scale by guiding their meals in accordance with the nutritional value of their foods. *See also* ANOREXIA NERVOSA; CANCER; DEFICIENCY DISEASES; FAT; NUTRITION; OBESITY *and* **medigraphs** ADDISON'S DISEASE; CELIAC DISEASE; DIABETES; HYPERPARATHYROIDISM; HYPERTHYROIDISM; LUPUS ERYTHEMATOSUS; THYROID HEART DISEASE; TUBERCULOSIS.

UNDESCENDED TESTICLES

MALE SEXUALITY IS BASED on the descent of the testicles into the scrotum at birth, since this is their natural environment. An undescended testicle is incapable of producing the sperm cells essential for reproduction, nor can it manufacture the hormones—especially *testosterone*—required for the development of secondary sex characteristics. It is extremely rare for both testicles to remain undescended; when this anomaly affects one, the descended testicle is sufficient to regulate normal sexuality.

causes

The testes remain quite high in the male fetus's abdominal cavity until late in its maturation, gradually lowering through the inguinal canal into the groin and into the scrotum by the time of delivery. Why this process fails to occur in some cases, or why one testicle does not descend and the other does, is still unknown. The condition is presumed due to a hormonal deficiency. This in turn may stem from an abnormal testicle's inability to produce sufficient amounts of testosterone.

Undescended Testicles

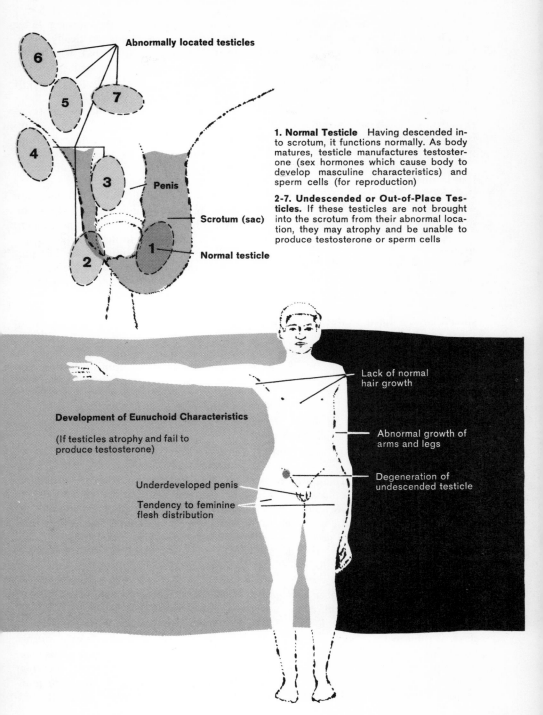

Abnormally located testicles

6

5

7

4

3   Penis

Scrotum (sac)

1

2

Normal testicle

1. Normal Testicle Having descended into scrotum, it functions normally. As body matures, testicle manufactures testosterone (sex hormones which cause body to develop masculine characteristics) and sperm cells (for reproduction)

2-7. Undescended or Out-of-Place Testicles. If these testicles are not brought into the scrotum from their abnormal location, they may atrophy and be unable to produce testosterone or sperm cells

Development of Eunuchoid Characteristics

(If testicles atrophy and fail to produce testosterone)

Underdeveloped penis

Tendency to feminine flesh distribution

Lack of normal hair growth

Abnormal growth of arms and legs

Degeneration of undescended testicle

symptoms

If the undescended testicle has not been brought down by surgery before the onset of male puberty, the boy's sexual development will proceed normally because of the normal descent of the other one. The site of the undescended testicle may or may not be painful, but the gland itself will probably shrink, and even if it is brought down after puberty, it may be permanently nonfunctioning.

In those rare instances where both testes remain undescended after puberty, the boy will be permanently sterile and will manifest the eunuchoid characteristics described in the illustration.

treatment

Child development specialists agree that because of psychological factors related to body comparisons at school, surgical correction of the undescended testicle should be scheduled between the ages of three and five. Although hormone treatments are sometimes recommended as a substitute for surgery, the results from this type of therapy have not proved as successful.

UNDULANT FEVER, *brucellosis, Malta fever,* an infectious disease contracted most often by drinking unpasteurized milk.

It was first recognized and studied by British army and navy officers stationed on the island of Malta. Scientists established that unpasteurized goat's milk can be contaminated by the germ *Brucella melitensis* (goat), causing the disease. Other species of the Brucella infect the hog (*B. suis*) and cattle (*B. abortus*). Meat of infected cattle, sheep and goats may also be sources of infection.

After an incubation period of 5–21 days, the illness may begin abruptly with chills, fever and sweats, or with extreme weakness, so that the slightest exertion induces fatigue and exhaustion. In the chronic form, the evening temperature rises to 104° or 105°F. (40° or 40.5°C.) and drops gradually in the morning. Later the fever occurs characteristically in repeated waves (undulations) with intervening remissions. Associated symptoms are headaches, vague body pains, loss of weight and anemia. In general, the symptoms are somewhat similar to those of malaria or typhoid fever. The most common physical signs are enlargement of the lymph nodes, liver and spleen, tenderness on pressure over the abdomen, and skin eruptions.

Possible complications of undulant fever include inflammation of the vertebrae, heart valves, liver, gallbladder, nerves, brain and testicles.

Pasteurization of milk is the best preventive measure. Antibiotics are used for treatment. *See also* INFECTIOUS DISEASES *and* **medigraph** ORCHITIS.

UNGUENT, *ointment,* a soft semisolid fatty mass for external application consisting of an active ingredient and a base composed of petrolatum or lanolin. *See also* LANOLIN; OINTMENT; SKIN CARE.

UNSATURATED FAT. *See* FAT, UNSATURATED.

UREA, the final product of the decomposition of proteins in the body, being the form in which nitrogen is eliminated. It is manufactured in the liver from amino acids and other compounds of ammonia, passed into the blood and lymph, and excreted in the urine. *See also* KIDNEY; LIVER; UREMIA; URINE AND URINATION.

UREMIA, accumulation in the blood of urea and other waste products normally excreted in the urine. The disturbance occurs in acute and chronic forms. Symptoms are headache, insomnia, nausea, vomiting, loss of appetite, muscular twitchings, darkening of the skin, puffiness of the face, shortness of breath, generalized itching and coma. The most prominent early signs of chronic uremia are lassitude and mental depression. Blood tests show increased amounts of urea and nonprotein nitrogen.

The causes of uremia include *nephritis* or other kidney diseases; *congestive heart failure;* the *crush syndrome* following extensive burns or transfusion reactions; *poisons* (especially mercury and carbon tetrachloride); and *sulfonamide drugs.* Unless the uremia is due to a remediable cause, the outlook for recovery is poor, particularly when the blood chemical readings are high. In chronic cases, convulsions accompanying high blood pressure may foretell an early death.

The most important part of treatment is to find a remedial cause of the uremia and correct it if possible. Symptomatic treatment is employed as various complications arise. Control of high blood pressure and maintenance of the balance of mineral salts in the blood are valuable adjuncts to therapy. The intake of water and salt often must be restricted. Sometimes intravenous injection of glucose 15 percent in water helps by reducing the protein breakdown and hence the development of uremia. Artificial kidney machines which act by *dialysis* (filtering the urea and other waste products out of the system) are prolonging many lives. Excellent results have followed transplantation of a kidney from a volunteer donor. *See also* DIALYSIS; KIDNEY; KIDNEY FAILURE; KIDNEY FUNCTION TESTS; ORGAN TRANSPLANTS *and* **medigraphs** DIABETES; ECLAMPSIA AND PREECLAMPSIA; HEART FAILURE; MERCURY POISONING; NEPHRITIS; URINARY TRACT PROBLEMS.

URETER, one of a pair of thick-walled muscular tubes extending from the pelvis of the kidney to the bladder. It is about 12 inches long, one-fifth inch in diameter, and starts in the kidney as a number of short cup-shaped tubes which merge into a single channel. The urine is collected continuously from the kidney and propelled in spurts along the ureter and into the bladder. The ureter may be twisted, infected, ruptured, or blocked by a stone which requires surgical removal. The diagnosis of diseases of the ureter is usually made under x-ray examination and study by a urologist. *See also* BLADDER; BLADDER DISEASES; KIDNEY; URETERITIS; URINE AND URINATION *and* **medigraphs** KIDNEY STONES; NEPHRITIS; URINARY TRACT PROBLEMS.

URETERITIS, inflammation of the *ureter,* resulting from infection carried downward from the kidney or the pelvis of the kidney, or upward from the bladder. The usual causes of *descending* ureteritis are *nephritis* or *pyelitis* (inflammation of the kidney pelvis); of *ascending* ureteritis, obstruction in the bladder as by a stone or an enlarged prostate. *Cystic ureteritis* is characterized by multiple protruding cysts in the lining membrane. *See also* URETER.

URETHRA, the passage tube for urine from the bladder and in the male also for semen from the prostate and seminal vesicles. The exit opening is called the *meatus.*

The *male urethra* is about eight inches long and has three portions. The *prostatic portion* runs through the prostate and is connected with the ejaculatory duct, which discharges semen into it from the seminal vesicle and prostate. The *membranous portion* connects with the *penile portion,* which continues inside the penis to the exit. The urethra is lined with mucous membrane dotted with a number of small pit-like recesses and lubricated near the end with *Cowper's (bulbourethral) glands.*

The *female urethra* is about one-and-a-half inches long and consists of one continuous tube lined with mucous membrane and lubricated with small glands.

The principal disease affecting the urethra in both sexes is gonorrhea (*urethritis*). Congenital deformities of the male penis are *hypospadias,* in which the opening is located on the underside, and *epispadias,* in which it is on the upper side. *See also* BLADDER; COWPER'S GLANDS; EJACULATORY SYSTEM; PENIS; PROSTATE; SEMEN; URETHRITIS; URINE AND URINATION; VULVA *and* **medigraphs** GONORRHEA; KIDNEY STONES; PROSTATE GLAND ENLARGEMENT; TRICHOMONAS; URINARY TRACT PROBLEMS.

URETHRITIS, inflammation of the urethra, often due to gonorrhea transmitted by sexual intercourse. When it is caused by other infectious organisms, it is termed *nonspecific urethritis.* In men, the first symptoms are burning urination and a milky discharge from the penis; in women, redness and swelling of the vulva and a profuse discharge of pus from the urethra and vulva. The diagnosis is confirmed by microscopical examination of the discharge. The principal complications of male urethritis are *epididymitis, prostatitis,* and *urethral stricture.* Effective treatment is with antibiotics. *See also* URETHRA.

RESEARCH REPORT

SOME CASES OF URETHRITIS CAUSED BY NEWLY ISOLATED BACTERIAL STRAIN

Medical researchers associated with the UNIVERSITY OF WASHINGTON in Seattle have tracked down one of the causes of *nongonococcal urethritis* (NGU), a genitourinary infection that differs from similar gonococcal disorders in that it does not respond to treatment with *penicillin.* NGU occurs more frequently among sexually active men than *gonococcal* urethritis, especially among more affluent whites. Its control until now has been hampered by lack of information about its cause.

The Seattle researchers report that the bacterial organism *Chlamydia trachomatis* caused half the cases of NGU studied recently. No other bac-terial or viral agents known to be responsible for various genitourinary infections were found to be factors in the patients who were investigated.

Three groups of sexually active men were evaluated: 118 with NGU, 58 without overt infection, and 69 with *gonorrhea.* The C. trachomatis organism was isolated from 42 percent of the first group, 7 percent of the men without symptoms, and 19 percent of the gonorrhea patients. The organism was also recovered from 15 sexual partners of 22 patients whose NGU was caused by it.

Although these studies have not yet designated C. trachomatis as the only cause of the infection, there appears to be no doubt that the organism is sexually transmitted. Therefore, in cases where symptoms appear, the Seattle researchers advise that both partners be treated with the antibiotic *tetracycline.*   NIH1215

URIC ACID, the end product of purine metabolism, present in the blood and urine. A high blood level is characteristic of *gout. See also* ACID; URINE AND URINATION *and* **medigraph** GOUT.

URINALYSIS, examination of the urine, a standard procedure in all medical examinations. The customary report covers the specific gravity and the presence of albumin, sugar, acetone, and casts (blood) in the urine. Other tests are made for special diagnostic purposes. *See also* DIABETIC TESTS; KIDNEY FUNCTION TESTS; TESTS.

URINARY INCONTINENCE, inability to control urination, usually caused by injury or disease of the nerve roots from the lower spinal cord. A special form of incontinence, *enuresis* (bed wetting), is common in children.

URINARY SYSTEM, the organs designed for excretion of urine. They consist of the *kidneys,* the *ureters,* the *bladder* and the *urethra. See also* BLADDER; KIDNEY; URINE AND URINATION.

URINARY TRACT PROBLEMS

U RINARY INFECTIONS CAUSED by bacteria are comparatively common, especially among diabetics and among females of all ages. Fortunately, most such infections can be cured by antibiotics before they do any irreversible tissue damage. *Pyelitis,* which may be acute or chronic, is an infection of the pelvic area of the kidney. *Cystitis* is the general term for various types of bladder infections. Tumors of the urinary tract are not very common. However, there is a rare kidney malignancy known as *Wilms' tumor* (*nephroblastoma*) which may occur in children under five. When kidney tumors do occur in adulthood, they are more often found in men than in women, and rarely before the age of forty.

causes

In its acute form, pyelitis is the most common of all kidney infections. It is caused by bacteria that invade the kidney from nearby structures or from the bladder. Bacteria may also accumulate if a kidney stone or a congenital obstruction causes the normal flow of urine to back up. During pregnancy or during catheterization for other reasons, bacteria may be introduced into the urinary tract by instruments that are not entirely sterile. During early childhood, infectious bacteria in fecal matter may enter the urethra because of improper habits of personal hygiene.

Cystitis is caused by bacteria that enter the bladder through the urethra from the outside, or that descend from an infection in the kidney. It may also be a secondary manifestation of enlarged prostate, bladder stones, tumor, or of neurological disorders of the bladder. The condition in women which is known as *cystocele* (in which part of the bladder protrudes through the vaginal wall) is another cause of cystitis.

The cause of all urinary tract tumors, including Wilms' tumor, is unknown.

symptoms

Pyelitis is characterized by sudden high fever, pain in the abdomen and back, rigidity and soreness of the abdominal area, nausea and vomiting.

Cystitis causes an increase in the need to urinate, during which there is a burning sensation. The urine may contain some blood.

Tumors of the kidney produce a mass in the abdomen, pain in the middle of the back, blood in the urine—usually with no fever and no pain during urination. In Wilms' tumor, there is visible swelling of the child's abdomen.

complications

Chronic *pyelonephritis* (infection of the kidney and the renal pelvis) may follow an original acute attack of pyelitis. It may appear and disappear, eventually leading to hypertension and cardiovascular involvement. As kidney function is progressively impaired, uremia may cause death.

Cystitis may become chronic, or the local infection may spread to the kidneys.

Any growth that impedes urinary function can cause fatal kidney failure. If a tumor has metastasized to other parts of the body—especially to the lungs —life expectancy is considerably reduced even if the tumor itself is removed.

treatment

Antibiotics, bed rest and catheterization are therapeutic measures for both acute and chronic infections of the kidney. Underlying causes such as kidney stones or primary infections must also be treated, and where an obstruction is the underlying cause, corrective surgery may be essential.

Antibiotics are prescribed for cystitis,

Urinary Tract Tumors and Infections

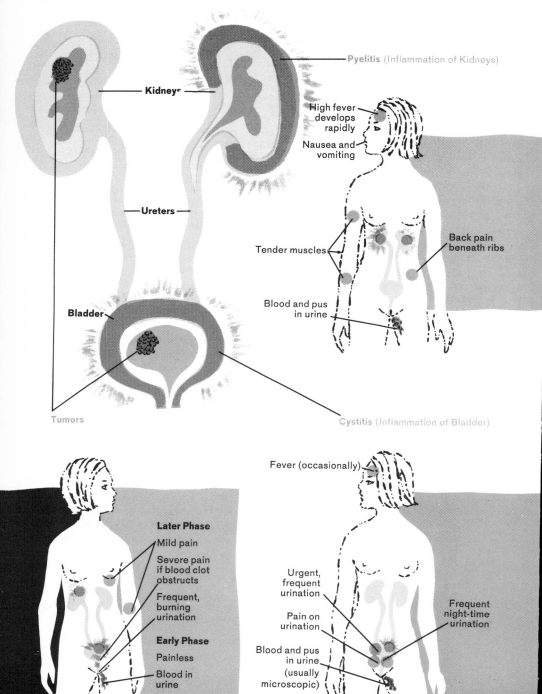

Pyelitis (Inflammation of Kidneys)

Kidney

High fever develops rapidly

Nausea and vomiting

Ureters

Tender muscles

Back pain beneath ribs

Blood and pus in urine

Bladder

Tumors

Cystitis (Inflammation of Bladder)

Later Phase

Mild pain

Severe pain if blood clot obstructs

Frequent, burning urination

Early Phase

Painless

Blood in urine

Fever (occasionally)

Urgent, frequent urination

Pain on urination

Blood and pus in urine (usually microscopic)

Frequent night-time urination

1448

together with analgesics and sedatives for the relief of acute discomfort. Treatment of underlying causes such as diabetes or pyelonephritis is undertaken. A regimen that eliminates alcoholic beverages and highly seasoned foods may also be recommended.

A malignancy diagnosed before metastasis has occurred is removed surgically together with the diseased kidney. In Wilms' tumor, surgery is followed by x-ray treatment; chemotherapy is undertaken for a period of about two years. The combination effectively cures about 90 percent of all cases. The cure rate drops to about 60 percent if metastasis has occurred.

prevention

Many urinary infections could be prevented by attending to any primary illness or disorder that might lead to bladder or kidney involvement. Extreme care in hospitals regarding sterilization of instruments, catheters and the like, would reduce the number of "staph" infections. Routine personal cleanliness for females should include wiping the anus toward the back after defecation rather than toward the front.

RESEARCH **R**EPORT

ANTIBIOTIC TAKEN ORALLY AFTER INTERCOURSE PREVENTS CHRONIC BLADDER INFECTIONS

Recurrent *bladder infections* in some women can be prevented by a single dose of an antibiotic immediately after sexual intercourse. This conclusion was the result of STANFORD UNIVERSITY research involving a group of women showing a high incidence of chronic or recurrent infection of the urinary tract. Such infections are often related to sexual intercourse, presumably because at such times, bacteria are afforded a means of entry from the urethra into the bladder. Varied methods for solving this problem have generally met with little success. Consequently, some patients with this chronic condition tend to curtail their sexual activity and find themselves having to deal with marital tension rather than localized infection.

The California study was based on 14 women attending a special clinic for patients with a recurrent history of urinary tract infections related to sexual intercourse. During a period of approximately six years, 90 infections occurred prior to treatment. In contrast, over a slightly longer period during which the same patients were instructed in the self-administration of antibiotics, only 19 infections occurred.

The antibiotics used in the study were *nitrofurantoin, cephalexin, nalidixic acid, sulfonamide,* and *penicillin G.* None of the patients had to discontinue treatment because of allergic reaction or drug intolerance. In cases where the bacterial organisms became resistant to one of the antibiotics, another was recommended and was equally effective.   NIH615

URINE AND URINATION. Urine is the clear amber-colored fluid extracted from the blood by the kidneys, stored in the bladder, and evacuated at intervals through the urethra. The average amount produced per day is 40–50 fluid ounces, though more is produced in cold weather and after drinking coffee or tea and less in hot weather and when not drinking fluids.

An increased volume of urine above 85 fluid ounces (*polyuria*) suggests chills, recovery from fever, diabetes mellitus or insipidus, or chronic nephritis. A reduced volume below 25 fluid ounces (*oliguria*) suggests fever, heart failure, disease of the kidney tubules (*nephrosis*), or loss of fluid from vomiting, diarrhea or hemorrhage.

The urine contains urea, uric acid, mineral salts, bile pigments, oxalic acid, and traces of other waste products dissolved in water. The chemical reaction is slightly acid. Abnormal ingredients of urine are *albumin* and microscopical *casts* (blood) in kidney disease, *sugar* in diabetes mellitus, *acetone* in impending

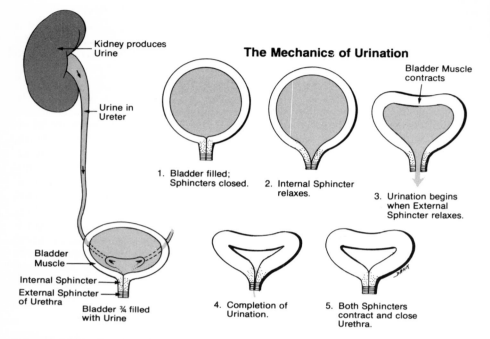

The Mechanics of Urination

Kidney produces Urine

Urine in Ureter

Bladder Muscle

Internal Sphincter

External Sphincter of Urethra

Bladder ¾ filled with Urine

Bladder Muscle contracts

1. Bladder filled; Sphincters closed.

2. Internal Sphincter relaxes.

3. Urination begins when External Sphincter relaxes.

4. Completion of Urination.

5. Both Sphincters contract and close Urethra.

Urine and Urination—The kidneys filter waste products from the blood and form urine. This fluid passes down the two ureters and is stored in the bladder. A full bladder causes the internal sphincter muscle to relax and make known the need to urinate. At urination, the external sphincter relaxes, the bladder contracts and urine is released through the urethra.

acidosis, and pus and blood in infections of the urinary tract. The normal specific gravity is 1015–1030; it is higher in diabetes mellitus and lower in diabetes insipidus. The most reliable specimen for urinalysis is the total urinated during a four-hour period.

The act of urination is begun under control of the brain but continues automatically. When the bladder is full, the desire to urinate leads to the usual preparation and then motor reflexes take over and contract the bladder and the associated muscles, at the same time relaxing the circular sphincter (closure muscle). The nervous regulation of urination is through a center in the spinal cord controlled by the brain. Involuntary urination may occur during a stroke, epileptic convulsion, in locomotor ataxia, or bed wetting in children.

The normal frequency of urination is three or four times a day. The most common causes of absent or reduced urination are kidney disease, obstruction of the bladder by an enlarged prostate, obstruction of the urinary tract by a kidney or bladder stone, and paralysis of the lower spinal cord. Failure to urinate may lead to uremia and ultimately death. *See also* ALBUMINURIA; ALKAPTONURIA; ANURIA; BED WETTING; BLADDER; DIABETES INSIPIDUS; DIABETIC TESTS; DYSURIA; EXCRETION; HEMATURIA; INCONTINENCE; KIDNEY; KIDNEY DIALYSIS; KIDNEY FAILURE; KIDNEY FUNCTION TESTS; NEPHROSIS; NOCTURIA; RETENTION OF URINE; UREA; UREMIA; URETER; URETHRA; URIC ACID *and* **medigraphs** DIABETES; KIDNEY STONES; NEPHRITIS; PROSTATE GLAND ENLARGEMENT; URINARY TRACT PROBLEMS. R{ESEARCH EPORT} *follows* KIDNEY STONES.

UROLOGY, the specialty of diseases of the urinary system including the male sexual organs. A specialist in that field is called a *urologist.*

URTICARIA. *See* HIVES.

UTERINE TUBES. *See* FALLOPIAN TUBES.

UTERUS, *womb,* the organ which receives the fertilized egg cell from the Fallopian tube and holds it during the nine months of its growth until the infant is expelled at childbirth. It is a hollow pear-shaped thick-walled muscular organ situated deep in the pelvic cavity between the bladder and the rectum. On its upper part the Fallopian tubes—one on each side—connect with the ovaries and below, the cavity opens into the vagina. The nonpregnant uterus weighs about 1–1⅓ ounces and measures three inches in length, two inches in breadth, and one inch in thickness. It has two portions: the *body* and the *cervix* (constricted neck). It is suspended in the pelvis by the broad and round ligaments. The uterus is lined with mucous membrane continuous with that of the vagina.

During pregnancy the uterus grows progressively to accommodate the embryo or fetus and after childbirth returns gradually to its normal size. About every 28 days, menstrual bleeding occurs and the mucous membrane peels off and is later replaced by a new growth.

Principal disorders of the uterus include *anteflexion of the cervix* (forward bending), *retroversion* (backward bending prolapse), lacerations at childbirth, fibroid tumors, cysts, polyps and cancer. *See also* ABORTION; AFTERBIRTH; AMNIOCENTESIS; BIRTH CONTROL; CANCER; CERVIX; CONCEPTION; ENDOMETRITIS; GYNECOLOGICAL EXAMINATION; HYSTERECTOMY; MENSTRUATION; OVARIES; OVULATION; PREGNANCY; PRENATAL DEVELOPMENT; REPRODUCTIVE SYSTEM; TIPPED UTERUS; VAGINA; VULVA *and* **medigraphs** CANCER OF THE CERVIX AND UTERUS; FIBROID TUMOR; MENOPAUSE; OVARIAN INFECTION; STERILITY.

UVEITIS, inflammation of the *uvea,* the colored vascular layer of the eye.

UVULA, the small fleshy conical mass which hangs loosely from the soft palate at the back of the mouth.

V

VACCINATION, production of immunity to infectious diseases by inoculation with killed or weakened germs or viruses of the disease or with those of a similar milder disease. Inoculation is usually performed by scratching the skin of the upper arm or thigh, applying the vaccine to the scratch, and putting on a protective dressing and bandage. When successful,

Vaccination—The simple act pictured here represents one of science's great triumphs. It is the conferring of immunity to certain infectious diseases by injection of a killed or weakened form of the organism responsible.

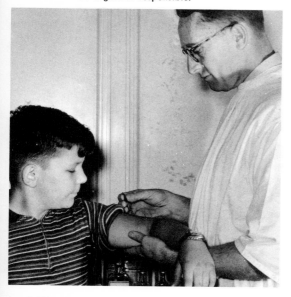

the procedure results in a mild local reaction followed by a long period of immunity. The most important vaccine is against *smallpox,* produced by inoculation with *cowpox,* which has virtually eliminated one of the most deadly of all infections. The *typhoid-paratyphoid triple vaccine* successfully protects against other deadly diseases. Other vaccines are available for protection from cholera, measles, German measles, polio, whooping cough, rabies and Rocky Mountain spotted fever.

An *autogenous vaccine* is one made from the germs contained in a patient's own blood or secretions. Effective vaccines have been developed for some strains of influenza. *See also* ANTIBODY; IMMUNITY; IMMUNIZATION; INFECTION; PREVENTIVE MEDICINE; SMALLPOX *and* **medigraphs** CHOLERA; DIPHTHERIA; FLU; GERMAN MEASLES; MEASLES; MUMPS; POLIOMYELITIS; RABIES; ROCKY MOUNTAIN SPOTTED FEVER; TETANUS; TYPHOID FEVER; WHOOPING COUGH.

R ESEARCH
E P O R T

○ **TOOTH DECAY MAY ONE DAY** ○
BE PREVENTABLE
BY VACCINATION

○ According to scientists at the NA- ○
TIONAL INSTITUTE OF DENTAL RE-
○ SEARCH, the concept of protecting ○
tooth enamel by a form of immuniza-
○ tion is not farfetched, since there ap- ○

pears to be a relationship between the prevalence of cavities and the levels of immunoglobulins and antibodies in saliva. The mechanism by which a vaccine might work would consist of a vaccination causing antibodies to enter the mouth through the salivary glands and gum tissues. The antibody could combine with the cavity-causing microorganisms in a way that would prevent their colonizing on the tooth surfaces. Antibody might also eliminate the formation of sticky substances formed in carbohydrate metabolism by preventing the interaction of bacterial enzymes and carbohydrates.

Another therapeutic possibility is based on the fact that microorganisms covered by a layer of antibody are highly susceptible to destruction by white blood cells. Since significant numbers of white blood cells are commonly found in saliva, they would be stimulated to kill off the decay-causing bacteria covered with antibodies.

Experiments in London have successfully reduced the numbers of cavities in monkeys by intravenous injection of live *Streptococcus mutans,* the bacteria responsible for tooth decay. The success of these tests is especially relevant, since monkeys who are fed a human diet develop cavities which are clinically and radiographically indistinguishable from those developed by people.

In the belief that more effective results might be achieved by using the secretory system as well as the serum system for immunization, researchers at the STATE UNIVERSITY OF NEW YORK in Buffalo injected a vaccine of killed S. mutans into the ducts of the salivary glands of anesthetized monkeys. The vaccine stimulated the production of salivary antibodies against the live bacteria and dramatically reduced their number on the tooth surfaces.

Since injections into human salivary glands are painful and might lead to infection, researchers are hoping to find an alternate site for administering the vaccine.   NIH814

VAGINA, the sheathlike sexual passage of the female, extends from the external

opening to the uterus and is situated behind the bladder and in front of the rectum. It is about 2½–3 inches long in front and 3½ inches in back. It is constricted in front, dilated in the middle, and narrowed near its uterine end. It has a recess behind called the *fornix,* forming the receptacle for the seminal pool during sexual intercourse. The vagina consists of an internal mucous membrane and a muscular coat separated by a layer of erectile tissue. It is lubricated by *Bartholin's glands,* situated at the opening in front.

The vagina is vulnerable to various infectious diseases, especially gonorrhea, but also scarlet fever, measles, and trichomoniasis—a protozoan infection causing diarrhea and a persistent discharge. *Vaginal mycosis (candidiasis)* is a fungus infection of the vagina (usually with *Candida albicans*) that causes intense itching. It is treated with a fungicidal antibiotic.

Vaginal bleeding is normal during menstrual periods. When it occurs irregularly, it is a significant symptom for which a doctor should be consulted. Excessive or prolonged bleeding associated with menstruation is called *menorrhagia* and requires a pelvic examination to diagnose its cause. Spotting of blood between periods—*metrorrhagia*—is a danger sign that may indicate fibroids, polyps, or cancer of the uterus. Bleeding during early pregnancy may be due to a threatened abortion.

Other disorders to which the vaginal passage is subjected are *vaginal fistulas*—abnormal openings connecting the vagina with the bladder and cavity of the uterus or with the rectum (resulting from damage to the lining of the vagina during childbirth), and *vaginal hernias*—protrusions of intestines and other abdominal contents into the vagina.

A persistent vaginal discharge is commonly known as *leukorrhea (the whites). Vaginismus* is a painful spasm of the muscles at the entrance to the vagina; it is common in newly-wed women during intercourse. *See also* BARTHOLIN'S GLANDS; FEMININE HYGIENE; FUNGUS; GYNECO-LOGICAL EXAMINATION; HYMEN; LEUKOR-RHEA; MENSTRUATION; MONILIASIS; PAP SMEAR TEST; RECTOCELE; REPRODUCTIVE SYSTEM; UTERUS; VAGINITIS; VULVA *and* **medigraphs** CANCER OF THE CERVIX AND UTERUS; ECTOPIC PREGNANCY; GONOR-RHEA; TRICHOMONAS.

VAGINITIS, infection of the vagina, most often gonorrhea. It may also be a complication of measles or scarlet fever. Other microorganisms that may infect the vagina include the *trichomonas vaginalis,* the *Candida albicans* fungus, and germs complicating various systemic diseases. The vagina can be contaminated from uncleanliness. *See also* VAGINA.

VAGUS NERVE, *pneumogastric (tenth cranial) nerve,* a *parasympathetic* nerve whose branches are widely distributed to various areas of the body, including those in the neck, thorax and abdomen. Its fibers are mixed: *autonomous, motor,* and *sensory.* In effect, the vagus is a regulating control of bodily functions. It restrains and slows the heartbeat (an

inhibitory action), regulates automatic breathing, activates the movements and secretions of the stomach and intestines during digestion, opposes sympathetic nerve actions, helps to regulate the action of the vocal cords through its recurrent laryngeal branch, and has many other diverse functions. Belladonna and atropine oppose many of the parasympathetic actions of the vagus. *See also* NERVOUS SYSTEM.

VALLEY FEVER. *See* COCCIDIOIDOMY-COSIS.

VANADIUM, a rare light gray or white lustrous powder often fused in hard lumps, used in the manufacture of rust-resistant steel. The dust irritates the lungs and causes a skin rash. *See also* DUST; METALLIC POISONS.

VARICELLA. *See* CHICKENPOX.

VARICES, dilated and twisted veins, commonly located on the inner sides of the thighs and the backs of the legs. They may be the sites of clots in the veins called *thrombi. See also* VEINS *and* **medigraphs** VARICOCELE; VARICOSE VEINS.

VARICOCELE AND HYDROCELE

TWO CONDITIONS THAT AFFECT the male genitals, varicocele and hydrocele, are rarely a threat to health, although they may cause a certain amount of discomfort and interfere with normal sexual activity. Both disorders may appear spontaneously and they may also disappear without treatment.
VARICOCELE is a varicocity of the network of veins that lies along the spermatic cord. This is a condition that may develop in the early teens after the onset of puberty.
HYDROCELE is a condition in which there

is a swelling of the scrotum caused by a collection of fluid between the layers of tissue that form the outermost covering of the testicles. Hydrocele is more likely to occur in older than in younger men.

causes
In most cases, neither of these conditions can be traced to a particular cause, although hydrocele is sometimes attributable to an underlying disorder that becomes apparent after the drawing off or analysis of the fluid.

Hydrocele and Varicocele

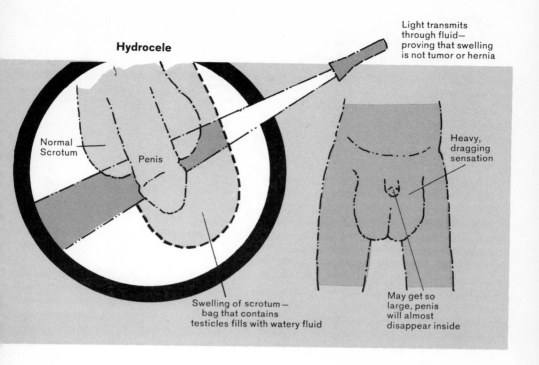

Hydrocele

Light transmits through fluid— proving that swelling is not tumor or hernia

Normal Scrotum

Penis

Swelling of scrotum— bag that contains testicles fills with watery fluid

Heavy, dragging sensation

May get so large, penis will almost disappear inside

Varicocele

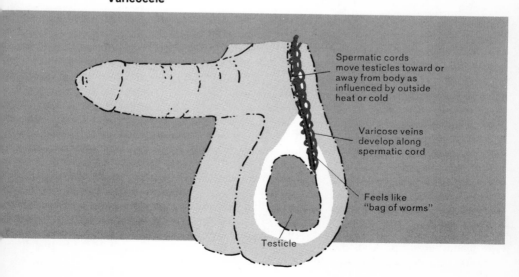

Spermatic cords move testicles toward or away from body as influenced by outside heat or cold

Varicose veins develop along spermatic cord

Feels like "bag of worms"

Testicle

symptoms

Varicocele may cause pain in the groin accompanied by a sensation of heaviness. For reasons not yet determined, it occurs most often on the left side.

Hydrocele may cause the testicle to appear to be twice its normal size. The enlargement of the scrotum is smooth and painless. The hydrocele is translucent—that is, when bright light is directed at it in the dark, the whole swelling illuminates, indicating that it is not a tumor or a hernia.

complications

Extreme discomfort or secondary symptoms may result from infection or hemorrhage.

treatment

Varicoceles that persist and cause discomfort are removed surgically.

Hydroceles that do not disappear without treatment may be drained or removed surgically. Either procedure is simple, but the latter is preferred since it precludes the possibility of recurrence.

VARICOSE VEINS

VARICOSE VEINS ARE SWOLLEN, knotted and distended veins visible below the skin surface. After the age of 40, they occur in the legs of about half the female population and a quarter of the male population. Young people in occupations which require motionless sitting or standing through most of the working day are more vulnerable to varicose veins than those who move around a great deal. A tendency to the disorder appears to be inherited.

causes

Because humans spend a great deal of time in an upright position, the blood returning from the leg veins to the heart must do so against the gravitational pull. This is accomplished by the contraction of the leg muscles which pump the blood upward through the veins. The blood is prevented from flowing backward by flaplike valves operating in pairs at frequent intervals within the vein. These valves are open when the blood flows toward the heart, and they close if the blood tries to flow backward, thus stopping its reverse movement.

Long periods of sitting or standing in one position cause the massaging action of the muscles to diminish so that the blood backs up. Also, the large abdominal vein that carries the blood from the

legs to the heart has no valves, causing an unsupported column of blood to press on the legs when the body is erect. The downward weight against the closed valves causes the veins to distend and lose elasticity. The valves then no longer close properly and the blood stagnates within the veins.

Among the individual circumstances that contribute to varicosity other than aging are pregnancy (during which the uterus 'puts extra pressure against veins of the legs) and occupations such as hairdressing, dentistry, easel painting, lecturing and typing.

symptoms

Even before the varicose veins become visible, the condition produces a feeling of fatigue and heaviness in the legs, cramps in the leg muscles at night and swollen ankles at the end of the day. Also the skin may itch and burn.

complications

Untreated varicosities may spread, the veins may thicken and harden, and the pain may intensify. Phlebitis and ulceration may develop, and skin rashes may appear. Ruptured veins cause subcutaneous hemorrhages, and in severe cases, the legs become so swollen and sore that the victim is immobilized.

testicle to the seminal vesicle. Inside the spermatic cord it passes through the *inguinal canal* and unites with the duct of the seminal vesicle to form the *ejaculatory duct,* contractions of which at the climax of sexual intercourse squirt the semen through the urethra. *See also* EJACULATORY SYSTEM; REPRODUCTIVE SYSTEM; TESTICLES; VASECTOMY *and* **medigraph** STERILITY.

VASECTOMY, a method of contraception by which a section of each *vas deferens* is removed surgically so that the exit of spermatozoa is blocked. The operation is simple and painless and does not interfere with sexual enjoyment. *See also* BIRTH CONTROL; STERILIZATION; VAS DEFERENS *and* **medigraph** STERILITY.

VASOCONSTRICTOR, causing tightening and narrowing of a blood vessel leading to a diminished flow of blood to the affected part of the body. The principal vasoconstrictive drug is *epinephrine,* which is used to control bleeding and also to raise blood pressure in cases of shock.

VASODILATOR, a drug or nerve causing dilatation (expansion) of a blood vessel, thereby lowering blood pressure and sending an increased supply of blood to the affected part, such as the heart. There are many peripheral vasodilative drugs including *nitroglycerin.*

VASOMOTOR, regulating the contraction (*vasoconstriction*) and relaxation (*vasodilatation*) of a blood vessel.

VEINS, the blood vessels which carry blood laden with carbon dioxide and metabolic wastes away from the tissues to the heart and lungs. Most veins are paired with arteries of the same name and follow the same general route.

Pulmonary veins return the oxygenated blood from the lungs to the left atrium

Vasectomy

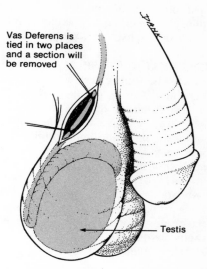

Vas Deferens is tied in two places and a section will be removed

Testis

Vasectomy—This relatively minor procedure is the most common method of making a man incapable of reproduction. A section of the duct (vas deferens) that transports sperm from each testicle is removed and the sperm are trapped.

of the heart. *Portal veins* drain the blood from the stomach, intestines, spleen, pancreas and gallbladder and carry it to the liver for purification. Two large veins return blood from the body to the heart. The *inferior vena cava* returns the blood from the trunk, pelvis, abdomen and lower limbs; the *superior vena cava,* from the head, neck, chest and upper limbs.

Veins have three thin inelastic coats. Many veins—especially those in the thighs and legs—have valves which open outward to prevent the backflow of blood. The *great saphenous vein* (the longest in the body) extends from the groin to the foot, running along the inner side of the thigh and leg. It is commonly the site of *varices* and of clots (*thrombi*).

Varicose veins are dilated and twisted, most often located on the inner side of the thigh or the back of the leg. In wounds of the veins, the blood oozes out in contrast to arterial wounds, which spurt. A wound of the large *jugular vein* in the neck is dangerous because of the rapid loss of blood and difficulty in controlling it. *See also* CIRCULATORY SYSTEM; VASCULAR SYSTEM.

VENEREAL DISEASE, *V.D.,* an infectious disease usually contracted by sexual intercourse with an infected person. The principal venereal diseases are *syphilis, gonorrhea, chancroid, trichomoniasis, granuloma inguinale* and *lymphogranuloma venereum.* Modern antibiotics combat most of these diseases effectively. *See also* ANTIBIOTICS; CHANCRE; CHANCROID; CONDOM; GRANULOMA INGUINALE; LYMPHOGRANULOMA VENEREUM; PREVENTIVE MEDICINE; PROPHYLACTIC *and* **medigraphs** GONORRHEA; SYPHILIS. RESEARCH REPORT *follows* URETHRITIS.

Vertebra—The body of each vertebra of the spine is the weight-bearing area. A layer of cartilage cushions one bone from the other and strong ligaments maintain the flexible structure. Projections at the rear form the ringlike opening that surrounds and protects the spinal cord. The vertebrae vary in size and details. The smallest are in the neck, the largest in the lower back.

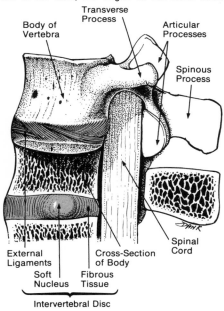

Transverse Process

Body of Vertebra

Articular Processes

Spinous Process

Spinal Cord

External Ligaments

Cross-Section of Body

Soft Nucleus

Fibrous Tissue

Intervertebral Disc

VENIPUNCTURE, puncture of a vein with a hypodermic needle to withdraw a specimen of blood or inject a drug for immediate action. *See also* INJECTION; INTRAVENOUS FEEDING.

VENTILATION, the supply of fresh air in enclosed areas such as rooms, offices and halls. Ventilation can be natural or artificial. Fresh air supplies needed oxygen for lungs and removes the noxious exhaled carbon dioxide. Good ventilation provides freedom from tobacco fumes, dust, smoke and the expired air of others. In a properly heated and ventilated room, the summer temperature is 70–85° F. (21.1-29.4°C.); winter, 68–70° F. (20-21.1°C.), with sufficient moisture to produce a relative humidity of 30–60 percent. The pollen count should also be acceptably low. The incidence of common colds in children is lowest in naturally ventilated rooms. *See also* AIR; AIR CONDITIONING; AIR POLLUTION; CARBON DIOXIDE; HUMIDITY; OXYGEN.

VERMIFORM APPENDIX. *See* APPENDIX.

VERTEBRA, one of 26 similar bones that form the *spinal column;* 7 in the neck, 12 in the thorax, 5 in the loin (lower back), the sacrum and the coccyx.

The individual vertebrae are buffered and separated from each other by a plate of cartilage called an *intervertebral disc.* The vertebra is shaped like a signet ring, with a large flat and semicircular body in front, an oval hole through the middle, a wing on each side (*transverse process*), and a spinous projection behind. Various ligaments and muscles are attached to the spinal column to support it and provide mobility. The spinal cord passes through the line of holes in the vertebrae, and the spinal nerves emerge from the openings near the wings. The first neck vertebra—called the *atlas* because it carries the weight of the skull—is flattened on top and has a circular opening behind the front arch for the pivot of the second neck bone (the *axis*) which turns the head from side to side.

The vertebrae are subject to various injuries and diseases. Broken back is common in war casualties and automobile accidents. A slipped disc is one of the most frequent causes of low backache, sacroiliac disease and sciatica. *Spondylolisthesis* (a forward displacement of the fifth lumbar vertebra upon the sacrum), broken neck (fracture of the cervical vertebrae), spinal cord tumors, tuberculosis of the spine (*Pott's disease*), and osteoarthritis are among the many disorders of the column of vertebrae.

A lack of calcium may soften the vertebrae; an excess may make the intervertebral discs brittle and nonresilient. *See also* SPINE.

VERTIGO, a sensation of whirling around in space, often called giddiness or dizziness, caused by a disturbance of the semicircular canals in the internal ear and often experienced as motion sickness. It is commonly felt by sensitive persons who travel by sea, air, train or bus, and it may be a sign of hardening of the arteries affecting the internal ear. Many cases of vertigo cause nausea and vomiting. The symptom is usually relieved by antihistaminic drugs. *See also* DIZZINESS; EAR; MOTION SICKNESS; NEUROLOGICAL AND NEUROMUSCULAR DISORDERS; VESTIBULAR DISORDERS *and* **medigraph** MÈNIÉRE'S DISEASE.

VESTIBULAR DISORDERS, most often refers to those conditions affecting the *aural vestibule* (bony chamber) which is situated between the *cochlea* (organ of hearing) and the *semicircular canals* (equilibratory apparatus) of the ear. The principal symptoms are vertigo, falling and *nystagmus* (horizontal movements of the eyes), which are usually relieved by antihistaminic drugs.

Inflammation of the nasal vestibule (an area just inside the nostrils) is referred to as *vestibulitis.* It can be caused by nasal discharge, nose picking and plucking hairs from the nose. *See also* EAR; NOSE.

VETERINARIAN, a specialist in diseases of animals, especially horses, dogs, cats and livestock. Veterinary science is concerned not only with the welfare of animals for their own sake, but also with their experimental use in human medicine and the safety of people who eat their flesh. *See also* ANIMAL RESEARCH; VIVISECTION.

VILLUS, a small elongated projection from the surface of a mucous membrane. The villi of the small intestine contain small blood and lymphatic vessels and absorb digested food products into the blood and lymph to support nutrition.

VINCENT'S ANGINA. *See* TRENCH MOUTH.

VIRILISM, *mannishness,* masculine traits in a woman, either physical or psychological or both. *Pseudohermaphroditism* is a condition in which the woman has ovaries and a uterus but also a rudimentary penis. Some virile women are *transvestites* and prefer to dress like and be accepted as a man. *See also* ACHARD-THIERS SYNDROME; ADRENAL GLAND DISORDERS; HERMAPHRODITE.

VIRUSES, the smallest of all infectious agents which can be seen only through an ultramicroscope and cannot pass through a porcelain filter. They consist of tiny particles which differ from each other in size, structure and stability.

Viruses differ from bacteria in the following essential respects: they are much smaller; they do not grow on ordinary artificial culture media but only in living tissue; many are subject to mutation with

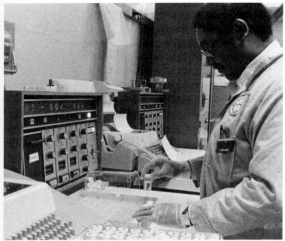

Courtesy, National Institutes of Health

Viruses—These most minute of infectious organisms are known to cause many contagious diseases. Effective vaccines have been developed to control some of them. Evidence that viruses can cause cancers in certain animals has spurred massive efforts to identify human cancer viruses. A technician stores viruses under study in a special cabinet at a cancer virus laboratory.

changes in their properties and virulence; and with few exceptions, they are not destroyed by antibiotic drugs.

There are more than 50 known virus diseases, including the *common cold, influenza, smallpox, chickenpox, poliomyelitis, measles, German measles, mumps, cold sores, herpes zoster* (shingles), *viral hepatitis, viral pneumonia, yellow fever, psittacosis* (parrot fever), *rabies, infectious mononucleosis, croup, viral encephalitis* (inflammation of the brain), and *foot-and-mouth disease.* Viruses are also suspected of being the cause of leukemia and many other diseases.

Virus diseases are transmitted by direct contact, inhalation of droplets expelled by sneezing or coughing, conveyance by insects, contamination of water, milk or food, and by blood transfusion. Virologists in research institutions are conducting extensive studies to determine the causes of many diseases, including can-

cer. Viruses which attack and destroy bacteria are known as *bacteriophages,* some of which have been used in medicine.

Some vaccines made from killed or weakened viruses succeed in producing a degree of immunity but, in general, virus vaccines are less effective than bacterial vaccines. The two vaccines for protection from poliomyelitis are the Salk killed vaccine, given by injection, and the Sabin weak living vaccine, given by mouth. *Gamma globulin* contains the essential antibodies against poliomyelitis and thus provides a measure of temporary immunity against the disease. Vaccines are useful in prevention and treatment of certain influenza strain viruses but not against other strains. Travelers to the tropics should be protected against such viral disorders as yellow fever, dysentery and many other infections which may be prevalent in the area where they will travel, and for which vaccines are available. *See also* IMMUNIZATION; IMMUNOGLOBULINS; INFECTION; INFECTIOUS DISEASES; INFECTIOUS DISEASES, CONTROL OF; PARASITES; VACCINATION.

RESEARCH REPORT *follows* IMMUNITY; MONONUCLEOSIS, INFECTIOUS.

RESEARCH REPORT

VIRUS ISOLATED FROM LAB-GROWN HUMAN LEUKEMIC CELLS

The isolation of a *virus* from the laboratory-grown diseased cells of a 61-year-old woman with one of the rarer types of leukemia is reported by NATIONAL CANCER INSTITUTE scientists. As a result of this advance, researchers are now provided with a human virus that may be useful in identifying the cause of leukemia as well as in detecting and treating it. The patient from whom the cells derived had acute *myelogenous leukemia,* a cancer of the blood in which precursor cells in the bone marrow do not mature properly into normal white blood cells.

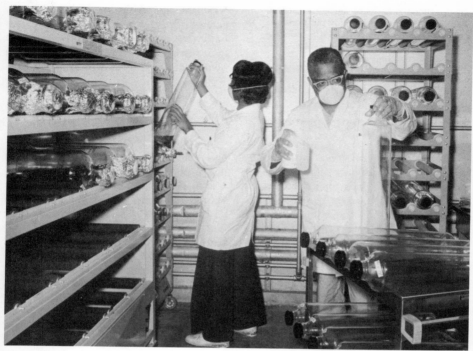

Viruses—These technicians are producing proven cancer-causing viruses in tissue culture for use in cancer virus studies. A small number of virus-infected cells are put with a liquid nutrient into bottles (*above*). Continuous growth and multiplication occur during several days of storage on rotating racks. The fluids, containing a large number of virus particles, are then harvested. In an ultracentrifuge (*right*) rotating at speeds up to 35,000 rpm, these fluids are concentrated a thousandfold, yielding nearly one billion virus particles per milliliter of fluid.

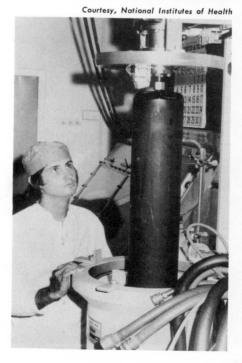

Investigators have not yet determined whether the isolated virus is the cause of various types of human leukemia. However, they have already demonstrated that it is biochemically and immunologically similar to two viruses that cause cancer in primates other than man.

Ongoing research is designed to find out whether the human virus is limited to one patient with one type of leukemia, or whether it can be found in a wide range of human subjects suffering from other forms of blood cancer.

○ Blood samples of leukemic patients are also to be tested for the presence
○ of *antibodies* to this virus in order to discover whether antibodies are pres-
○ ent during only one stage of the disease or throughout its course. NIH315

○ **VISION,** the ability to see. Light rays
○ entering the eye are focused by the lens onto the retina, which converts them
○ into nerve impulses relayed to the brain by the optic nerve. *See also* EYE.

VITAMIN A DEFICIENCY

P RESENT IN ITS NATURAL form only in animal food sources, vitamin A is an essential nutrient. It is manufactured by man and animals from the plant pigments known as carotenes and is found in such vegetables as carrots, squash, broccoli, sweet potatoes, kale and spinach. Vitamin A is obtained directly from such animal products as liver, eggs, cheese, whole milk and cream. Deficiency of this vitamin causes disease of the bones, skin and teeth, defects of vision, and susceptibility of epithelial and bone tissue to infection.

causes
The chief cause of vitamin A deficiency is just as likely to be ignorance as pov-- erty. It is calculated, for example, that

Vitamin A Deficiency—This type of dry and pimply skin is a sign of vitamin A deficiency. Foods rich in vitamin A should be eaten daily to avoid the condition. These include green leafy and yellow vegetables, liver, eggs, and dairy products such as milk, butter and cheese.

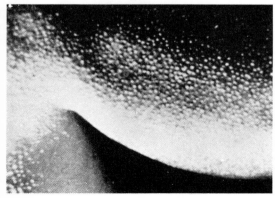

less than .0001 ounce of vitamin A a day is enough to activate the light-sensitive eye cells, yet in many parts of the world where the vegetable sources are available, infants go blind because their diet is deficient in the proper foods. Vitamin A deficiency may occur because of adherence to a fad diet. It may also result from malabsorption syndromes such as celiac disease and cystic fibrosis, or from a metabolic failure caused by diseases of the liver, glandular disorders, or diabetes. In children, temporary vitamin A deficiency may follow infections such as pneumonia, influenza, or strep throat.

symptoms
Symptoms of the deficiency depend on the age of the victim. In infants, the skin and the eye membranes (especially the cornea) are affected. Youngsters in whom the deficiency is chronic are retarded in their skeletal growth. In all ages, tooth decay, night blindness and thickening and drying out of the skin are apparent. Resistance to secondary infection is low.

complications
In early childhood, the chronic deficiency may lead to blindness. In adults, the hair falls out; skin becomes bumpy and discolored; the cornea dries as epithelial tissue falls off; tear ducts and conjunctiva fail to function; and corneal ulceration leads to secondary eye infections.

treatment
Therapeutic doses of vitamin A are administered over a supervised period, fol-

Vitamin A Deficiency

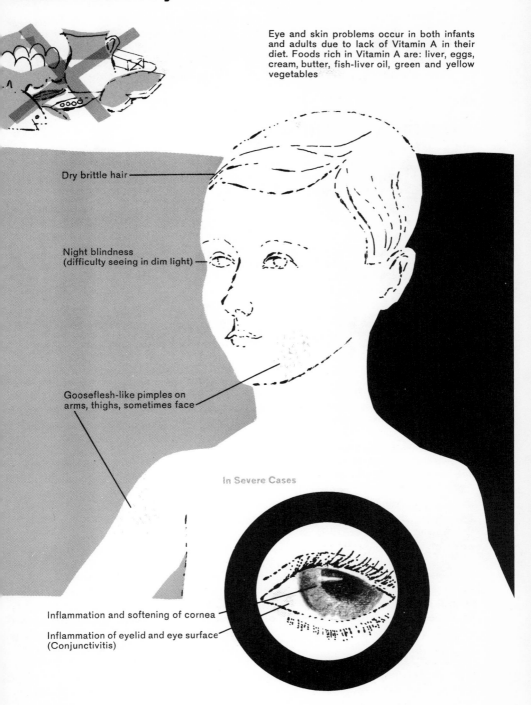

Eye and skin problems occur in both infants and adults due to lack of Vitamin A in their diet. Foods rich in Vitamin A are: liver, eggs, cream, butter, fish-liver oil, green and yellow vegetables

Dry brittle hair

Night blindness (difficulty seeing in dim light)

Gooseflesh-like pimples on arms, thighs, sometimes face

In Severe Cases

Inflammation and softening of cornea

Inflammation of eyelid and eye surface (Conjunctivitis)

1465

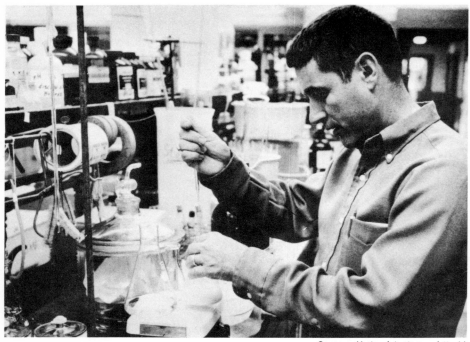

Courtesy, National Institutes of Health

Vitamins—Vitamin D is studied by a biochemist researching the function and uses of its various forms. Investigation has revealed that the vitamin must be converted in the body to activated forms. Certain activated forms of vitamin D₃ have been isolated and the compounds produced chemically. They are used successfully to treat bone diseases formerly difficult to manage, in cases of kidney failure, and to help calcium absorption in people lacking parathyroid glands.

lowed by maintenance doses as the symptoms are corrected. Amounts depend on age and severity of symptoms. Where malabsorption is the underlying cause, the disorder requires special treatment. Generally, vitamin A therapy in large doses over a long period is avoided in favor of a correction in eating habits.

prevention

Most cases of this deficiency can be prevented by proper diet. Infants may be given cod liver oil or a synthetic substitute as recommended by the doctor.

VITAMIN DEFICIENCIES. The definitely known results of vitamin deficiencies are as follows: vitamin A—*night blindness* and *xerophthalmia* (dryness and thickening of the conjunctiva); vitamin B_1—*beriberi* and *multiple neuritis;* vitamin B_2—*cheilosis* (inflammation of the lips and corners of the mouth); niacin—*pellagra;* vitamin C—*scurvy;* vitamin D—*rickets;* vitamin K—*bleeding tendency.*

Other suspected or contributory results are as follows: vitamin A—dryness of the skin and low resistance to infection, especially of the bronchi and lungs; vitamin B_1—poor appetite, weak muscles, and heart symptoms; vitamin B_6—metabolic disorders; vitamin B_{12}—anemia; vitamin C—gingivitis (sore gums); vitamin D—dental decay and poorly calcified bones; vitamin E—susceptibility to polysaturated fats; niacin—high cholesterol. **R**ESEARCH **R**EPORT *follows* AIR POLLUTION.

VITAMINS, accessory food substances present in small amounts which are indispensable to normal functioning of the body. A balanced diet contains all essential vitamins (A, B complex, C, D, E and K) in adequate amounts. However, some of them are lost by the heat of cooking, and dieters and whimsical eaters may need a multivitamin supplement. Such supplements are available which supply the recommended daily allowances (RDA) of all essential vitamins.

Vitamins help transform other food substances into bone, skin and other tissue. The lack of one or more vitamins from the diet can cause deficiency diseases such as *scurvy, beriberi* and *rickets.*

The B complex vitamins and vitamin C are soluble in water; the rest are fat-soluble. If the vitamins were not soluble, they could not be absorbed into the body. *See also* ASCORBIC ACID; AVITAMINOSIS; BIOTIN; BOWLEG; CAROTENE; CHEILOSIS; DEFICIENCY DISEASES; FOLIC ACID; GUMS; HYPERVITAMINOSIS; LIVER EXTRACTS; MALNUTRITION; NIACIN; NIGHT BLINDNESS; NUTRITION; PANTOTHENIC ACID; PYRIDOXINE; RIBOFLAVIN; THIAMIN; VITAMIN DEFICENCIES; XEROPHTHALMIA *and* **medigraphs** BERIBERI; CELIAC DISEASE; NEURITIS; PELLAGRA; PERNICIOUS ANEMIA; RICKETS; SCURVY; VITAMIN A DEFICIENCY.

R_{EPORT}ESEARCH *follows* ANEMIA; ASCORBIC ACID.

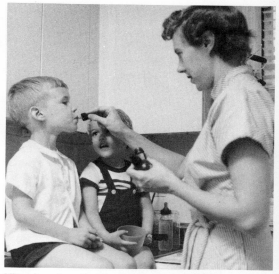

Vitamins—A mother feeds her children vitamins in liquid form—a safe and simple way. Supplementary vitamin intake is often prescribed for children, especially poor eaters. Sufficient amounts of vitamins C and D are especially important during the years of growth.

R_{EPORT}ESEARCH

○ ACTIVATED FORM OF VITAMIN D BENEFICIAL FOR BONE LESIONS

○   An activated form of *vitamin D* isolated by UNIVERSITY OF WISCONSIN scientists in 1971 is now being used in small quantities for the treatment of various bone diseases related to kidney failure. MAYO FOUNDATION researchers report that a group of patients with *uremic osteodystrophy* (defective bone formation) have responded favorably to the treatment.

○   Vitamin D, which is changed to 25-hydroxy vitamin D₃ in the liver, is then converted by the kidney into its most active form: 1,25 dihydroxy vitamin D₃ (1,25 DHCC). When it is orally administered in this form to patients with advanced renal failure, it improves calcium and phosphate balance, calcium absorption by the intestines, and increases the amount of calcium in the bloodstream. Until the present studies, the effects of this therapy on the skeletal lesions that characterize uremic osteodystrophy had not been known.

○   The latest Mayo Foundation findings indicate that the eight patients with skeletal abnormalities resulting from renal failure who were treated with 1,25 DHCC showed sufficient improvement in the lesions of *osteomalacia* (soft bones) to warrant continuing studies of the effects of prolonged therapy.   NIH515X

VITILIGO, a disfiguring skin disease with mottled patches of black and white of various sizes and shapes due to a lack of

Vitiligo

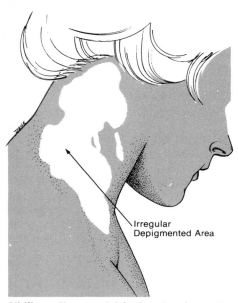

Irregular
Depigmented Area

Vitiligo—These unsightly but harmless white patches on the skin are due to a lack of pigment in those areas. Because of this, they are more sensitive to the sun. The cause of vitiligo is unknown. The face, backs of hands, armpits and around body openings are among the most common sites. Masking with specially prepared cosmetics is the most practical remedy.

the normal *melanin* pigment in the white areas. The distribution of the patches is more or less symmetrical, located mostly on the backs of the hands, the sides of the neck, and the trunk. The cause of the disease is unknown, and it occurs mostly in blacks. Except for causing emotional distress, vitiligo is harmless. Researchers report that in about 15 percent of cases the use of chemical substances isolated from the fruits of the Egyptian plant *Ammi majus,* in conjunction with sunlight or sunlamps, promotes repigmentation of the white patches. Cosmeticians have used various other dyes including Bismarck brown, henna and carmine to mask the disfigurement. Exposure to the sun may severely burn unpigmented skin. *See also* PIGMENTATION; SKIN.

VITREOUS FLOATERS. The *vitreous humor* is the transparent gelatinous substance that fills the greater part of the inside of the eyeball, situated between the lens in front and the retina in back. A vitreous floater is a small loose concretion of vitreous substance which floats around and causes spots before the eyes. It is of no significance but must be differentiated by the eye specialist from the dangerous retinal hemorrhage. *See also* EYE.

VIVISECTION, *animal experimentation,* the cutting of, or operation on, a living animal for physiological or pathological investigation. Every measure to reduce the pain and suffering is required by law. Much of our knowledge of physiology and medicine has been acquired by animal experimentation. For example, the determination of the safety and efficacy of new drugs would be impossible without it. *See also* ANIMAL RESEARCH.

VOCAL CORDS AND VOICE. The vocal cords are two strong bands of yellow elastic tissue inside the *larynx* (voice box) which vibrate during speaking or singing. They are longer in the male— hence his deeper voice. The sound comes out in the opening between the cords called the *glottis* and is also affected by the tongue, mouth and palate. The vocal cords are irritated by tobacco fumes, colds and excessive use, producing a hoarse voice. *See also* GLOTTIS; HOARSENESS; LARYNX; SPEECH.

VOMITING, the forceful ejection of stomach contents through the mouth, due to various causes. At the onset, the *pylorus* (through which the food normally passes from the stomach into the small intestine) closes, the wave of stomach contractions moves in reverse, the subject takes a deep breath, and the climax is a powerful contraction of both the midriff and the stomach muscles.

Mirror Image of the Vocal Cords

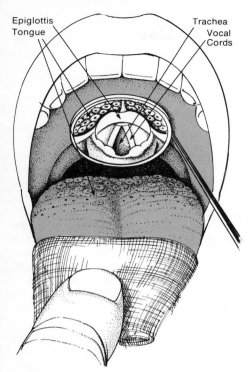

Epiglottis
Tongue
Trachea
Vocal
Cords

Vocal Cords and Voice—Sound comes as air is forced through the elastic vocal cords when they are drawn close together, causing them to vibrate. The tongue, palate and lips contribute to the articulation of the vocal sound into words. Voice texture and tone are affected by the resonating cavities in the head and chest as well as the size and shape of the vocal cords.

The principal causes of vomiting are overeating, nausea, spoiled food, and poisons or toxic drugs. Persistent vomiting, especially when the vomited matter is blood-tinged, suggests the possibility of ulcer or cancer of the stomach, the diagnosis of which may require an x-ray examination. *See also* HEMATEMESIS; NAUSEA; RETCHING.

VULVA, composite of the female external sexual organs, consisting of various parts situated at the front bottom of the abdomen and between the thighs. The *mons pubis (mons veneris, mount of Venus)*—a rounded prominence in front of the junction of the two pubic bones—is formed by a collection of fat beneath the skin which from puberty on is covered with hair. The *vaginal opening* lies behind the urethra and in front of the anus. It is irregular in size and covered in virgins by a thin membrane called the *hymen* (maidenhead), which is ruptured by sexual intercourse, masturbation, or vaginal examination. The area surrounding the urethra and vaginal opening is called the *vestibule*. It is covered by two folds of skin—the *labia majora* (thick lips) outside and the *labia minora* (thin lips) inside. The *clitoris,* an erectile organ, is at the apex of the vestibule, partly covered by the labia minora, and causes sexual excitement when rubbed by the penis or an object during masturbation. *Skene's ducts,* which open just below the clitoris, drain tiny glands similar to the male prostate. *Bartholin's glands,* located near the vaginal opening, lubricate it with a mucous secretion to facilitate the entrance of the penis. *See also* ACCESSORY SEX ORGANS; BARTHOLIN'S GLANDS; CLITORIS; REPRODUCTIVE SYSTEM; URETHRA; VAGINA *and* **medigraph** TRICHOMONAS.

VULVOVAGINITIS, inflammation of the vulva and vagina. *See also* VAGINA; VULVA.

W

WALLEYES, dense white opacity of the cornea caused by prolonged untreated syphilis, corneal ulcer or trachoma; or a cross-eyed condition in which the eyes are turned away from each other, also called divergent strabismus. The latter condition can be due to defective eye muscles, disease or heredity. The best hope for preventing impaired vision lies in early treatment. *See also* EYE.

WARTS

WARTS ARE NONCANCEROUS infectious swellings of the skin that may spread from one part of the body to another and from one person to another. They are especially common among children and the majority of them disappear without treatment. *Plantar warts,* which occur on the soles of the feet and grow inward because of pressure, can cause great discomfort.

causes

Warts are caused by the human papilloma virus which has an incubation period ranging from three weeks to six months. They are spread by scratching, shaving, or in the case of plantar warts, by going about barefooted in locker rooms and near swimming pools.

symptoms

Common warts usually start as tiny bumps on the skin that gradually become larger, rough-surfaced and brownish. They are painless except when they occur at the base of the fingernails and develop fissures. Plantar warts are likely to appear in conjunction with calluses. They are extremely painful when they are forced inward by the pressure of body weight.

treatment

If a common wart is neither painful nor aesthetically displeasing, it need not be treated in any way. A doctor should be consulted about warts that appear near the fingernails or on the scalp. Methods of removing troublesome or unwanted warts include electrocauterization, freezing with liquid nitrogen (*cryosurgery*), or the application of medications that cause the warts to shrink and vanish. Plantar warts should not be disturbed unless they are causing continuous discomfort, since many treatments involve considerable pain and inconvenience to the victim.

Warts

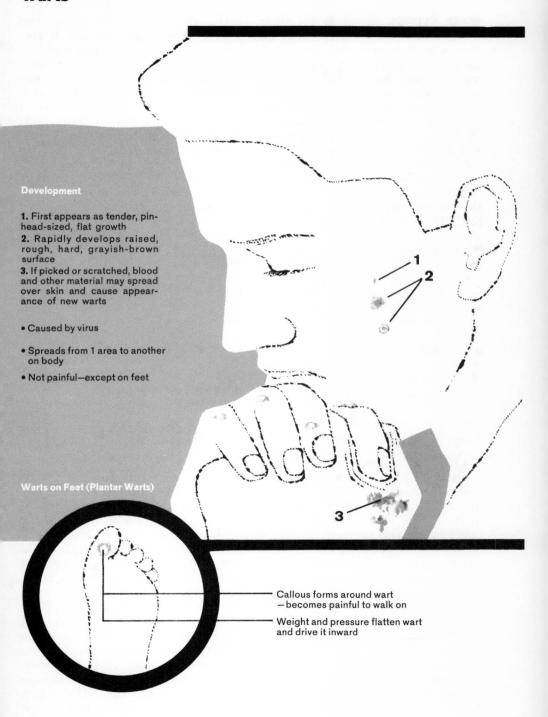

Development

1. First appears as tender, pin-head-sized, flat growth

2. Rapidly develops raised, rough, hard, grayish-brown surface

3. If picked or scratched, blood and other material may spread over skin and cause appearance of new warts

• Caused by virus

• Spreads from 1 area to another on body

• Not painful—except on feet

Warts on Feet (Plantar Warts)

1

2

3

Callous forms around wart —becomes painful to walk on

Weight and pressure flatten wart and drive it inward

WASP STINGS, similar to bee stings and sometimes fatal. The venom of the wasp, when injected into the skin, causes an allergic reaction with swelling and redness. Unlike the honeybee, the female wasp does not have a barbed stinger and therefore can inflict multiple stings upon its victim. The systemic reactions of shock may be so severe as to require administration of oxygen. The popular local application is vinegar. Drugs may be administered to combat the allergy and inflammation. *See also* BEE STINGS; INSECT BITES; STINGS.
R ESEARCH *follows* INSECT BITES.

WASSERMANN TEST, the generally recognized blood test to determine the presence and degree of active syphilis, as measured by complement fixation reactions. Various modifications of the original method are used. False positives sometimes result from reactions to other related diseases. The tests are repeated at frequent intervals during the course of treatment to evaluate its progress. When the central nervous system is affected, the test is made on the spinal fluid. *See also* KAHN TEST; PREMARITAL CHECKUP; TESTS *and* **medigraph** SYPHILIS.

WATER, H_2O, comprises about two-thirds of the weight of the body and 75 percent of protoplasm. Water is also a natural constituent of many foods. It is essential to life, comprises about 80 percent of the blood, and is eliminated by the kidneys, sweat glands and lungs together with dissolved waste products. An excessive amount of water in the body causes *edema* (dropsy); a deficiency, *dehydration*. The recommended amount of water to be drunk by a healthy person is 2–8 glasses daily, but more is needed in hot weather. In some illnesses the amount of water should be increased; in others, reduced. Diabetics suffer from constant thirst and drink a great deal of water.

Our water supply comes mainly from springs, wells, rivers and lakes. If contaminated by sewage, it may carry typhoid fever, dysentery, cholera, and other water-borne diseases which in the past occurred in epidemics. Many large cities receive their water supply from distant sources through a system of pipes, tanks and reservoirs; water is sterilized by addition of *chlorine*. In the home, tap water may be sterilized by boiling. Many communities add *fluoride* to the water to prevent dental cavities in children and adolescents. Other impurities sometimes found in tap water coming from corroded pipes are small amounts of lead and mercury. Persons with disorders of the kidneys or bladder should drink only pure spring water, which is free from chlorine, fluorine, and other impurities which are harmful to the urinary organs. *See also* ALGAE; CHLORINE; DEHYDRATION; EDEMA; EUTROPHICATION; FLUORIDATION; NUTRITION; POLYCHLORINATED BIPHENYLS; WATER POLLUTION.

WATER ON THE BRAIN. *See* HYDROCEPHALUS.

WATER ON THE KNEE. *See* KNEE.

WATER POLLUTION, defilement of the water supply by germs or harmful chemicals. Filthy streams and their tributaries carry water-borne infections, especially *typhoid fever, paratyphoid, cholera* and *dysentery*. Sanitary precautions have largely eliminated water-borne infections in the United States but water pollution due to dumping industrial wastes into the rivers and lakes has poisoned and killed millions of fish and added injurious elements to public water supplies. The United States Environmental Protection Agency has taken active steps to protect the purity of natural waters and eliminate pollution. *See also* DETERGENTS; POLYCHLORINATED BIPHENYLS; WATER *and* **medigraphs** AMEBIASIS

AND AMEBIC DYSENTERY; CHOLERA; MERCURY POISONING; TYPHOID FEVER.

WATER PURIFICATION, the production of a hygienically safe and pleasant-tasting drinking water from a potentially polluted source. Water-borne infections include typhoid and paratyphoid fevers, cholera, dysentery and other bacterial diseases. In reservoirs the water is sterilized by *chlorination* and *filtration;* in the home, by *boiling.* Other purification processes include *aeration* to remove obnoxious tastes and odors, *coagulation* for turbidity (muddiness) and coloration, sedimentation, filtration and softening.

Purified water is free from germs but contains small amounts of chlorine and fluorine and traces of lead, mercury and other metals. Recent studies of United States drinking waters have focused on chemical and mineral contaminants. Two studies of municipal drinking waters released by the U.S. Environmental Protection Agency in 1974 added to the list about 60 organic chemicals, including chloroform, carbon tetrachloride, cadmium, polyvinyl chloride, and other known or suspected cancer-causing agents. Health officials in a number of large American cities reported that their drinking water contained small amounts of potentially carcinogenic (cancer-causing) chemicals formed by the combination of chlorine with contaminating substances. It was suggested that a substitute for chlorine in water purification should be sought.

The only pure water is that bottled at the springs under sanitary conditons. *See also* WATER; WATER POLLUTION.

WEIGHT. Measurement of the weight is a standard procedure in every medical examination, both at the first visit and at later visits to determine change. Overnutrition and undernutrition are constant medical problems. Extreme overweight (*obesity*) shortens life and predisposes to atherosclerosis and coronary heart disease. Diabetes is four times as common in obese as in lean persons. Obesity also makes people susceptible to gallbladder and gallstone diseases and to accidents because of hampered agility, and it lowers resistance in case of pneumonia. Undernutrition leaves one vulnerable to tuberculosis.

Due to modern living habits, recent life insurance statistics provide new weight standards for men and women in developed nations. Automation and the easy life have decreased the energy expenditure for men, and greater physical activity has increased it for many women. The most important weight factor, however, is the diet.

The accompanying tables summarize the desirable weights for men and women, measured with shoes and clothing.

Weight—A woman is weighed at the start of a physical examination. Any excessive loss or gain since the previous visit will alert her physician to a possible organic cause. Severe weight fluctuation can also have an emotional basis. Extremes of weight loss or gain are usually damaging to health and should be investigated.

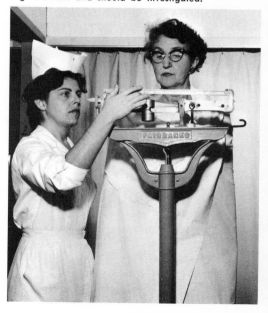

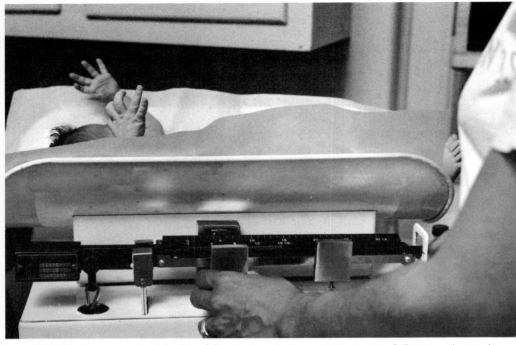

Weight—Checking a tiny infant's weight at regular intervals helps to monitor its condition. A steady weight gain after the first few days of life indicates good progress. Failure to gain may be the first indication of a digestive problem or other internal abnormality.

Although the control of body weight is not easily achieved, it is of vital importance for health and long life. It requires a proper balance between food intake in terms of calories and energy expenditure in comparable units. For a large and increasing proportion of people, the daily tasks both on the job and at home have been greatly lightened by labor-saving devices. Accordingly, fewer calories in the diet are needed, since the excess is stored as fat. Statistics emphasize the disadvantage of overweight in people of middle and older age. As a rule of thumb, if persons of any particular age keep their weight down to their average in the early 20s, it would be fairly close to the desirable weight at ages over 25.

Hereditary factors in overweight. Just about everybody has seen families in which both parents and all of the children are fat. In other families, the reverse is true. The Jack Spratt type (after the nursery-rhyme character who could eat no fat and whose wife could eat no lean) often results in some fat and some lean children. These observations suggest—but do not prove—that overweight may be hereditary.

Some authorities have suggested that inherited characteristics in the glands of internal secretion may be partly responsible for extreme overweight. Thus an overproduction of insulin may lead to hunger and overeating, deficient thyroid hormone to low basal metabolism, and lack of anterior (front) lobe pituitary hormone to slow mobilization of fat from its depots. The obesity of eunuchs suggests that absence of the male sex hormone is a cause.

DESIRABLE WEIGHTS FOR MEN
(Aged 25 and Over)

Height (with shoes on) 1-inch heels		Weight in Pounds (in indoor clothing)		
Feet	Inches	Small Frame	Medium Frame	Large Frame
5	2	112–120	118–129	126–141
5	3	115–123	121–133	129–144
5	4	118–126	124–136	132–148
5	5	121–129	127–139	135–152
5	6	124–133	130–143	138–156
5	7	128–137	134–147	142–161
5	8	132–141	138–152	147–166
5	9	136–145	142–156	151–170
5	10	140–150	146–160	155–174
5	11	144–154	150–165	159–179
6	0	148–158	154–170	164–184
6	1	152–162	158–175	168–189
6	2	156–167	162–180	173–194
6	3	160–171	167–185	178–199
6	4	164–175	172–190	182–204

DESIRABLE WEIGHTS FOR WOMEN
(Aged 25 and Over)

Height (with shoes on) 2-inch heels		Weight in Pounds (in indoor clothing)		
Feet	Inches	Small Frame	Medium Frame	Large Frame
4	10	92– 98	96–107	104–119
4	11	94–101	98–110	106–122
5	0	96–104	101–113	109–125
5	1	99–107	104–116	112–128
5	2	102–110	107–119	115–131
5	3	105–113	110–122	118–134
5	4	108–116	113–126	121–138
5	5	111–119	116–130	125–142
5	6	114–123	120–135	129–146
5	7	118–127	124–139	133–150
5	8	122–131	128–143	137–154
5	9	126–135	140–155	149–168
5	10	130–140	132–147	141–158
5	11	134–144	136–151	145–163
6	0	138–148	144–159	153–173

Note: Girls between 18 and 25 subtract 1 pound for each year under 25.

The modern belief is that family environment, psychological causes and acquired habits play a more important part in the development of overweight than heredity. Many people frustrated in love or bored with their jobs feel a sense of emptiness and make up for it by filling their stomachs. Then again there is the acquisition of certain habits. Those who like meat and potatoes and eat them regularly are apt to become fat, while the fastidious salad eaters remain slim. Alcoholic beverages before or with meals increase appetite and weight by adding extra empty calories, a habit that one often learns from parents. Smoking diminishes appetite and many weight conscious people resort to that unhealthy and harmful habit.

Certain exercises are acquired habits which are practiced in the popular desire to slim the figure. A long brisk walk may take off a pound, but the hearty appetite that follows more than makes up for it. Horseback riding reduces the weight of the horse more than the rider. As a result, doctors tell their patients about one exercise that never fails: push yourself away from the table three times a day. *See also* CALORIE; CARBOHYDRATES; DIET, REDUCING; FAT; NUTRITION; OBESITY; UNDERWEIGHT PROBLEMS.

WEIL'S DISEASE. *See* LEPTOSPIROSIS.

WELLS' FACIES, an anxious expression of the face observed in certain ovarian diseases.

WEN. *See* SEBACEOUS CYST.

WHEAL, a temporary swollen bump in the skin, varying in size, often accompanied by intense itching, tingling and burning. They occur after insect bites and physical injuries, and as hives in *urticaria. See also* ALLERGY *and* **medigraph** HIVES.

WHEAT SENSITIVITY. *See* ALLERGY.

WHIPLASH INJURY OF THE NECK

THANKS TO THE FACT THAT automobile seats are now designed with headrests and the increased use of safety belts by drivers and passengers, there has been a significant decrease in the number of whiplash injuries resulting from head-on and rear-end collisions. Unfortunately, whiplash injury is not an unusual cause of death of battered infants who have been fiercely shaken in an effort to make them stop crying.

causes
When, because of a sudden and powerful force, the head jerks backward and then flicks forward like a whiplash, the vertebrae in the cervical area of the spine and the surrounding tissues can be severely injured. Ligaments may tear, internal hemorrhaging may occur, bones may fracture and nerve ends may become inflamed. There may also be damage to the brain and its coverings, the meninges.

symptoms
Although consequences of the injury may not be immediately apparent, a day or so later the victim may complain of a stiff neck, an inability to move the head backward or forward, the onset of dizziness, vertigo and severe headache. The pain may extend into the shoulders and arms.

complications
Pain may be so acute as to be immobilizing. Alleviation of constant headaches and dizziness may require medication heavy enough to prevent routine activities. A slipped disc is a possible complication of fracture.

Whiplash Injury of the Neck

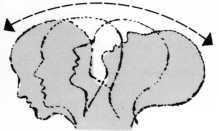

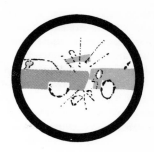

1. Accident As result of sharp impact, head snaps back and forth with great force

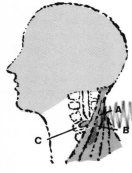

2. Damage
A. Stretching and tearing of ligaments
B. Bleeding around injured area
C. Occasionally goes on to severe nerve injury. Herniation of cervical disc, fracture or dislocation may be accompanying injuries

3. Initial Reaction
May be slight neck pain and limitation of head movement—or little noticeable pain

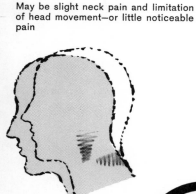

5. Next Several Weeks
Pain and weakness in neck, shoulders, arms during lifting or other strain producing activities

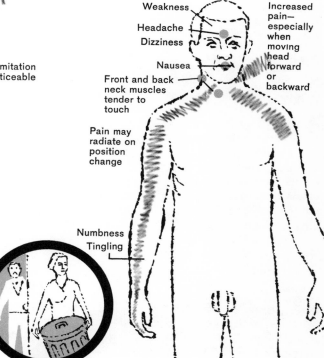

4. After 24 Hours

Weakness

Headache
Dizziness

Nausea

Front and back neck muscles tender to touch

Increased pain— especially when moving head forward or backward

Pain may radiate on position change

Numbness
Tingling

1477

treatment

Immobilization is essential to the healing process. A surgical neck brace with supportive collar has its discomforts, but it performs the same function as a cast on a broken arm or leg. Damaged neck muscles and stretched ligaments thus begin to recover at the same time that the victim is given pain-relievers. The supervised use of tranquilizers, sedatives, or antidepressants may be indicated during the early stage of healing if the person is too uncomfortable to engage in any routine activities. As recovery proceeds, physiotherapy is recommended to reestablish muscular vigor.

prevention

Habitual use of all safety devices when driving, and strict attention to the business of driving are the two best ways to prevent the accidents ordinarily responsible for whiplash injuries.

WHIRLPOOL BATHS combine the action of heat with that of gentle massage. In this form the average subject can tolerate a water temperature of 115° F. (46.1° C.). The whirlpool bath warms the skin by causing a heavy flow of blood. The bath should start with a temperature of 100° F. (37.7° C.) increasing gradually to tolerance. It is one of the measures employed at health spas. This treatment to relieve pain and promote healing can be given to individual limbs or the entire body. There are special tubs for immersion of an arm, a leg, the lower body or the whole body. *See also* BATHING; PHYSICAL THERAPY.

Whirlpool Baths—The therapist is lowering an arthritis sufferer into a whole-body whirlpool bath. The heat and gentle massage of the agitated water will bring relief to the man's painfully inflamed joints. This type of therapy is also used to relax the muscle spasms of low back pain, sprains and strains. Treatment can be given to individual limbs as well as the entire body.

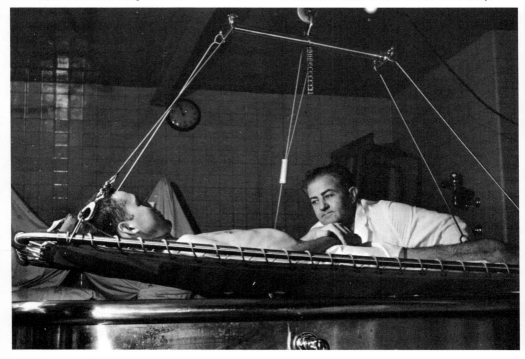

WHITE BLOOD CELLS. *See* LEUKO-CYTES.

WHITE BLOOD CELLS, diseases of. The average normal white blood cell count is 8000 per cubic millimeter. An increase in the number is called *leukocytosis;* a decrease, *leukopenia.*

There are six different types of normal white blood cells: *polymorphonuclear neutrophiles,* 70 percent; small *lymphocytes,* 20–25 percent; large *mononuclears* 4–8 percent; *eosinophiles* (stain red), 1–3 percent; *basophiles* (stain blue), ½ percent; and *transitional cells.*

The principal diseases of the white blood cells are *lymphatic* and *myelogenous leukemia,* in acute and chronic forms, and *infectious mononucleosis.*

Acute lymphatic leukemia occurs more commonly in children and is characterized by a growth of primitive white blood cells in the bone marrow. The suspected cause is a virus. The onset is sudden with high fever, joint pains, ulcers in the mouth and bleeding spots in the skin. The lymph nodes, spleen and liver are usually enlarged. The diagnosis is made by finding the abnormal primitive white blood cells in the blood smear. The white blood cell count is increased in 60 percent of cases. There is no cure for leukemia but remissions have been induced by corticosteroid drugs and drugs that inhibit abnormal cell growth. Irradiation and bone marrow transplants have proved unsuccessful in this type of leukemia.

Chronic leukemia, which seldom occurs in children, is much milder and the victim may survive as long as 15–20 years. In *chronic myelogenous leukemia* the white blood cell count is increased enormously, from 25,000 to 500,000 with the large polymorphonuclear neutrophiles predominating. Drugs that repress new growth of abnormal cells are used in this form of leukemia. The average length of life is 3–4 years but about 20 percent of patients survive longer than five years.

Infectious mononucleosis (kissing disease) occurs mainly among young people. It is believed to be due to a virus transmitted by kissing. It begins with sore throat, enlargement of the lymph nodes in the neck and tenderness on the left side of the abdomen due to enlargement of the spleen. The blood test shows an increased number of lymphocytes. The length of the illness varies from one week to several months, with natural recovery in most cases. The treatment includes bed rest, abundant water and aspirin to reduce high fever. Sore throat may be relieved by a soothing gargle or lozenges. *See also* AGRANULOCYTOSIS; AMINOPTERIN; BLOOD; BLOOD CONDITIONS; LEUKOCYTES; SPLEEN *and* **medigraphs** LEUKEMIA; MONONUCLEOSIS, INFECTIOUS.

WHITFIELD'S OINTMENT, *salicylic acid* and *benzoic acid,* removes superficial horny skin tissue and checks the growth of fungi. It is useful in the treatment of *athlete's foot* and *ringworm. See also* FUNGUS.

WHITLOW. *See* PARONYCHIA.

WHOOPING COUGH

MEDICALLY KNOWN AS *pertussis,* whooping cough is a highly contagious bacterial disease endemic everywhere, and now controllable by immunization and antibiotics. Half of all reported cases occur before the age of two, and of the acute infectious diseases of childhood, it is thought to be the one causing the largest number of infant deaths. When the disease occurs for the first time

Whooping Cough

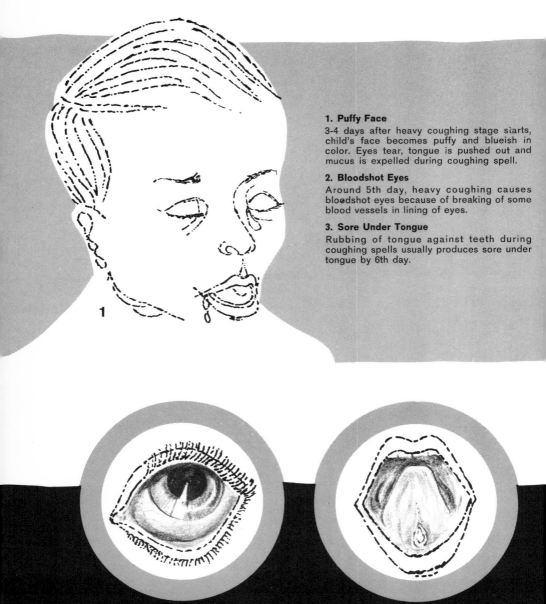

1. Puffy Face
3-4 days after heavy coughing stage starts, child's face becomes puffy and blueish in color. Eyes tear, tongue is pushed out and mucus is expelled during coughing spell.

2. Bloodshot Eyes
Around 5th day, heavy coughing causes bloodshot eyes because of breaking of some blood vessels in lining of eyes.

3. Sore Under Tongue
Rubbing of tongue against teeth during coughing spells usually produces sore under tongue by 6th day.

in adulthood, it is likely to be comparatively mild. One attack is presumed to confer immunity for a lifetime.

causes

Whooping cough is caused by the bacillary agent *Hemophilus pertussis* which inflames the mucous membranes of the respiratory tract—nose, pharynx, trachea and bronchi. The bacterial invasion results in an increase of mucus secretion which in turn causes the characteristic cough. The disease is spread by the airborne germs expelled during coughing. The likelihood of contagion is highest during the first few weeks of the disease. Where infant immunization is not the standard practice, epidemics are likely to occur among children under four. Incubation following infection takes from 1–2 weeks.

symptoms

The disease gets its popular name from its characteristic symptom—the "whooping" sound of the intake of breath following a prolonged coughing spell. Onset of infection is signaled by sneezing, bleary eyes with considerable tearing, loss of appetite, and a dry and persistent cough. This stage, called *catarrhal,* lasts for about ten days. It is followed by the *paroxysmal* stage, during which prolonged coughing spasms—interspersed with whooping—may succeed in loosening and expelling some of the congestive mucus. Instead of expectorating the mucus, infants and young children are likely to swallow or gag on it and throw up. Vomiting is typical, especially during night seizures. During the *convalescent* stage, coughing and vomiting decrease, but they may be triggered months later by a respiratory infection from some other source.

complications

In infancy, the coughing can lead to asphyxiation, convulsions and death. Pneu-monia is the most likely fatal complication in children under four and in the aged. Cerebral involvements caused by intracranial pressure may lead to internal hemorrhaging.

treatment

The treatment depends on the age of the victim and the acuteness of the symptoms. School-age children and adults who are otherwise in good health are usually given antibiotics and watched for possible complications. Infants and old people may require hospitalization for proper medical attention, nursing care and isolation from the rest of the family.

prevention

Because infants are highly vulnerable to whooping cough, child care experts recommend that immunization begin at no later than eight weeks. Preferred procedure consists of three vaccinations at two-month intervals with DPT serum which protects the baby against diphtheria, pertussis and tetanus. Booster shots are given at eight months and at entry into school. The pertussis vaccine does not confer lifetime immunity, but it does ensure that infection in later life will cause only mild symptoms. A doctor should be consulted for immunization procedure for anyone exposed to infection who has neither been immunized nor has had the disease.

WILMS' TUMOR, a malignant growth on a kidney occurring in infancy or childhood, due to embryonic misplacement of tissues and containing foreign tissues such as teeth, hair or other material. It travels to the lungs, brain and other distant organs. The chief symptom is blood in the urine, accompanied by a mass in the flank (side), dull pain, anemia and wasting. Early diagnosis, restriction of palpation, immediate removal of the kidney, plus pre- and postoperative irradiation and chemotherapy have

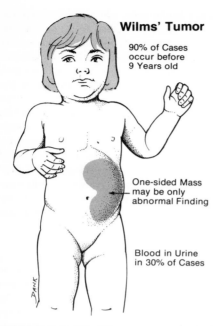

Wilms' Tumor

90% of Cases
occur before
9 Years old

One-sided Mass
may be only
abnormal Finding

Blood in Urine
in 30% of Cases

Wilms' Tumor—This kidney cancer occurs in infants and young children. Often it is not suspected before an abdominal lump is noticed. Since it is a fast-spreading malignancy, prompt removal of the involved kidney, drug therapy and irradiation are necessary. However, even if the tumor spreads, the cure rate is good.

dramatically reduced the formerly 90 percent death rate from this malignancy. *See also* KIDNEY; TUMOR.

WINDPIPE. *See* TRACHEA.

WISDOM TOOTH, the last or back tooth of the full set on the upper and lower jaw of each side. It grows from the late teens to the early twenties. The wisdom tooth is subject to decay and impaction and is often the last to come and the first to go. *See also* TEETH.

WITCH HAZEL, a liquid extract of the shrub *Hamamelis virginiana,* used as a mild and soothing astringent. *See also* ASTRINGENT.

WOMB. *See* UTERUS.

WOOD ALCOHOL POISONING. *Methanol, methyl alcohol* (wood alcohol), is an industrial solvent used in antifreeze liquids. It is highly poisonous and may cause blindness and death. The symptoms of methanol poisoning are drunkenness, blurring of vision, headache, dizziness and vomiting. The emergency treatment is to induce vomiting. A physician and the local poison control center should be notified for advice. *See also* AMAUROSIS; FIRST AID.

WOOD TICK BITES, caused by degenerate parasites in bushes which cling to the bare skin on contact. They may carry rickettsiae which transmit certain diseases such as *Rocky Mountain spotted fever.* The local symptoms are swelling, redness and bleeding into the skin. *See also* TICKS.

WORMS, various parasitic invertebrate animals which may cause infestations, especially of the gastrointestinal tract, usually when the eggs are swallowed.
Roundworm (Ascaris lumbricoides) may reach a length of 10–15 inches in the female, half that length in the male. The eggs hatch in the intestines and a female may produce up to 200,000 eggs a day. The larvae burrow through the intestine wall, reach the liver and lungs, and are coughed up and swallowed again. The main symptoms are colicky pains, diarrhea, swelling of the abdomen and loss of weight with hunger. Intestinal obstruction may occur as a complication. An anthelmintic (drug destructive to worms) is administered; it expels the worm in about 95 percent of cases.
Trichinella spiralis, the pork roundworm that causes *trichinosis,* may be contracted by eating uncooked or undercooked pork or bear meat. The main symptoms are fever, upset stomach, diarrhea and sore muscles. The worms may become encysted in the muscles and cause pain for years. Pork products are

inspected by governmental authorities but should be cooked thoroughly as an additional precaution.

Hookworm (*Necator americanus*) is transmitted by its larvae, which penetrate the skin of bare feet, are carried to the lungs and then coughed up, swallowed, and implanted in the duodenum (first part of the small intestine). The mature parasite attaches itself to the mucous membrane with its hooks and sucks human blood, causing a severe anemia. The main symptoms are cough, voracious appetite and anemia. The disease is prevented by wearing shoes outdoors.

Tapeworms (*Taenia saginata, solium, Diphyllobothrium latum*) are of three types: beef, pork and fish. They are transmitted by eating raw or under-cooked meat or fish. The principal symptoms are abdominal discomfort, diarrhea or constipation, and the finding of segments of the growing worm in the stools. The standard treatment is with worm-destroying drugs.

Pinworm (*Oxyuris vermicularis*) is transmitted particularly to children by unclean toilet seats and habits. The main symptom is itching around the anus. Certain anti-worm drugs are the effective treatment.

Whipworm (*Trichuris trichiura*) causes *trichuriasis* and lives primarily in the cecum and colon, causing abdominal pain, distention and flatulence, and nausea and vomiting. Repeated oral doses of certain worm-destroying drugs have been effective in some cases.

There are many other worm infestations which are prevalent in tropical countries with poor sanitary conditions. *See also* ASCARIASIS; FILARIASIS; FLAT-WORMS; FLUKE; INFECTION; PARASITES *and* **medigraphs** HOOKWORM; PINWORM; ROUNDWORM; SCHISTOSOMIASIS; TAPE-WORM; TRICHINOSIS.

WOUNDS, injuries that break the skin or other surfaces of the body. Among the most common wounds are those inflicted in battle by bullets, bayonets, or shell or shrapnel fragments. An *incised wound* is a slash or slit made by a sharp instrument such as a razor or a surgical scalpel; a *lacerated wound* is one in which the edges are torn; an *open wound* has a free external opening; a *contused wound* is made by a blunt weapon; a *penetrating wound* is one that pierces an organ or the walls of a cavity; a *punctured wound* is made by a pointed instrument.

The principal dangers of a wound are hemorrhage and infection.

Bleeding may come from a cut artery —which spurts, or from a vein—which oozes. Moderate bleeding is usually controlled by application of a gauze dressing and bandage. Severe bleeding requires direct pressure on the wound. Using a gauze pad over the wound, press with palm of hand. The victim should be kept lying down and quiet; the head lowered to prevent shock. Do not use a tourniquet unless these measures fail and you have been properly trained in its use. Serious tissue damage can result from improper use of a tourniquet.

Every wound requires immediate application of an effective antiseptic to prevent infection. Deep punctured wounds may be infected with *tetanus* spores and require active immunization with tetanus toxoid. A punctured wound by a dog bite may harbor the *rabies* virus and therefore require anti-rabies injections. *See also* FIRST AID.

WRIST, the part of the body between the lower end of the forearm and the hand. It contains eight bones arranged in two rows and forms a rounded joint with the two bones of the forearm above, and a connecting joint with the thumb and four hand bones below. The wrist is a frequent site of a sprain, due to wrenching of the joint. The pulse can be felt and counted on the outer side of the wrist in front. *See also* HAND.

WRYNECK, *torticollis,* a spasmodic turning of the head to one side due to jerky contractions of the large *sterno-cleidomastoid muscle* on the side of the neck. Often torticollis is a symptom of hysteria, along with other psychogenic (mind-induced) signs such as anxiety, blinking and facial twitches. Though seen at all ages, it most often occurs during the thirties through the sixties and runs a variable course. Excessive exposure to draft, a minor twisting injury to the neck and occasionally glandular or lymph node inflammation are other causes. It may be due also to a short sternocleidomastoid muscle, present at birth or resulting from an injury.

Rheumatic torticollis is a *myositis*— inflammation of a voluntary muscle or its covering sheath. Temporary relief is provided by antispasmodic drugs. In hysterical torticollis, there is a need for psychotherapy. Light exercises help to relax the spastic muscle. As a last resort, the nerves in the neck which stimulate the sternocleidomastoid muscle may be blocked by injections of *procaine. See also* MUSCLE.

Wryneck (Torticollis)

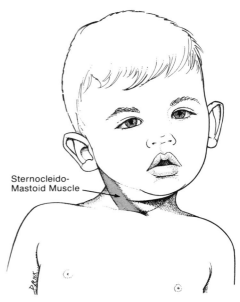

Sternocleido-
Mastoid Muscle

Wryneck—Involuntary twisting of the neck involves the sternocleidomastoid muscle, extending from behind the ear to the junction of the collarbone (clavicle) and breastbone (sternum). It may be abnormally shortened, or it may go into spasms due to hysteria, inflammation or injury.

XYZ

XANTHEMIA, *carotinemia,* presence of yellow coloring matter in the blood derived from green and yellow vegetables such as carrots, sweet potatoes, yellow corn, and string beans. *Carotene* is converted to *vitamin A* in the liver. *See also* CAROTENE.

XANTHOMA, a benign flat yellow tumor, containing a deposit of a fatty substance, commonly located on the inner side of the lower eyelid. Multiple xanthomata may be located in the skin of other parts of the body. When they are disfiguring, the tumors may be removed and do not recur in the same location. *See also* TUMOR.

XENOPHOBIA, a morbid fear of strangers or foreigners. *See also* PHOBIAS.

XERODERMA PIGMENTOSUM, a rare and fatal skin disease beginning in childhood, characterized by brown spots, ulcers, and dilated clumps of blood capillaries. *See also* FISH-SKIN DISEASE.

XEROMAMMOGRAPHY (also *Xerography*), a diagnostic technique for the location of breast tumors. An alternative image to the more conventional mammogram is produced by the x-ray machine displayed on a xerox selenium plate, and subsequently transferred to a special paper instead of film. Specialists are finding a xerogram of the breast more detailed and easier to read than an x-ray picture. *See also* **medigraph** BREAST CANCER.

XEROPHTHALMIA, *xeroma,* dryness and thickening of the *conjunctiva* (eye membrane) due to deficiency of vitamin A, accompanied by night blindness and lack of tears. The treatment is large amounts of vitamin A given daily under medical supervision. *See also* EYE; VITAMIN DEFICIENCIES *and* **medigraph** VITAMIN A DEFICIENCY.

XEROSIS, abnormal dryness, as of the skin or front of the eye. *See also* EYE; SKIN.

XEROSTOMIA, dryness of the mouth due to lack of saliva, usually temporary. It may be due to fever, nervous anxiety, the use of *atropine* to dilate the pupils for eye examinations, or a stone in one of the salivary gland ducts. In chronic cases caused by a stone, the mouth becomes rough and dry, with painful cracks that bleed easily. This obstruction causes pain and swelling and interferes with

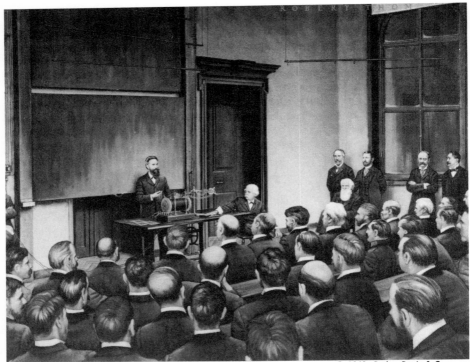

X-rays—The invisible rays that save lives were discovered in 1895 by the German physicist Wilhelm Roentgen. He is portrayed here astounding scientists at the first public demonstration of the rays. Within a year, x-rays were being used worldwide as a diagnostic tool. Later research revealed many therapeutic and industrial applications, as well as the hidden dangers, of x-rays.

eating. The stone should be removed surgically. *See also* **medigraph** HEAT STROKE.

X-RAYS, *roentgen rays,* short-wave radiation produced in a vacuum tube, similar to light but with power to penetrate beneath the skin and surface tissues. They were discovered by the German physicist Wilhelm Konrad Roentgen in 1895 and have become a very important diagnostic tool in medicine and surgery.

The diagnosis of fractures and the exact location of the fragments—as well as confirmation of the correctness of their position when set—are facilitated by taking x-ray pictures from different angles. The use of x-rays in dentistry is invaluable for showing the precise extent of decay and locating impactions, and also for determining the presence and extent of an abscess.

The size of the heart is outlined by the x-ray shadow, and spots of tuberculosis or lung cancer are clearly shown. After a *barium meal* (swallowing a barium sulfate mixture), the stomach and small intestines stand out in silhouette and x-rays will show the presence of an ulcer or cancer of the stomach or duodenum. A *barium enema* is used to diagnose the condition of the colon and rectum.

Special dyes which are opaque to x-rays are used for the diagnosis of gallstones, disorders of the uterus and vagina and of the bladder and ureters, and the location of brain and spinal cord tumors. A combination of iodine and poppyseed oil provides a good contrast medium, and radioactive minerals and isotopes have special valuable uses. A new x-ray diagnostic technique reported in 1974, known as *computerized tomography* (CT), shows more and earlier tumors than conventional brain scans. It was claimed to be the first method to distinguish tumors from normal tissue and one type of tumor from others.

X-rays as well as radium are useful in delaying the progress and extension of cancer and other malignant diseases and are used extensively in the treatment of many different conditions.

Excessive exposure to x-rays damages the various tissues of the body, especially the sexual organs. Early radiologists often allowed the rays to pass through

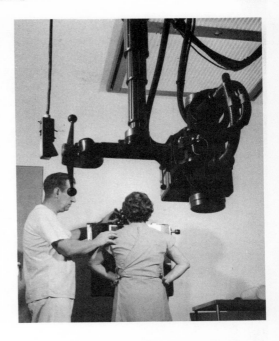

X-rays—The remarkable rays discovered by Roentgen penetrate skin and surface tissue to show the body skeleton and inner organs. The heavily shaded area in this x-ray of a child's chest (*below*) indicates disease within the lung.

X-rays—A technician positions a woman (*above*) for x-rays of her chest. X-ray pictures of that area detect diseases of the heart and aorta, as well as lung conditions such as tuberculosis, cancer, edema or abscess.

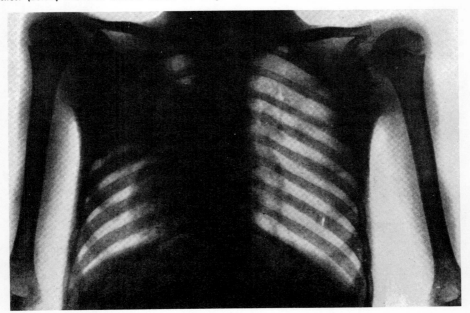

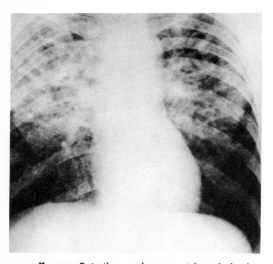

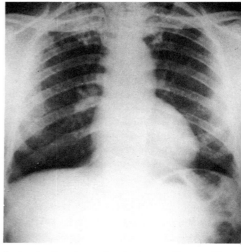

X-rays—Detecting pulmonary tuberculosis has long been one of the best-known areas of x-ray diagnosis. The closeup x-ray picture (*left*) shows extensive tuberculous infection in both lungs.

During treatment, regular chest x-ray films enable physicians to follow the course of the tuberculosis. The lungs at the right are responding to drug therapy and beginning to clear.

X-rays—A mobile unit takes free chest x-rays on a New York City street, a service that is available at most municipal health departments. Early TB diagnosis in this easy way means more certain recovery and greater protection for the uninfected.

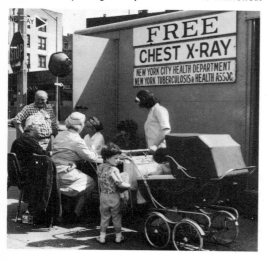

their own hands and arms, unaware of the danger. The tragic development of skin cancers in those areas prompted research which revealed the lethal hazards of x-rays. For this reason, operators wear protective devices and often work from a separate compartment. The United States Environmental Protection Agency reports that high dosage x-ray operation may contaminate the atmosphere dangerously. Mobile x-ray units have been used to take routine chest films of schoolchildren and the public for early diagnosis of tuberculosis. *See also* ANGIOGRAPHY; BARIUM SULFATE; FLUOROSCOPE; IRRADIATION; LYMPHOGRAPHY; MEDICAL INSTRUMENTATION; NUCLEAR MEDICINE; RADIATION INJURIES; RADIATION SICKNESS; RADIATION THERAPY; RADIOACTIVITY; RADIOGRAPHY.

YAWNING, a deep inhalation of air through the wide-open mouth, often as an involuntary sign of fatigue or boredom, but it can also be a symptom of certain diseases such as *encephalitis*.

YAWS, a spirochetal disease closely related to syphilis, prevalent in the West Indies and other tropical countries. It is caused by the *Treponema pertenue,* related to the *Treponema pallidum* of syphilis, and transmitted by close personal contact. The characteristic signs are raspberry-colored growths on various parts of the body, especially the face, feet, hands, legs and genital organs. The growths join to form large masses and ulcerate. After several years from the date of infection, skin eruptions similar to those of syphilis and deep growths like *gummas* (syphilitic tumors) develop. The Wassermann test for syphilis is usually positive. It is, however, classified as a nonvenereal disease. As for syphilis, antibiotics are used in the treatment of yaws. *See also* INFECTIOUS DISEASES.

YEAST, the cells of yeast fungi, used for leavening bread and producing alcoholic fermentation. Dried brewer's yeast, a byproduct of brewing, is in compressed form with a starchy or absorbent base available in tablets for medicinal use. Brewer's yeast is rich in the vitamin B-complex, including vitamins B_1, B_2, B_6, niacin and pantothenic acid. It is often fortified with other B-complex vitamins. Some nonmedicinal yeasts, other than brewer's yeast, are toxic.

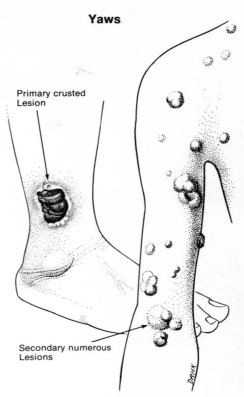

Yaws

Primary crusted Lesion

Secondary numerous Lesions

Yaws—These raised sores are the most frequent eruptions of yaws. It is a highly contagious disease, common in tropical areas where living conditions are primitive. A parasitic microorganism which usually enters the body through broken skin is the infecting agent. Without early antibiotic treatment, the ulcerating lesions of yaws can destroy tissue and deform bones and joints.

YELLOW FEVER

YELLOW FEVER—ALSO CALLED *yellow jack*—is an acute disease of the tropics of South America and Central Africa. During the late eighteenth century, the United States was swept by many epidemics. The last one of major proportions occurred in Philadelphia in 1793. The disease was brought in by ship from the West Indies and was fatal to 5000 of those afflicted with it.

causes

Yellow fever is caused by a virus transmitted into the bloodstream of the human victim by the bite of a mosquito which has previously bitten a person already infected. The time of transmission from one human to another takes about 12 days, since this is the period necessary for the incubation of the virus within the mosquito. In most cases, the insect vector

Yellow Fever

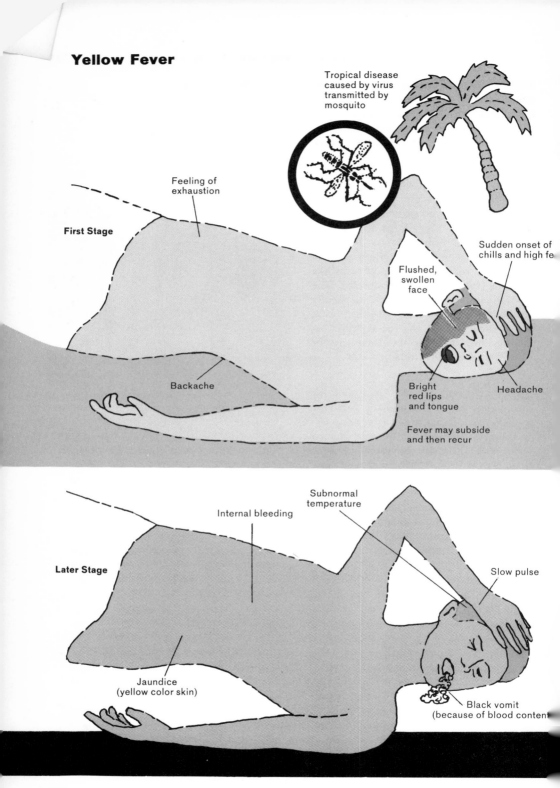

Tropical disease caused by virus transmitted by mosquito

First Stage

Feeling of exhaustion

Backache

Flushed, swollen face

Sudden onset of chills and high fe[ver]

Bright red lips and tongue

Headache

Fever may subside and then recur

Later Stage

Internal bleeding

Subnormal temperature

Slow pulse

Jaundice (yellow color skin)

Black vomit (because of blood conten[t]

is *Aedes aegypti.* Other types of mosquitoes found in the jungle forests of Brazil and parts of Africa can also transmit the disease, both to forest workers and to tree monkeys who become additional reservoirs for human infection.

symptoms
The disease is called "yellow" fever since it interferes with liver functioning and causes jaundice, the condition in which excess bile pigment is released into the blood. At the onset—which is sudden and acute—the victim suffers prostration caused by high fever, severe headache and crippling muscle pains. Pulse drops, and in addition to the yellowing of the skin, urine darkens, bleeding occurs in the mucous membranes and blood is apparent in the vomit.

complications
Yellow fever in and of itself is almost never fatal. In about 5 percent of all cases, death is caused by failure of the liver, kidneys, or heart.

treatment
There is no treatment for yellow fever other than bed rest and alleviation of symptoms by painkillers, sedatives and aspirin to control the victim's temperature. Medical supervision of diet can speed convalescence.

prevention
Anyone planning to visit a part of the world where yellow fever is endemic must be vaccinated against it. One injection of the vaccine provides immunity beginning seven days following inoculation and lasting for about six years. Control of the disease is based on the efforts of the World Health Organization and of government public health authorities to wipe out the mosquitoes that spread it. Customs authorities in those countries where the disease is nonexistent usually have quarantine regulations on monkeys

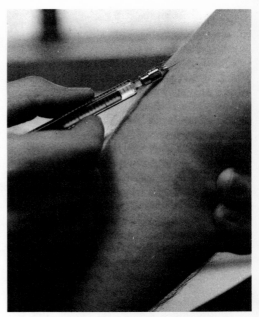

Yellow Fever—A vaccine is being administered against this acute tropical disease that is spread by mosquitoes. Several years' immunity is gained from one inoculation.

and marmosets that come from yellow fever territory and may therefore be sources of human infection.

YELLOW JAUNDICE. *See* JAUNDICE.

YOGA, a Hindu discipline recommending consciousness training in the form of directing attention exclusively to an object, abstract or concrete, for the purpose of identification with the object. Various postural and controlled physical exercises, such as control of breathing and other physiological functions, are included in the practice. Complete control of one's own body is the basic idea of yoga, which has many followers in the United States and Europe as well as in India.

YOGURT, semisolid milk fermented and acidified by addition of lactic acid bacilli.

The Russian biologist Elie Metchnikoff (1845–1916) theorized in 1906 that lactic acid bacilli counteract the harmful putrefactive (causing decomposition) bacteria in the intestines and thereby prolong life. Yogurt is often recommended in cases of intestinal sluggishness and to replace the lactic acid bacteria when they are destroyed by administration of certain antibiotics. *See also* MILK.

YOLK SAC, in embryology, a spherical membranous sac attached to the embryo and containing food yolk for its nutrition.

ZINC, a bluish-white lustrous metal, many salts of which are used in medicine, including the bacitracin, chloride, oxide, peroxide, stearate, sulfate and undecylenate. Some of them are ingredients of ointments and dusting powders. *Zinc phosphide* is a toxic rat poison. *See also* METALLIC POISONS.

ZOONOSIS, an animal disease such as rabies or malaria that is communicable to man.

ZOOPHOBIA, an irrational fear of animals. *See also* PHOBIAS.

ZYGOMA, the arch formed by the union of the *zygomatic process* of the temporal bone of the skull, the *upper jawbone,* and the *zygomatic* (cheek) *bone.* A high zygomatic arch is characteristic of Orientals and American Indians. *See also* SKULL.

ZYGOTE, the fertilized ovum produced by the union of the female egg and the male spermatozoon, before its cell division. *See also* REPRODUCTIVE SYSTEM.

ZYME, an organized ferment or a harmful agent that develops an infectious disease by promoting the growth of bacteria.

INDEX

Bold face numbers indicate major point of reference.

INDEX

INDEX

INDEX

INDEX

dumping syndrome, 505
 in peptic ulcer, 1147
duodenal ulcer, 1438-1440
duodenum, 505-506
 and bile, 206-207
 in the bowel, 252
 peptic ulcer of, 1146-1147
Dupuytren's contracture, 390-391, 506
dura mater, 506
 brain, 253
dust, 506-507
 in conjunctivitis, 385-387
 and emphysema, 531
 and hay fever, 714
dusting powders, 198
dwarfs, 507-508
 achondroplasia, 31
dyschezia, 387
dyscratic autointoxication, 174
dysentery, 508
dysmenorrhea, 508
dyspareunia, 508-509
 and frigidity, 654
dyspepsia, 819-820
dysphagia, 137, 509
dysplasia, 509
dyspnea, 509
dystrophy, 509
dysuria, 509

E

ear, 510-514
 in aero otitis media, 63
 in deafness, 422-428
 and decibels, 429
 fenestration of, 604-605
 and foreign bodies, 650
 keratosis obturans of, 875
 lop ear surgery, 922
 otosclerosis of, 1113
 otoscope examination, 1113
 perforated eardrum, 1147
 ringing in, see ringing in the ears
 specialization, 1113
 stapes operation, 1350
 stuffiness, 514-515
 tympanic membrane of, 1432
 tympanoplasty of, 1432
ear infection, 953, 1113
ear pressure, 290
earwax, 515
Eastern spotted fever, 1275
eating habits
 appetite, 145
 tachyphagia, 1381
Eberth, Carl J., 180
ecchymosis, 515
ECG, 515-516
 see also electrocardiogram
echolalia, 516
eclampsia, 516-517
 convulsion in, 391-392
 jaundice in, 865
ecthyma, 518
ectoderm, 1198
ectomorph, 1001
ectopic pregnancy, 518-520
 and abortion, 22
eczema, 520
 Kaposi's varicelliform eruption in, 547
edema, 521
 in ascites, 160
 in beriberi, 203-205
 in congestive heart failure, 385
 in coronary thrombosis, 397
 and diuretics, 486-487
 fluid retention, 642-643
 in glomerulonephritis, 694
 in heart failure, 733
 in kala-azar, 873
 in kwashiorkor, 893
 in nephritis, 1038
 in nephrosis, 1040
 in pericarditis, 1149

EEG, 521
 see also electroencephalogram
effort syndrome, 1050-1051
eggs in the diet, 521-522
ego, 522
ejaculation, 522
ejaculatory ducts, 522
 in prostatism, 1209
ejaculatory system, 522
EKG, see electrocardiogram
elbow, 522-524
electric shock
 asphyxia, 162-163
 in electrical injuries, 524
 treatment, 525
electrocardiogram, 515-516
 in computerized medicine, 380
 in coronary thrombosis, 396-397
 in heart murmur diagnosis, 735
 in heart trouble symptoms, 749
electrocardiograph, 525
electrocoagulation
 diathermy, 470
 in electrolysis, 526
electroencephalogram, 521
 in computerized medicine, 380
electroencephalograph, 525-526
electrolysis, 526
 as a depilatory, 445
electrolytes, 526
electromyography, 1016
electronic medical aid, 526-527
electroshock therapy, 525
elephantiasis, 527
 filiariasis, 612-614
elixir, 527
Ellsworth-Howard test, 1211-1212
emaciation, 527
 in sprue, 1349
embolism, 527-528
 in apoplexy, 139
 in phlebitis, 1162
embryo, 528
emergencies, medical, 615-636
emetic, 529-530
 alum, 92
 mustard as, 1018
emission, 530
emollient, 530
 castor oil as, 315-316
emotion, 530
 anxiety, 135-136
 and impotence, 818-819
 and indigestion, 820
emotional disturbances, 530-531
 and bed wetting, 198-199
 behavior, 199-200
 in chorea, 359
 compulsion, 380
 and dyspareunia, 508
 and dysphagia, 509
 and exhaustion, 557-558
 in middle age change, 991
 neurosis, 1053-1054
 in premenstrual tension, 1197
emphysema, 531-533
 and asthma, 164
 in bronchiectasis, 272
 in bronchitis, 275
 and the death rate, 429
 and dust, 506-507
 and mortality, 1001
 in pneumoconiosis, 1178
 pulmonary heart disease in, 1218
 in silicosis, 1310
empyema, 533
 from lung abscess, 926
emulsion, 533
enamel, 533
 and dental caries, 436-437
encephalitis, 534-535
 from carbuncles, 310-312
 delirium in, 433
 from folliculitis, 310-312
 from furuncles, 310-312
 from mumps, 1006-1008
 narcolepsy in, 1035
encephalogram, 535
encephalomyelitis, 535-536

encopresis, 536
encounter groups, 536
endarteritis, 536
endemic, 536
endocarditis, 536
endocarditis, subacute bacterial, 536-538
endocardium, 538
endocrine glands, 538-539, 690
endogenous, 539
endometrial cancer, 300-303
endometriosis
 hormone therapy for, 785
endometritis, 539-540
endometrium, 539-540
endomorph, 1001
endotoxin, 180
enema, 540
enophthalmia, 541
enteric fever, 541
 paratyphoid, 1137
 typhoid, 1432
enteritis, 541
enterocele, 541
enteroptosis, 541
entoderm, 1198
enuresis, 198-199
environment
 and birth defects, 218-219
 and emphysema, 531-533
 and mental health, 974
 and weight, 1474
environmental health, 1218
enzyme, 541-542
 amylase, 101
 and fermentation, 605
eosinophilia, 542, 235-236
ephedrine, 542
 for asthma, 164
 in decongestants, 429
epidemic, 542
 and immunization, 814-815
epidemic pleurodynia, 454, 456
epidemiology, 542
epidermis, 1321
epidermolysis bullosa, 542
epididymis, 542-543
 and accessory sex organs, 24
 and ejaculatory system, 522
epididymitis, 543
epiglottis, 543-544
epilepsy, 544-546
 and Dilantin, 482
 in cerebral palsy, 326
 first aid for, 627
epinephrine, 546
 and blood pressure control, 239
 for burn shock, 280
 for cardiac arrest, 313
 vasoconstrictor, 1459
episiotomy, 343, 546
epispadias, 1146
epistaxis, 1062
epithelial tissue, 546
epithelioma, 546
 in bladder tumor, 231
Epsom salts, 546-547
 for blepharitis, 233
epulis, 547
equilibrium, 547
 in airsickness, 75-76
 and the auditory nerve, 171
 and the cerebellum 326
 and the ear, 510-514
equine encephalomyelitis, 535
Erb's paralysis, 253
erection, 1250
ergot, 547
ergotamine, 547
ergotism, 547
 gangrene in, 667
errors of metabolism, inborn, see metabolism, inborn errors
errors of refraction, see refraction, errors of
eruption, 547
erysipelas, 547
 and tattoo, 1384
erythema, 547-548

1503

INDEX

erythremia, 548
erythroblastosis foetalis, 548
erythrocytes, 235, 548
see also red blood cells
erythromelalgia, 548
erythromycin, 127
erythropoietin, 878
Escherichia coli
 in bacteremia, 179
 in cystitis, 230
esophagoscope, 549, 551
esophagus, **548-549**
 in cardiospasm, 313-314
 in digestion, 477-478
 diseases of, 549-551
 diverticulum of, 487
 foreign bodies in, 650
 in hiatus hernia, 768-770
 in scleroderma, 1291
ESP, 559
essential amino acids, 97
estrogens, **551**
 in birth control, 212-213
 and breast cancer, 262
 in cosmetics, 400
 and menstruation, 974
 in menopause, 970-972
 and uterine cancer, 300
ether, **552**
 and anesthesias, 108
 in asphyxiation, 163
ethmoid bone, 402
ethology, 552
ethylene, 109
ethylenediamine, 97
etiology, 552
eucalyptus oil, 552
eugenics, 552
eunuch, 552
 and castration, 316
eunuchoidism, 552
euphoria, 552
 in paresis, 1137-1138
European relapsing fever, 197
Eustachian tube, **552**
 in aero otitis media, 63
 in deafness, 422
 and the ear, 510, 512
 in ear stuffiness, 514-515
 and nasopharynx, 1035
 and the nose, 1060
euthanasia, 553
eutrophication, 553
Ewing's sarcoma, 553
exacerbation, 553
exanthem, 553
excess hair, **553-554**, 708
 and feminine hygiene, 602
 hypertrichosis, 797-798
exchange transfusion, 246
excision, 554
excoriations, 554
excretion, **554**
 feces, 595
 perspiration, 1157
 urine, 1449
exercise, **554-557**
 and ache, 30
 conditioning, 382
 and fibromyositis, 610-611
 for fibrositis, 612
 isometrics, 862-863
 after mastectomy, 950
 in postnatal care, 1186
 postural drainage, 1187
exfoliation, 557
exfoliative dermatitis, 388
exhalation, **557**
 in breathing, 267
 and carbon dioxide, 309
exhaustion, 557-558
exhibitionism, 558
exocrine glands, 689-690
exophthalmic goiter, **558**, 697-698
 basal metabolism in, 194-195
 heartbeat in, 726, 729
exophthalmos, 558-559
expectorant, **559**
 in bronchial asthma, 271

expectoration, 559
extended care facility, 1068-1075
extrasensory perception, 559
extrovert, 559
exudation, 559
eye, **559-582**
 adaptation of, 43-44
 aqueous humor of, 146
 astigmatism, 165-166
 bank, 579-580
 in Bell's palsy, 202
 care, 580-581
 cataracts of, 316-318
 cornea of, 392-393
 and corneal transplantation, 393
 in exophthalmos, 558
 foreign bodies in, 650
 habit spasm of, 706
 and headache, 719
 in high blood pressure, 772
 injuries, 583
 lens of, 902
 macula of, 938
 photosensitivity of, 1163
 protrusion of, 558-559
 pupil of, 1221
 in sandfly fever, 1283
 specialist, 1091
 spots before, 1347
 in vitamin A deficiency, 1464
 vitreous floaters in, 1468
eye disorders
 amblyopia, 94
 asthenopia, 164
 blepharitis, 232
 conjunctivitis, 385
 in cystic fibrosis, 417
 enophthalmia, 541
 glaucoma, 691
 glioma, 694
 iritis, 858
 ophthalmia, 1091
 paralysis, 1091-1092
 retinitis, 1258
 retinitis pigmentosa, 1258
 retinoblastoma, 1259
 retrolental fibroplasia, 1259
 trachoma, 1419
 ultraviolet keratitis, 1441
 uveitis, 1451
 xerophthalmia, 1485
 see also vision impairment
eyeglasses, 581-583
 bifocals, 206
 contact lenses, 390
eyelash, 362
 in conjunctivitis, 385-387
 hair of, 707
 in trichiasis, 1424
eyelids, **583-584**
 in Chagas' disease, 334
 hordeolum of, 785
 in myasthenia gravis, 1019
 in ragweed dermatitis, 1236
 sty on, 1369
 in trichinosis, 1424
 xanthoma of, 1485
eyestrain, **574-575**
 and eye care, 580-581

F

face, **585-586**
 cranial nerve of, 402
 paralysis in Bell's palsy, 200
 plastic surgery on, 1175
 Wells' facies, 1476
facial neuralgia, 1410
facial paralysis, 200
fainting, **586-587**
 in bradycardia, 253
 in polycythemia, 1185
fallen arches, 587-588
Fallopian tubes, **588-589**
 in conception, 380
 ectopic pregnancy in, 518-520
 in gonorrhea, 700
 and salpingitis, 1283

Fall's test, 1191
false pregnancy, 589
Fanconi syndrome, 138
farmer's lung, 507
farsightedness, **589**
 and astigmatism, 166
 presbyopia, 1199
fasciectomy, 506
fasting, 589-590
fat, **590-591**
fatigue, **591**
 in amphetamine withdrawal, 101
 in beriberi, 203-205
 furuncles from, 660
 headache from, 719
fats
 in digestion, 477-478
 in the liver, 916-917
 in nutrition, 1076
 unsaturated, 591-593
fats, saturated
 in arteriosclerosis, 151
 in atherosclerosis, 168
 and cholesterol, 358, 592
 and low-cholesterol diet, 475
fauces, 593
favus, 593
fear, **593-595**
febrile, 595
fecal incontinence, 536
feces, **595**
 impaction of, 816
feeblemindedness, 980-982
feet, **595-599**
 in arctic health, 148-149
 care in diabetes, 463
 podiatry, 1180
 see also foot disorders
fellatio, 782
felon, 599
female sex hormones, 599-600
feminine hygiene, 600-604
femoral
 arteries, 151
 vein, 1404
fenestration, 604-605
fermentation, 605
fertile period, 380
fertility, 605
fetus, **605**
 and bag of waters, 183
 in childbirth, 341-344
 and chorion, 359
 in ectopic pregnancy, 518
 impaction of, 816
 in prenatal development, 1198
fever, **605-607**
 blackwater, 229
 blisters, 374-376
 and breathing, 267
 in child care, 345
 and chill, 353
 dehydration in, 433
 and delirium, 433
 dengue, 435
 furuncles from, 660
 in heat stroke, 750
 ice bag for, 808
 in infection, 828
 in leukemia, 904
 in lung abscess, 926
 in lung cancer, 928
 in malaria, 940
 Q fever, 1224
 rat-bite, 1237
 relapsing, 1244
 rheumatic, 1260
 Rocky Mountain spotted, 1275
 in roseola infantum, 1278
 sandfly, 1283
 scarlet, 1284
 scrub typhus, 1292
 trench, 1422
 tularemia, 1430
 typhoid, 1432
 typhus, 1434
 undulant, 1444
 of unknown origin, 1221
 yellow, 1489

1504

INDEX

germicide, **688**
  and disinfection, 486
germs, 688
gerontology, 66-71
gestalt groups, 688
gestation, 688
giantism, 35
Gilchrist's disease, 232
gingivitis, 688-689
GI series, 551
glanders, 689
glands, **689-690**
  adrenal, 58
  apocrine, 139
  Bartholin's, 194
  Cowper's, 401
  endocrine, 538
  lacrimal, 894
  liver, 916
  ovaries, 1115
  pancreas, 1128
  parathyroid, 1136
  pineal, 1167
  pituitary, 1170
  prostate, 1206
  thymus, 1406
  thyroid, 1406
glandular fever, 691
  see also mononucleosis, infectious
glans, 1146
glassblower's cataract, 691
glass eyes, 691
glaucoma, **691-693**
  as a birth defect, 214, 219
  in genetic counseling, 679
  iridectomy for, 858
  night blindness in, 1055
gleet, 693-694
glioma, **694**, 989
globulin, 1210
globus hystericus, 806
glomerulonephritis, **694**, 1038
  in impetigo, 818
  in polyarteritis nodosa, 1183
glomerulus, 694
glossitis, 694
glossopathy, 694
glossopharyngeal nerve, 402
  and taste, 1382
glossopharyngeal neuralgia, 694
glottis, **695**
  and epiglottis, 543-544
  in hiccups, 770
glucagon, 695
glucocorticoids, 59
glucose, **695**
  and diabetes, 456-464
  for jaundice, 865-866
  in the liver, 916-918
glucose tolerance test, 464-465, 695
glues, sniffing of, 695-967
gluteal muscles, 288
gluten, 324-325
glycerin, 697
  as an emollient, 530
glycogen, 697
  in exercise, 556
  and the liver, 917-918
glycosuria, 697
goat fever, 1444
goat's milk, 994-995
goiter, 697-698
gold, 698
gonads, 1250-1255
gonococcus
  in bacteremia, 179
  in gonorrhea, 698-700
gonorrhea, **698-700**
  birth defects from, 220
  chronic cystitis from, 230
  bubo in, 277
  cervicitis from, 333
  chordee from, 359
  and Fallopian tubes, 588
  gleet, 693
  ovarian infection from, 1113
  premarital checkup for, 1191

gonorrheal epididymitis, 543
gout, **700-703**
  and arteriosclerosis, 151
  as a birth defect, 222
  and bursitis, 286-288
  colchicine for, 373
  low-purine diet for, 476-477
  meat intake in, 957
grafting, 703
Gram-negative bacteria, 180
Gram-positive bacteria, 180
grand mal, **703**, 544
granulation, 703
granulocyte, 235
granulocytopenia, 72-73
granuloma annulare, 703
granuloma inguinale, 703
granulopenia, 72
Graves' disease, 796
gravity, 704
gray matter, 253, 254
green sickness, 355
greenstick fracture, 651
grinder's rot, 1310
gristle, 314
groin, 704
ground itch, 783-785
group therapy, 704
growing pains, 704
growth
  in adolescence, 53
  hormone, 753
growth retardation, **704**
  achondroplasia, 31
  in celiac disease, 324
  dwarfs, 507
  from goiter, 697
  in Hand's disease, 711
  in hookworm infestation, 783
  in kwashiorkor, 893
guilt, 595
gullet, 548-549
gumma, 704
gums, **704-705**
  epulis on, 547
  gingivitis of, 688-689
  pyorrhea of, 1223
  in trench mouth, 1422
Guterman test, 1191
gynecologic examination, 705
gynecologist, **705**, 489
  and douche, 492
  and ovarian infection, 1115
gynecomastia, 705

H

habits, **706**
  head banging, 719-720
  and longevity, 921-922
  nail-biting, 1033
  thumb-sucking, 1405
Haemophilus influenzae, 968
hair, **707-708**
  care of, 708-709
  in trichotillomania, 1427
hair follicles, **645**
  in baldness, 183-190
  in electrolysis, 526
  in folliculitis, 310-312, 645
hair loss
  alopecia, 91
  baldness, 183-190
  in exfoliative dermatitis, 388
hair removal, 445, 526
Hale, Stephen, 238-239
halitosis, **709-710**
  and dentifrices, 442
hallucination, **710**
  in amphetamine abuse, 99
  aura, 171
  in barbiturate poisoning, 194
  in deadly nightshade poisoning, 420
  in delirium, 433
  in glue sniffing, 695
  in LSD abuse, 924-926
  in paranoia, 1135

hallucinogenic drug, 488
  LSD abuse, 924-926
  mescaline, 987
halothane, 109
hammertoe, 710
hand, 710-711
  abnormality, 506
  skill, 945
Hand's disease, 711
hangnail, 711
hangover, 711
Hansen's disease, 711-713
hardening of the arteries
  arteriosclerosis, 151
  atherosclerosis, 167
  and cholesterol, 358
  claudication in, 366
  congestive heart failure from, 385
  coronary thrombosis from, 394
  insomnia in, 847
  ischemia in, 861
  and mortality, 1001
  night cramps in, 1055
  peripheral arteriosclerosis, 1152
  and pulseless disease, 1221
harelip, **713**
  as a birth defect, 214, 222, 223
  and cleft palate, 367
  in genetic counseling, 674, 681
harvest mite, 341
hashish, **713**
  and marijuana, 947
Haverhill fever, 1237
Haversian canals, 1319
hay fever, **714-716**
  in children, 90-91
  and climate, 368
  and decongestants, 429
  in food allergy, 647
  and histamine, 774
head, **718**
  growth of in children, 347
  lice, 912-914
head abnormality
  brachycephaly, 253
  in cretinism, 403-405
  hydrocephalus, 788
  microcephaly, 990
  in myxedema, 403-405
headache, **718-719**
  in acidosis, 32
  and acupuncture, 43
  in apoplexy, 139
  in astigmatism, 166
  and brain tumor, 258
  and glioma, 694
  in hangover, 711
  in heat exhaustion, 749
  in hypoglycemia, 800
  migraine, see migraine headache
  in whiplash injury, 1476
head banging, **719-720**
  in autism, 173
head injuries, **720-722**
  and convulsion, 391-392
  and deafness, 422
  first aid for, 628
health
  and appetite, 145
  care of, 722
  foods, 722
  neurosis, 799-800
hearing, 722
  aids, 427, **722-723**
  hardness of, see deafness
  tests, 723, 1275
hearing impairment
  in cerebral palsy, 326-328
  deaf mutism, 421
  deafness, 422
  earwax, 515
  in head injuries, 722
  and intelligence, 851
  in otosclerosis, 1113
  paracusis, 1134
  from perforated eardrum, 1147
  in poisoning, 309, 985
  presbycusis, 1199

INDEX

kidney stones, **889-891**
 calculus, 291
 colic in, 376
 in hyperparathyroidism, 792
kinesiology, 1010-1011
kissing disease, 998-999
Klebs, Edwin, 180
Klebsiella pneumoniae, 275-276
kleptomania, 891
Klinefelter's syndrome, 891
knee, 891-892
kneecap, 1141
knee jerk, 893
 in tabes dorsalis, 1381
knock-knee, 893
knockout drops, 354
Koch, Robert, 180
Koller, Karl, 108
Koplik's spots, 956
Korsakoff's psychosis, 79, 965
Kupffer cells, 919
Kussmaul-Maier disease, 1183
kwashiorkor, **893**, 963
kymograph, 241
kyphosis, 893

L

labia, 894
labor, **341-344**
 induction of, 821
laboratory tests, 1395-1398
labyrinthine disease, 513
labyrinthitis, 966-967
laceration, **894**
 in head injuries, 722
lacrimal glands, **894**
 and the eyes, 565
lacrimal sac, 419
lactation, 895
lacteals, 935
lactic acid, 31
 and dental caries, 435-437
lameness, 366
laminectomy, 895
 for slipped disc, 1326
Landry's acute ascending paralysis, 1225
Landsteiner's classification, 242
Langerhans, Paul, 861
lanolin, 504-505
laparoscopy, 895, 1354
large intestine, 855
 cecum, 324
 colon, 378
 in dysentery, 508
laryngeal spasm, 355
laryngectomy, 505
laryngismus stridulus, 407
laryngitis, 895
laryngoscope, 895
larynx, **895-896**
 bruises of, 277
 and croup, 407
 in myasthenia gravis, 1019
 in sicca syndrome, 1305
 in stuttering, 1367
laser, 896
lateral sclerosis, 896-897
laudanum, 897
laughing gas, 1057
laughter, 897
laxatives, **897-898**
 cascara sagrada, 315
 cathartics, 323
 magnesium citrate, 938
 in medicine chest, 961
 milk of magnesia, 995
 mineral oil, 995
lazy eye, **898**
 amblyopia, 94
L-dopa
 for cerebral palsy, 328
 for Parkinson's disease, 1140
lead poisoning, **898-900**
 hemolytic anemia in, 105-106
 and industrial health, 822
 neuritis in, 1048

learning disability, **900,** 995
lecithin, 900
left-handedness, 900
leg, 900-901
 ulcers of, 901
leg cramps
 in atherosclerosis, 168
 claudication, 366
 night cramps, 1055
 in peripheral arteriosclerosis, 1152
leishmaniasis, **902,** 1100
lens, **902**
 cataracts on, 316-322
 in presbyopia, 1199
leprosy, 711-713
leptospirosis, 902-904
 jaundice in, 865
lesbianism, 904
lesion, 904
leukemia, **238, 904-909**
 gingivitis from, 688
 purpura in, 1222
 from radiation injuries, 1230
 radium treatment for, 1236
leukocytes, **909**
leukocytosis, 235, 911
leukopenia, 235, 909, 911
leukoplakia, 910-911
leukorrhea, **911**
leukotomy, 911
libido, 911
lice, **912-914**
 and relapsing fever, 1244
 and trench fever, 1422
lichen planus, 914
lichen simplex, 914
ligaments, **914**
 in dislocation, 486
 and joints, 868
 and posture, 1189
ligation, 914
lightning injuries, 524
light reactions, 915
light sensitivity, 1163
limping, 915
 intermittent, 366
liniment, 915
lipase, 207, 478
lipids, 915
 in serum, 1298
 in Tay-Sachs disease, 1384
lipoic acid, 915
lipoma, 915
liposarcoma, 1283
lipotropic, 900
lips, 915-916
liquid petrolatum, 995
lisp, 1334
listlessness, 985
Lister, Joseph, 133, 833
lithium, 916
lithotomy, 916
livedo reticularis, 916
liver, **916-919**
 and alcohol, 78
 in Chagas' disease, 334-335
 cirrhosis, *see* cirrhosis of the liver
 congestion of, 385
 diseases of, 919-921
 extracts, 921
 and fibrinogen deficiency, 608
 and fluke infestation, 643
 in glue sniffing, 695
 gumma of, 704
 in heat stroke, 750
 hepatitis, 760
 in histoplasmosis, 774
 in hypoglycemia, 800
 in kala-azar, 873
 and lymphosarcoma, 937
 in Niemann-Pick disease, 1054
 radiation injuries to, 1229
 rupture of, 277
 in schistosomiasis, 1286
 spots, 921
 in undulant fever, 1444
 in yellow fever, 1491

loa loa worm disease, 612-614
lobotomy, 911
local anesthesia, 108-111
lochia, 921
locked elbow, 523
lockjaw, 1398-1400
locomotor ataxia, 1381
 paraplegia in, 1135
Loeffler's syndrome, 921
loiasis, 614
longevity, 921-922
lop ears, 922
lordosis, 922
low back pain, 922
low birth weight, 826
low blood pressure, 923-924
 in Simmonds' disease, 1313
low blood sugar, 800-802
low body temperature, 803-804
low-cholesterol diet, 475-476
low-purine diet, 476-477
low-residue diet, 476
low-salt diet, 472
lozenges, 924
LSD abuse, 924-926
lumbago, **926**
 fibromyositis, 610-611
 fibrositis, 612
lumbar, 926
lumbar puncture, 1344
lump
 ganglion, 667
 Heberden's nodes, 752
 in rheumatoid arthritis, 1266
lumpy jaw, 37-38
lung cancer, **928-930**
 and the death rate, 429
 in pneumoconiosis, 1178
 from radioactive contamination, 1233
 smoking and, 1329
lungs, **930-932**
 abscess of, 926
 aerosols for, 928
 alveoli of, 93
 in atelectasis, 167
 and carbon dioxide, 309
 in chromoblastomycosis, 360
 compression of, 380
 congestion in, 385
 in congestive heart failure, 385
 diseases of, *see* pulmonary diseases
 and dust, 506
 and Ewing's sarcoma, 553
 examination of, 276
 excretion by, 554
 fluke infestation of, 643
 foreign bodies in, 650
 in glanders, 689
 in glue sniffing, 695
 in infectious mononucleosis, 998
 in scleroderma, 1291
lunula, 932
lupus erythematosus, **932-934**
 agranulocytosis in, 72
 fever in, 1221
 fibromyositis in, 610-611
 nephrosis in, 1040
lupus vulgaris, 934
lymph, 935
lymphadenoma, 778-780
lymphatic system, **935**
lymphatic vessels
 and circulatory system, 362-364
 in elephantiasis, 1178
 in filiariasis, 612-613
lymphedema, 936
lymph node inflammation
 in Asian flu, 162
 in bubo, 277
 in bubonic plague, 277
 in Chagas' disease, 334-335
 in glandular fever, 691
 in gonorrhea, 700
 in Hodgkin's disease, 778-780
 in plague, 1173
 in rat-bite fever, 1237
 in undulant fever, 1444

1510

INDEX

INDEX

spastic paralysis
  cerebral palsy, 326
  in congenital defects, 382
  hemiplegia, 754
speech, 1334
speech impairment
  aphasia, 137
  in apoplexy, 140
  in autism, 173
  in cerebral palsy, 326
  in cleft palate, 367
  in deaf mutism, 421-422
  in deafness, 427
  dumbness, 505
  in Friedreich's ataxia, 654
  in multiple sclerosis, 1006
  in myasthenia gravis, 1019
  in myxedema, 402
  in paresis, 1137
  stuttering, 1334
sperm, **1339**
  in birth control, 209-214
  in conception, 380-381
  and the scrotum, 1292
  in semen, 1297
  and spermatogenesis, 1339
  and undescended testicles, 1442
spermatic arteries, 151
spermatic cords, 1339
  varicocele of, 1454
spermatogenesis, 1339
sphenoid bone, 1316, 1325
sphincter, **1339**
  of the anus, 135
  of the bladder, 229-230
sphingolipidosis, 1054
sphygmomanometer, **1339**
  for blood pressure, 238-239
spider bites, 1339-1340
spina bifida, **1341**
  in genetic counseling, 674, 681
  plastic surgery for, 1175
spinal
  bulb, 256
  column, see spine
  curvature, 1342-1343
  disc, 485
  injuries, 1343
  manipulation, 354
  surgery, 895
  tap, 1344
spinal cord, **1341-1342**
  in broken neck, 1037
  in the nervous system, 1042-1046
  in paraplegia, 1135-1136
  in tabes dorsalis, 1381
spine, **1345**
  and backache, 177
  in broken neck, 1037-1038
  intervertebral discs of, 852
  in spina bifida, 1341
  vertebra of, 1460
spleen, 1345-1346
  in Chagas' disease, 334
  in Gaucher's disease, 671
  in infectious mononucleosis, 998
  in kala-azar, 873
  in polycythemia, 1185
  in relapsing fever, 1244
  in schistosomiasis, 1286
  in thalassemia, 1401
  in thrombocytopenia, 1404
  in undulant fever, 1444
splenectomy, 1404
splenic disease, 1346
splenomegaly, 1346
spirilla, 180
splinters, 1346
splints, 1346
split personality, 1288
split spine, 1341
spondylitis, ankylosing, 1346
spondylolisthesis, 1346
spontaneous abortion, 22
  see also miscarriage
sporotrichosis, 1346
spots before the eyes, 1347
sprains, 1348-1349
  first aid for, 632

sprays, sniffing of, 695-697
sprue, **1349-1350**
  celiac disease, 324-325
sputum, **1350**
  expectoration of, 559
  from lung abscess, 926
  postural drainage of, 1187
  after thoracentesis, 1403
squint, 1350
stammering, 1367
Stanford-Binet test, 1350
stapes, 510
  surgery, 1350
staphylococcus, **1350**
  in bacteremia, 179
  in blepharitis, 232
  in cellulitis, 326
  in food poisoning, 647
  in sty, 1369
starvation, 1350
steatorrhea, 1351
Stein-Leventhal syndrome, 1351
stenosis, 1351
sterility, 1351-1353
  in cystic fibrosis, 418
sterilization, 1353
steroids, 1354
stertor, 1354
stethoscope, 1354
  in blood pressure, 239
stiff neck
  in encephalitis, 535
  in encephalomyelitis, 535
  in poliomyelitis, 1182
  in septic sore throat, 1298
  in tetanus, 1398
  in whiplash injury, 1476
stigma, 1354
stilbestrol, 452
stillbirth, 1354, 220
stimulants, **1355**
stings, **1355**
  bee, 199
  insect bites, 845
  wasp, 1472
stomach, **1355-1356**
  and abdominal pain, 18-19
  ache, 18-19
  and alcohol, 78
  diverticulum of, 487
  foreign bodies in, 650
  gastrectomy of, 668
  and gastritis, 668
  and gastroenteritis, 670
  in gastroptosis, 671
  gastrostomy of, 671
  pylorus of, 1223
stomach cancer, 1356-1358. .
stomach ulcer, 1146-1147
stomatitis, 1358
  gingivitis, 688
  glossitis, 694
stonecutter's cough, 1310
stools, 595
strabismus, 1350
strains, 1348-1349
  first aid for, 632
strangulated hernia, 764
strangulation, 1358
strawberry marks, **1358**
  birthmark, 227
  hemangioma, 118
strep throat, **1358**
  and influenza, 642
streptococcus, **1358**
  in bacteremia, 179
  in cellulitis, 326
  in chorea, 359
  in impetigo, 816
  in ovarian infection, 1113
  in septic sore throat, 1298
  in strep throat, 1358
streptomycin, **128, 1358**
  for bronchopneumonia, 276
  and infection, 833
stress, 1359
  incontinence, 819
  testing, 1024, **1359-1364**
stretch marks, 1364

stricture, 1364
stridor, 1364
stroke, **1364-1366**
  in hypertensive heart disease, 794
  oxygen therapy for, 1118
strontium-90, 1229-1230
strychnine, 1367
  in rat control, 1237
stupor, 1367
stuttering, 1367
sty, 1368-1369
  hordeolum, 785
styptic, 1369
subconscious, 1369
sublingual gland, 689, 1282
submaxillary gland, 689, 1282
submucous resection, 454
sudden infant death syndrome, 1369
  and congenital heart disease, 384
suffocation, 162
suicide, **1371**
  and depression, 447
  and mortality, 1001
suicidal impulse, 944
sulfa drugs, 1372
sulfonamide drugs, **1372**
  and cyanosis, 414
  and uremia, 1444
sulfur dioxide, 1372
sulfuric acid, 31
  chemical burns, 336-337
sunbathing and cancer, 304
sunburn, 1372
sunglasses, 1373
sunstroke, 750-752
superior vena cava, 1459
suppository, 1373
suppression, 1373
suppuration, 1373
suppurative labyrinthitis, 967
suppressive cure, 131-132
suprarenal capsules, 690
  see also adrenal gland
surgeon, 489-490
surgery, **1373-1375**
  and acupuncture, 38-43
  in angina pectoris, 117
  for birth defects, 223
  for breast cancer, 262, 304, 948
  for cataracts, 318
  for deafness, 422
  dental, 442
  for dislocation, 653
  hypothermia in, 803
  for inguinal hernia, 841
  and older people, 1375
  oral, 443
  orthopedic, 1106-1107
  oscilloscope in, 1107
  and patchy baldness, 184
  plastic, see plastic surgery
  shock during, 1304
surgical procedures
  appendectomy, 141
  circumcision, 364
  corneal transplantation, 393
  coronary by-pass, 397
  cryosurgery, 407
  diathermy, 470
  dilatation and curettage, 483
  fasciectomy, 506
  gastrostomy, 671
  hysterectomy, 806
  ileostomy, 810
  iridectomy, 858
  laminectomy, 895
  mastectomy, 948
  nephrectomy, 1038
  nephrostomy, 1041
  nephrotomy, 1041
  oophorectomy, 1091
  psychosurgery, 1217
  resection, 1255
  stapes operation, 1350
  thoracoplasty, 1403
  tubal ligation, 1428
  tympanoplasty, 1432
  vasectomy, 1459

1520

INDEX

suture, 1375
swab, 1375
swallowing, 1375
swallowing impairment
aphagia, 137
in Bell's palsy, 202
in botulism, 251
in cleft palate, 367
in deadly nightshade poisoning, 420
in dermatomyositis, 448
dysphagia, 509
in mumps, 1006
in myasthenia gravis, 1019-1021
in rabies, 1227
in septic sore throat, 1298
in tetanus, 1398
sway-back, 922
sweat, 1157
sweat glands
apocrine, 139
and boils, 310
swelling, 1376
in ascites, 160
compress for, 380
of glands, *see* swollen glands
hydrocele, 787
ice bag for, 808
in inflammation, 837
intumescence, 856
lymphedema, 936
in varicose veins, 1456
swelling of ankles
in cirrhosis of the liver, 364-365
in erythremia, 548
heart trouble symptoms, 748
in pericarditis, 1149
in preeclampsia, 516
swelling of joints
in arthritis, 155-157
in hemophilia, 755-757
in rheumatic fever, 1260
in rheumatoid arthritis, 1266
swineherd's disease, 902-904
swollen glands, 1376
in diphtheria, 483
in German measles, 688
in Hodgkin's disease, 778
in infectious mononucleosis, 998
in leukemia, 904
in mumps, 1006-1008
in scarlet fever, 1284
in toxoplasmosis, 1417
in trench mouth, 1422
sycosis vulgaris, 191
Sydenham's chorea, 359
sympathectomy, 324
sympathetic nervous system, 1042
neuroblastoma of, 1051
sympathetic ophthalmia, 576-577
sympathetic pain, 1376
symptom, 1376
abatement, 1244
chill, 353
circadian rhythm, 362
cough, 400
diarrhea, 469
dizziness, 488
double vision, 492
dysphagia, 509
emaciation, 527
eyelid edema, 583
fever, 605
headache, 718
in hypochondriasis, 799
lumbago, 926
pain, 1126
periodic syndrome, 1152
rale, 1236
remission of, 1244
vomiting, 1468
synapse, 1042
syncope, 586-587
syndrome, 1377
synovial
fluid, 868
membranes, 1377
synovitis, 870-871
in tennis elbow, 1393

syphilis, **1377-1379**
aneurysms in, 112
aphonia from, 138
bubo in, 277
bursitis from, 286
cirrhosis of the liver from, 364
deafness from, 422
gumma in, 704
iritis from, 858
Kahn test for, 873
leukoplakia in, 911
and the lymphatic system, 935
orchitis from, 1095
paresis in, 1137
premarital checkup for, 1191
and tattoo, 1384
tongue in, 1412
Wassermann test for, 1472
and yaws, 1489
syringe, 1380
systole, 725
systolic pressure, 238-239

T

tabes dorsalis, **1381**
paraplegia in, 1135
in paresis, 1137
tachycardia, 1381
tachyphagia, 1381
talipes, 1382
clubfoot, 368
tampons, 1382
tannic acid, 1382
tapeworm, **1382-1383**
Atabrine for, 166
and rat control, 1237
tartar, 1382
taste, 1382
taste impairment, 202
tattoo, 1384
Tay-Sachs disease, **1384-1386**
amniocentesis for detection, 99
as a birth defect, 215, 218
in genetic counseling, 680, 682
tear
gas, 1386
glands, 894-895
tearing eyes, 504
teeth, **1386-1390**
bicuspid, 260
in cystic fibrosis, 417
deciduous, 429
dental caries, 435
dental hygiene, 440
dental research, 441
dentifrice for, 441
dentistry, 442
enamel of, 533
and fluoridation, 643
and gums, 704
impaction of, 816
malocclusion of, 943
occlusion of, 1086
orthodontia for, 1100
in rickets, 1273
in scurvy, 1292
and tartar, 1382
and thumb-sucking, 1405
toothache, 1415
and trench mouth, 1422
in vitamin A deficiency, 1464
wisdom, 1482
telangiectases, 1391
telemetry, 1391
and brain tumor, 258
telescopic vision, 1258
temporal bones, 1316
mastoid of, 951
petrositis of, 1158
temporal lobe, 253-256
temperature, **1392**
in fever, 605
in sleep, 1325
inversion, 1393
thermometer for, 1402
temporomandibular joint, 866-867
syndrome, 992

tendinitis, 523
tendon, **1393**
Achilles, 30
inflammation of, 523
in sprains, 1349
and voluntary muscles, 1009
tenesmus, 1393
tennis elbow, 523, **1393**
and bursitis, 286-288
tension, **1394**
furuncles from, 660
headache from, 718
stripes, 1394
teratogens, 1394
teratogenicity, 211
teratoma, 1394
Terramycin, 128, 1394
testes, *see* testicles
testicles, 1394
in castration, 316
in crytorchism, 412
and the endocrine system, 538
and epididymitis, 543
and gonorrhea, 700
hydrocele of, 787
in hypogonadism, 802
inflammation of, 1095
in mumps, 1006-1008
orchitis, 1095
spermatic cords of, 1339
tumors of, 1395
undescended, 1442
testosterone, **786, 1395**
and baldness, 184
in middle age change, 991
tests, **1395-1398**
amniocentesis, 99
Aschheim-Zondek, 160
biopsy, 208
BMR, 194
diabetic, 464
Dick, 470
Ellsworth-Howard, 1211
glucose tolerance, 695
intelligence, 852
Kahn, 873
kidney function, 888
Pap smear, 1134
placebo use in, 1173
pregnancy, 1191
PSP, 888
Rinne, 1275
Rorschach, 1277
Schick, 1286
Stanford-Binet, 1350
urinalysis, 1446
Wassermann, 1472
tetanus, **1398-1400**
oxygen therapy for, 1118
in snake bites, 1330
opisthotonos in, 1093
tetany, 1136
tetracycline, 31, 128, 1400
tetrahydrocannabinol, 1400
tetralogy of Fallot, 1400
in congenital heart disease, 382
thalamus
and basal ganglia, 194
and emotion, 530
thalassemia, **1400-1401**
as a birth defect, 218
in genetic counseling, 680
thalidomide, 1402
theophylline, 97
therapy
chemotherapy, 337
cryotherapy, 412
diathermy, 470
electric shock, 525
exercise as, 556
heliotherapy, 753
insulin shock, 849
massage, 948
occupational, 1086
whirlpool baths, 1478
x-rays, 1487
thermal pollution, 1402
thermography, 1402
in breast cancer, 262

INDEX

ultrasonography, 222, 1441
 and foreign bodies, 650
ultraviolet
 keratitis, 1441
 therapy, 660
umbilical
 cord, 1441
 hernia, 1036
umbilicus, 1036
unconsciousness, **1441**
 catalepsy, 316
 coma, 379
 first aid for, 633
 in skull fracture, 651
underweight problems, 1441-1442
undescended testicles, 1442-1444
undulant fever, 1444
unguent, 1444
unsaturated fat, 591
urea, 1444
uremia, 1444
 in high blood pressure, 772
ureter, 1445
ureteritis, 1445
urethra, **1445-1446**
 foreign bodies in, 650
 in prostatism, 1209
 urethritis, 1446
urethritis, 1446
 in Reiter's syndrome, 1244
uric acid, 1446
 and gout, 700-702
urinalysis, 1446
urinary
 acidification, 889
 calculus, 889-891
 cast, 315
 incontinence, 1446
 tract problems, 1447-1449
urinary system, 1446
 and urology, 1451
urination, **1449-1450**
 in bladder diseases, 230-232
 difficult, 509
 in gout, 702
 in nocturia, 1057
 in prostatitis, 1209
 in tabes dorsalis, 1381
 in trichomonas infection, 1427
 in urethritis, 1446
urine, **1449-1450**
 in alkaptonuria, 83
 absence of, 134
 in Aschheim-Zondek test, 160
 in bladder diseases, 230
 in cholera, 356
 in diuresis, 486
 hematuria, 754
 in hepatitis, 760
 in porphyria, 1186
 in preeclampsia, 516
 and the ureter, 1445
 urinalysis, 1446
 in Wilms' tumor, 1481
urolithiasis, 889-891
urologist, 490
urology, 1451
urticaria, 776-778
uterine tubes, 588
uterus, **1451**
 in abortion, 22
 and backache, 177
 cancer of, 300
 cervix of, 333
 in childbirth, 341-344
 choriocarcinoma of, 359
 in conception, 380-381
 in dilatation and curettage, 483
 in dysmenorrhea, 508
 in endometritis, 539-540
 fibroid tumors of, 608
 in gynecologic examination, 705
 hysterectomy, 806
 metritis of, 990
 mole in, 997
 polyp in, 1185
 prolapse of, 1205
 removal of, 806
 tipped, 1411

uveitis, 1451
uvula, 1451

V

vaccination, **1452**
 birth defect prevention, 224-225, 328
 booster dose, 249
 in immunity, 811
 in infant care, 825
 and infection, 832
 see also immunization; vaccines
vaccines,
 Asian flu, 162
 BCG, 196
 birth defect prevention, 224
 booster dose, 249
 cholera, 358
 German measles, 688
 measles, 954
 mumps, 1008
 rabies, 1227
 rickettsial diseases, 1273
 Sabin, 1281
 typhoid, 1434
 from viruses, 1462
vagina, **1453**
 in bisexuality, 228
 in childbirth, 341
 colpotomy of, 379
 douche for, 492
 foams for, 210
 in gynecologic examination, 705
 jellies for, 210
 odor from, 602-604
 pessary for, 1158
 and puerperal fever, 1218
 in trichomonas infection, 1427
 in vaginitis, 1454
vaginal bleeding
 in abortion, 22
 in abruptio placentae, 23
 in ectopic pregnancy, 518
 in miscarriage, 996
 in prenatal care, 1198
vaginal discharge
 leukorrhea, 911
 lochia, 921
vaginismus, 508
vaginitis, 1454
vaginoplasty, 228
vagus nerve, **1454**
 in bradycardia, 253
 in fainting, 586
valley fever, 372
vanadium, 1454
varicella, 339
varices, 1454
varicocele, 1454-1456
varicose ulcers, 901-902
varicose veins, **1456-1458**
 in fibroid tumor, 611
 hemorrhoids, 758-760
variola, 1328
vascular system, 1458
vas deferens, 1458
 in vasectomy, 1459
vasectomy, 213, 1459
vasoconstrictor, 1459
vasodilator, 1459
vasomotor, 1459
veins, **1459**
 in the circulatory system, 362
 inflammation of, 1160-1162
 varicose, 1456
Velpeau's bandage, 366
vena cava, 1459
venereal disease, **1460**
 chancroid, 336
 gonorrhea, 698-700
 granuloma inguinale, 703
 and homosexuality, 782-783
 lymphogranuloma venereum, 936
 and sex education, 1299
 and sterility, 1351
 syphilis, 1377
venipuncture, 1460

venom
 in bee stings, 199
 in snake bites, 1330
ventilation, **1460**
 in air conditioning, 73-74
 and carbon dioxide, 309
 and carbon tetrachloride, 310
ventricular fibrillation, 608
 defibrillators for, 430
venules
 and capillaries, 308
 in the circulatory system, 362
vermiform appendix, 144
Veronal, 191
vernal conjunctivitis, 1169
vertebra, **1460**
 and backache, 177-179
 and intervertebral discs, 852-853
 and slipped disc, 1326
 in spondylolisthesis, 1346
 in whiplash injury, 1476
vertigo, **1461**
 in benzene poisoning, 203
 in caisson disease, 290
 in ear disorders, 513
 in Ménière's disease, 967
 in whiplash injury, 1476
vestibular
 disorders, 1461
 nerve, 171
vestibule, 1469
vestigial organ, 248
veterinarian, 1461
villus, 1461
Vincent's
 angina, 1422
 organisms, 872
viomycin, 128
viral pneumonia, 1178-1180
 acranulocytosis in, 72
virilism, **1461**
 in Achard-Thiers syndrome, 29
 in adrenogenital syndrome, 61
viruses, 1461-1463
vision, 1464
 in children, 577-578
 see also eye
vision impairment
 aniseikonia, 120
 asthenopia, 164
 astigmatism, 165
 in beriberi, 205
 cataract, 316
 in cerebral palsy, 326-328
 in dermatomyositis, 448
 in diabetes mellitus, 458
 double vision, 492
 eyeglasses for, 581
 farsightedness, 589
 glassblower's cataract, 691
 in glaucoma, 691-693
 in head injuries, 722
 hemianopsia, 754
 and intelligence, 851
 nearsightedness, 1036
 in poisoning, 309, 420, 985
 in polycythemia, 1185
 presbyopia, 1199
 in retinitis pigmentosa, 1258
 in snake bites, 1330
 in trachoma, 1419
 in vitamin A deficiency, 1464
 see also blindness; eye disorders
vitamin A deficiency, 1464-1466
 xerophthalmia, 1485
vitamin B2, 1271
vitamin C, 160
 deficiencies, 107, 1466
vitamin deficiencies, **1466**
 bowleg from, 252
 deficiency diseases, 430
 gait in, 661
 gastritis from, 668
 glossitis from, 694
 and jungle rot, 872
 liver extracts for, 921
 ophthalmoplegia from, 1091
 spontaneous abortion from, 22
 see also deficiency diseases

1523